Vaccinology and Immunizations

Vaccinology and Immunizations

Jahangir Moini, MD, MPH
Professor of Science and Health (Ret)
Science and Health
Eastern Florida State College
Palm Bay, Florida, United States

Obehi Enabulele, PharmD, MBA, MS
Pediatric Clinical Pharmacist
Children's Hospital Colorado
Aurora, Colorado

Mandana Naderi, PharmD, MPH, BCIDP
Medical Science Director in pharmaceutical industry
Former Assistant Professor of Practice
R. Ken Coit College of Pharmacy at the University of Arizona
Los Angeles, CA

ELSEVIER

Academic Press is an imprint of Elsevier
125 London Wall, London EC2Y 5AS, United Kingdom
525 B Street, Suite 1650, San Diego, CA 92101, United States
50 Hampshire Street, 5th Floor, Cambridge, MA 02139, United States

ISBN: 978-0-443-23915-1

For Information on all Academic Press publications
visit our website at https://www.elsevier.com/books-and-journals

Publisher: Peter Linsley
Acquisitions Editor: Emms Sykes
Editorial Project Manager: Surbhi Tyagi
Publishing Services Manager: Deepthi Unni
Production Project Manager: Surya Narayanan Jayachandran
Cover Designer: Greg Harris

Typeset by MPS Limited, Chennai, India

Printed in Great Britain by CPI Group (UK) Ltd,
Croydon, CR0 4YY

Last digit is the print number: 9 8 7 6 5 4 3 2 1

Dr. Moini:
To my precious grandchildren, Artemis, Anastasia, Anabelle, and Laila.

Dr. Enabulele:
This project is dedicated to my husband, Eseosa Enabulele, and my son, Nehizena Enabulele, who supported me throughout the development phase. I could not have done this without you both.

Dr. Naderi:
To the younger me, whose perseverance made dreams become reality, and to my family, who made it all possible.

Contents

For additional information on the topics covered in the book, visit the companion site: https://shop.elsevier.com/books/book-companion/9780443239151

For additional materials for qualified instructors, please visit the instructor site: https://www.educate.elsevier.com/book/details/9780443239151

Contributors

Jahangir Moini, MD, MPH
Professor of Science and Health (Ret)
Science and Health
Eastern Florida State College
Palm Bay, Florida, United States

Obehi Enabulele, PharmD, MBA, MS
Pediatric Clinical Pharmacist
Children's Hospital Colorado
Aurora, Colorado

Mandana Naderi, PharmD, MPH, BCIDP
Medical Science Director in pharmaceutical industry
Former Assistant Professor of Practice
R. Ken Coit College of Pharmacy at the University of Arizona
Los Angeles, CA

About the Authors

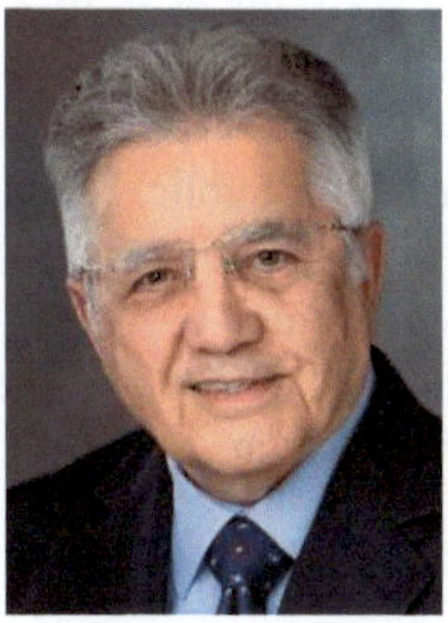

Dr. Moini was an assistant professor at Tehran University Medical School, Department of Epidemiology and Preventive Medicine, for nine years. He was also practicing medicine. For 18 years, he was the Director of Epidemiology for the Brevard County Health Department. For 15 years, he was the Director of Science and Health for Everest University in Melbourne, FL. He was also a Professor of Science and Health at Everest for 24 years. He was a Professor of Science and Health at Eastern Florida State College for six years but is now retired. Dr. Moini has been actively teaching for 39 and 24 years and is an international author of 57 books. His "Anatomy & Physiology for Healthcare Professionals" was translated and released in Japan and South Korea in 2020. His Complications of Diabetes Mellitus are translated into the Spanish language.

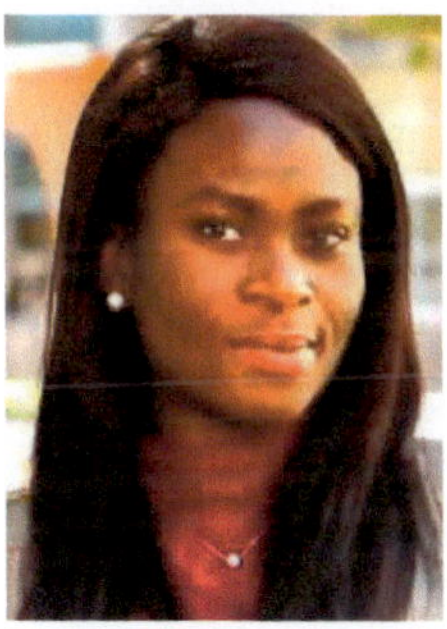

Dr. Enabulele is a pediatric clinical pharmacist currently working in clinical research focused on therapies for children's diseases, including rare diseases. Her career spans over eight years of experience in retail and hospital pharmacy settings, with a significant proportion being in sterile compounding. As a well-rounded pharmacist, Obehi actively develops standards and procedures that guide pharmacy operations in different locations.

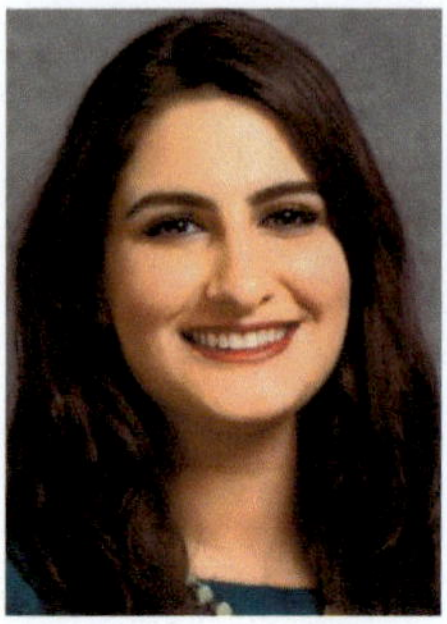

Dr. Naderi is an infectious diseases pharmacist and an Assistant Professor of Practice at the R. Ken Coit College of Pharmacy at the University of Arizona. She also serves as the Lead Antimicrobial Stewardship Expert and Co-chair of the Antimicrobial Stewardship Subcommittee at the Arizona Department of Health Services (ADHS) in Phoenix, Arizona. Her role with ADHS also included serving as a Clinical Therapeutics Lead during the COVID-19 and Mpox public health emergency response efforts. Before her public health role, Dr. Naderi worked as an inpatient clinical infectious diseases pharmacist, and she continues to maintain her clinical skills as an acute care hospital staff pharmacist. She earned her Bachelor of Science in Public Health from the University of Washington, her Doctor of Pharmacy degree from Washington State University, and her Master of Public Health degree from the University of Arizona. She completed post-graduate pharmacy residency training at Geisinger Wyoming Valley Medical Center in Wilkes-Barre, Pennsylvania, and a specialized residency in infectious diseases at the University of Arizona/Banner University Medical Center in Tucson, Arizona.

Preface

“Vaccinology and Immunizations” is an essential topic for healthcare providers. Updated vaccines become available regularly, and new vaccines enter the market to prevent infectious diseases. All healthcare professionals must be familiar with the available vaccines and understand how to store and administer them. Since the development of vaccine technology, millions have been saved from many infectious diseases.

This book is organized into “Immunity and Immunizations” and “Vaccinology”. Unit I contains two chapters, while Unit II contains 10. The first unit includes chapters that discuss the immune system and integrative immunology. Part II covers vaccine history, preparation, approval, infectious disease prevention and eradication, vaccine safety and errors, preventable childhood infections, pediatric and adult immunizations, immunology in older adults, and vaccines for travelers.

The chapters contain an outline, keywords, learning objectives, overview, figures, tables, highlighted “You Should Remember” boxes that focus on essential aspects of the text, Test Your Knowledge review questions, bolded key terms that are defined in the Glossary at the back of the book, and lists of other books for further reading. Some chapters feature case studies that include critical thinking questions, which help readers understand real-life scenarios related to the subject matter. The answers to the essential thinking questions appear in an Answer Key at the end of the book. Additional ancillaries include abstracts for each chapter, a test bank with an answer key, and PowerPoint presentations. Finally, there is an index of essential terms.

Acknowledgments

The authors appreciate the contributions of everyone who assisted in creating this book: Katey Birtcher (Publishing Director), Peter B. Linsley (Publisher), Surya Narayanan Jayachandran (Senior Project Manager), Emma Hayes (Senior Acquisitions Editor), Bathsheba Lockwood Brook (Editorial Product Manager), and Greg Vadimsky.

Unit I

Vaccinology and Immunizations

Chapter 1

The Immune System

Chapter Outline

Learning Objectives

After study of this chapter, readers should be able to:

1. Describe the functions of the five different leukocytes and their characteristics.
2. Discuss the role of cytokines and interferons in immunity.
3. Explain factors that affect the innate defense system.

Vaccinology and Immunizations. http://doi.org/10.1016/B978-0-443-23915-1.00001-9

4. Describe humoral and cellular immunities.
5. Explain the activation and differentiation of B cells.
6. Define "antigen" and describe how antigens affect the adaptive defenses.
7. Describe the structures and functions of the five antibodies.
8. Compare active and passive humoral immunity.
9. Describe the roles of different types of T cells.
10. Discuss primary and secondary immunodeficiency.

OVERVIEW

The immune system is a complex network of cells, organs, and proteins. It defends the body against infection and "remembers" each microorganism that has intruded into the body before and has been defeated. Therefore it can recognize and destroy the microbe quickly if it enters the body again. Immune system abnormalities can lead to infections, allergic diseases, immunodeficiencies, and autoimmune disorders. An autoimmune disorder can develop when there is a malfunction of the immune system. Common autoimmune disorders include Addison disease, celiac disease, dermatomyositis, Graves disease, Hashimoto thyroiditis, multiple sclerosis, myasthenia gravis, pernicious anemia, reactive arthritis, rheumatoid arthritis, Sjögren syndrome, systemic lupus erythematosus, and type 1 diabetes.

LYMPHOID CELLS, TISSUES, AND ORGANS

The immune system is a complex network of organs, cells, and proteins that defend the body against infection while protecting the body's cells. The immune system records every microorganism it has defeated to recognize and destroy the microbe quickly if it enters the body again. Therefore the immune system has a vital role in the human body. It also protects against cell changes in the body that can cause cancers. The immune system comprises various cells, tissues, and organs. The primary lymphoid organs of the immune system include the thymus and bone marrow, as well as secondary lymphatic tissues, including the spleen, tonsils, lymph vessels, lymph nodes, adenoids, skin, and liver.

Leukocytes and Lymphoid Cells

The immune system cells include neutrophils, basophils, eosinophils, monocytes, and lymphocytes. The lymphoid cells contain the immune system and supporting cells, forming a scaffold-like tissue structure. T lymphocytes (T cells) and B lymphocytes (B cells) protect against **antigens**. Activated T cells coordinate the immune response. **Macrophages** are vital because they phagocytize foreign substances and help activate T cells. They are assisted by the **dendritic cells** (stellate macrophages), which capture antigens and return them to the lymph nodes. The **reticular cells** are similar to fibroblasts and produce the reticular fiber stroma, a network that supports other cells in the lymphoid organs and tissues. These cells will be discussed in detail later in this chapter.

Neutrophils

Neutrophils are the most abundant **leukocytes** in circulation, accounting for about 70% of all leukocytes. Neutrophils have been regarded as the first line of defense in the innate arm of the immune system. They capture and destroy invading microorganisms through phagocytosis and intracellular degradation, the release of granules, and the formation of neutrophil extracellular traps after detecting pathogens. Neutrophils also participate as mediators of inflammation. Neutrophils are the primary mediators of the rapid innate host defense against most bacterial and fungal pathogens that occur before the complex humoral and lymphocyte cellular processes of acquired immunity can be brought to bear on an infection. The number of neutrophils in blood circulation remains relatively constant due to a strict balance between their production and elimination. Neutrophils also actively change to be able to perform particular functions at different times or places.

Neutrophils are the primary mediators of the rapid innate host defense against most bacterial and fungal pathogens before acquired immune processes can occur. Neutrophils, also called polymorphonuclear leukocytes, play the primary role in the clearance of bacteria and fungi while shaping the host response to infection and immune system **homeostasis**. They capture and destroy invading microorganisms via **phagocytosis** and **intracellular degradation**, release granules, and form extracellular traps once pathogens are detected. They are also mediators of inflammation and immune responses. Every day, the bone marrow produces approximately 100 billion neutrophils. When homeostasis is normal, neutrophils enter the circulation, move to the tissues, execute their functions, and are eliminated by macrophages within 1 day. Neutrophils respond to many different signals and produce **cytokines**, other inflammatory factors that influence and regulate inflammation and the immune system's actions.

Basophils

Basophils are the rarest type of white blood cells (WBCs), accounting for only 0.5% to 1% of WBCs. They are the primary effector cells in hypersensitivity reactions. Basophils express a high-affinity immunoglobulin E (IgE) receptor, contain granules, and release histamine. Basophils mediate allergic reactions, play essential roles in **immunomodulation**, and are responsible for the onset of allergic, autoimmune, and infectious diseases. These cells do not proliferate after maturation and have a lifespan of up to 60 hours.

Eosinophils

Eosinophils develop in the bone marrow, migrate into the bloodstream, and comprise about 2% to 4% of WBCs. They are associated with allergic diseases and parasitic infections, with multiple roles in innate and adaptive immunity. As effector cells in **innate immunity**, eosinophils have a proinflammatory and destructive role in immune responses. They can be recruited by "warning" signals released by pathogenic infections or tissue injury, inducing host defenses against parasitic, fungal, bacterial, or viral diseases or promoting tissue repair and remodeling. Additionally, eosinophils function as **antigen-presenting cells** (APCs) responding to allergens or helminth infections. They actively regulate or interact with T lymphocytes and dendritic cells.

Monocytes

Monocytes account for 3% to 8% of WBCs. They are the largest leukocytes. They enter tissues in the body and become *macrophages* or *dendritic cells*. Monocytes have a very short circulating lifespan of 1 to 22 hours. Unlike short-lived neutrophils, the lifespan of a macrophage ranges from months to years. Monocytes are critical components of the innate immune system. They play a role in the inflammatory and antiinflammatory processes during an immune response. Macrophages surround and kill microorganisms, ingest foreign material, remove dead cells, and boost immune responses. During inflammation, dendritic cells encourage immune responses by showing antigens on their surface to other immune system cells. Macrophages are also significant in immunity and immune responses. They can phagocytize parasites and microbes. They regulate lymphocyte activation and proliferation and are essential in the activation process of B and T lymphocytes by antigens and **allogeneic cells**. Increased bactericidal activity of activated macrophages is based on immunologically linked factors involving lymphocytes. Macrophages kill ingested microbes, though this occurrence is not entirely understood. The common types of macrophages and their locations and functions are as follows:

- **Alveolar macrophages:** located in the lung alveoli; they phagocytize small particles of dust, dead cells, or bacteria; they also initiate and control immunity to respiratory pathogens. The alveolar macrophages are also called **dust cells**.
- **Kupffer cells:** located in the liver; they initiate immune responses and remodeling of liver tissues.
- **Microglia:** located in the brain; they eliminate old or dead neurons and control immunity within the brain.

Lymphocytes

Lymphocytes account for 25% of WBCs. They are the smallest WBCs in size. The two main types of lymphocytes are B lymphocytes and T lymphocytes. B lymphocytes make **antibodies**, and T lymphocytes help kill tumor cells and help control immune responses. They are found in blood circulation, lymphoid tissues, and organs. Most lymphocytes are short-lived, with an average lifespan of a week to a few months, but a few live for years. Some lymphocytes migrate to the **thymus**, where they mature into T cells. Others remain in the bone marrow, where they develop into B cells.

In the thymus, T cells multiply and differentiate into helper, regulatory, or **cytotoxic T cells** (T_C cells), or they become **memory T cells**. They are then seeded to the peripheral tissues or lymphatic system. Once stimulated by the appropriate antigen, T_H cells secrete chemical messengers called cytokines, which facilitate the differentiation of B cells into **plasma cells**, thereby promoting antibody production. **Regulatory T cells** act to control immune reactions. T_C cells, activated by various cytokines, bind to and kill infected and cancer cells.

You Should Remember

Mast cells and basophils are the most relevant sources of histamine in the immune system. Mast cells can be found in connective tissues, especially under the skin near blood vessels, lymph vessels, nerves, and the lungs and intestines. They are essential in how the immune system responds to certain bacteria and parasites. Basophils form in the bone marrow and travel to damaged tissues once they mature to help heal them after an injury.

You Should Remember

Several cells, such as mast cells, macrophages, neutrophils, and eosinophils, produce leukotrienes during an asthma attack, which are primarily responsible for bronchoconstriction.

TEST YOUR KNOWLEDGE

1. What are some of the cells of the immune system?
2. What are the functions of neutrophils?
3. What are the functions of lymphocytes in the immune system?

Lymphoid Tissues

The lymphoid tissues are organized structures that support immune responses. The most highly organized lymphoid tissues are in the thymus and lymph nodes, which are well defined. There are two types of collections of lymphoid tissue, as follows:

- **Diffuse lymphoid tissue:** a loose grouping of lymphoid cells with reticular fibers present in most body organs; larger groups are in the **lamina propria** of the mucous membranes.

- **Lymphoid follicles:** solid round structures made up of tightly packed lymphoid cells and reticular fibers; they often have lighter-staining germinal centers where quickly dividing B cells predominate; the germinal centers enlarge significantly when B cells are rapidly dividing and producing plasma cells.

Lymphoid Organs

The lymphatic system is commonly divided into the primary lymphoid organs, which are the sites of B- and T-cell maturation, and the secondary lymphoid organs, in which further differentiation of lymphocytes occurs. Primary lymphoid organs include the bone marrow and thymus. These are the key players in immune function. All lymphocytes derive from stem cells in the bone marrow. **Stem cells** destined to become B lymphocytes remain in the bone marrow as they mature, while prospective T cells migrate to the thymus for further growth. Mature B and T lymphocytes exit the primary lymphoid organs and are transported via the bloodstream to the secondary lymphoid organs, activated by contact with foreign materials. Secondary lymphoid organs include the tonsils, lymph nodes, spleen, small masses of Peyer patches, and the appendix. They serve two essential functions: a site of further lymphocyte maturation and to efficiently trap antigens for exposure to T and B cells.

Bone Marrow

Bone marrow is a spongy substance found in the center of the bones. It manufactures bone marrow stem cells and other substances, producing blood cells. Each type of blood cell the bone marrow makes has an important job. There are two types of bone marrow: red and yellow. Red bone marrow contains blood stem cells that can become red blood cells, WBCs, or **platelets**. Yellow bone marrow is made mainly of fat and contains stem cells that can become cartilage, fat, or bone cells.

Red blood cells carry oxygen to tissues in the body. WBCs work to help the body fight off infections. Platelets help the blood clot and prevent uncontrolled bleeding.

Thymus Gland

The *thymus gland* is located behind the **sternum bone** in the inferior neck, extending into the superior thorax. The gland has two lobes and partly overlies the heart. T-lymphocyte precursors mature in the thymus, becoming immunocompetent lymphocytes, which can defend the body against specific pathogens. The gland is prominent in newborns and infants, increasing in size during the first year of life. However, it is only active until puberty. After puberty, the thymus starts to shrink slowly and is replaced by fat and fibrous tissue by the time of old age. Even though the thymus atrophies, it does continue to produce immunocompetent cells, much less than before. **Thymosin** is the hormone secreted by the thymus.

It stimulates the development of disease-fighting T cells. The mature T cells in the thymus differ from the secondary lymphoid organs.

Tonsils

The **tonsils** are small masses of lymphatic tissue located in the pharynx wall at the rear of the throat. These are a pair of oval-shaped masses protruding from each side of the oral pharynx. Humans are born with four types of tonsils. The **adenoid** is just behind the nasal passages and helps the body prevent or fight infections by trapping bacteria and other microorganisms. The **palatine tonsils** are two round, fleshy masses in the throat's back. They are the most enormous tonsils and the most likely to become infected. The two tiny **tubal tonsils** surround the openings of the **auditory tubes** into the throat. The **lingual tonsil** is a lumpy collection of lymphoid follicles at the base of the tongue. Collectively, the tonsils form a ring around the entrance to the throat. They help to filter out bacteria and other germs to prevent infection in the body. A bacterial or viral infection can cause tonsillitis.

Lymph Nodes

The lymph nodes are small bean-shaped structures that filter substances passing through the lymphatic fluid. There are hundreds of lymph nodes throughout the body. They are connected by lymph vessels. Clusters of lymph nodes are found in the neck, axilla, chest, abdomen, and groin. In comparison, the brain lacks them. There are 20 to 40 lymph nodes in the axilla. The lymph nodes are the only lymphoid organs that cleanse the lymphatic fluid. Besides the lymph nodes, the other secondary lymphoid organs usually have efferent lymphatics that drain them and lack afferent lymphatics.

Spleen

The **spleen** is an organ inside the left side of the rib cage, just above the stomach. It is part of the lymphatic system and part of the immune system. It is the largest lymphatic organ in the body. Surrounded by a connective tissue capsule, which extends inward to divide the organ into lobules, the spleen consists of two types of tissue: white and red. It stores and filters blood and hosts lymphocytes and all primary mononuclear phagocytes, including macrophages and monocytes, which protect the body from infection. The spleen controls the level of WBCs, red blood cells, and platelets. White pulp produces lymphocytes, which produce antibodies to fight infection. Red pulp acts as a filter, removing waste from the blood and removing old or damaged blood cells; it also destroys bacteria and viruses.

Peyer Patches

Peyer patches are large clusters of lymphoid follicles that resemble the tonsils. They are within the wall of the distal portion of the small intestine. The Peyer patches keep the intestinal flora at appropriate levels and reduce the number of pathogens, preventing many infections. As a part of the **pathogenesis** of food allergies, the Peyer patches and vasculature of the lamina propria allow the circulation of inflammatory cells to reach the immune structures.

Appendix

The *appendix* is a tubelike structure attached to the first portion of the large intestine (cecum). It contains many lymphoid follicles. Like Peyer patches, the appendix is positioned to prevent bacteria from getting through the intestinal wall, generating many "memory" lymphocytes to provide long-term immunity.

You Should Remember

While the central nervous system lacks lymphatic vasculature and is considered immune privileged, a network of lymphatics in the meninges runs beside the dural venous sinuses. It extends upon the dura mater surrounding the brain. However, there are no lymph nodes in the brain or spinal cord.

TEST YOUR KNOWLEDGE

1. What are the two types of collections of lymphoid tissue?
2. What are the primary and secondary lymphoid organs?
3. What are the functions of the white and red pulp of the spleen?

CYTOKINES, INTERFERONS, AND INTERLEUKINS

Cytokines consist of many different small proteins. They primarily stimulate the migration of leukocytes. Therefore cytokines are essential for the development and homeostasis of the immune system. They are implicated in all protective or destructive immune and inflammatory responses. Cytokines stimulate many other migratory behaviors, including **haptotaxis**, **chemokinesis**, and hypokinesis.

Interferons (IFNs) are a broad class of cytokines elicited on challenge to the host defense and are essential for mobilizing immune responses to pathogens. IFNs possess several important properties, including antiviral, anticancer, and immunomodulatory properties. Protein envelopes surround viruses that do not have the cellular mechanics needed to generate ATP or synthesize proteins (Figure 1.1). Instead, viruses function in the body by invading tissue cells and then taking control of cellular metabolic activities to reproduce themselves. Infected cells cannot combat viruses to any significant degree. However, some infected cells secrete small proteins known as IFNs. These help protect cells that have not yet been virally infected.

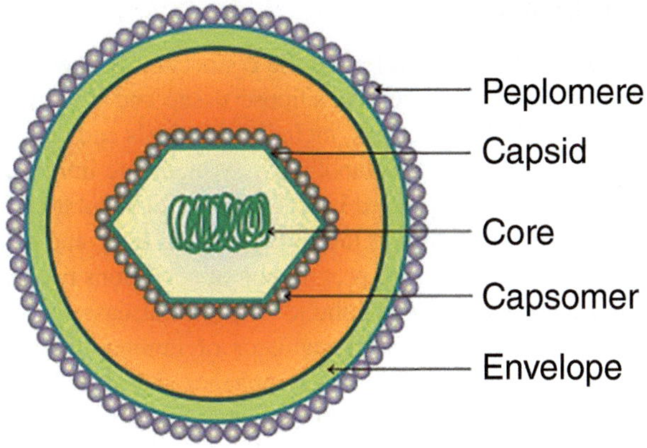

FIGURE 1.1 The structure of a virus.

There are three types of IFNs: alpha, beta, and gamma. IFN-alpha and -beta have antiviral effects while activating natural killer cells. Lymphocytes secrete IFN-gamma or immune IFN with wide-ranging immune mobilization effects, including macrophage activation. The IFNs indirectly combat cancer because macrophages and natural killer cells act directly against cancerous cells. They are used to treat disorders that include hepatitis C, **multiple sclerosis**, and **genital warts**.

Interleukins (ILs) are a group of cytokines with inflammatory or antiinflammatory functions. They are essential for immune cell proliferation, maturation, migration, activation, and differentiation. They work by interacting with high-affinity cell surface receptors. There are many types of ILs with distinct cellular functions. IL-1, secreted by macrophages, **fibroblasts**, B cells, granular lymphocytes, endothelium, and **astrocytes**, triggers immune and inflammatory responses by activating lymphocytes and macrophages and increasing the hepatic release of acute-phase proteins.

IL-2, secreted by T cells, triggers the proliferation and differentiation of B and T cells and the synthesis of cytokines and antibodies. T cells also secrete IL-3, which functions as a multilineage colony-stimulating factor. IL-4, IL-5, IL-6, and IL-7 mainly act on B cells and promote the activation and differentiation of B cells and antibody production. Some ILs, such as IL-10, IL-11, and IL-13, inhibit the action of proinflammatory cytokines. In contrast, ILs (IL-17, IL-31, and IL-32) increase the release of proinflammatory cytokines.

You Should Remember

Approximately 19 different chemokine receptors are divided into four families based on the type of chemokine they bind (CXC, CC, CX_3C, and XC receptors). They function in signal transduction and infection control.

IMMUNOMETABOLISM

The term **immunometabolism** refers to the connection between immunology and metabolism. Immune cells in the adipose tissue and liver regulate tissue homeostasis and metabolic functions, including **lipolysis** and the roles of insulin. Nutrient intake and related metabolism may modulate immune responses. Metabolic inflammation is regulated by cellular and molecular components of the immune response, which affects the adipose tissue, liver, and pancreas. This contributes to pathogenesis and the progression of conditions related to obesity, including type 2 diabetes and nonalcoholic fatty liver disease.

Cellular metabolism is a central regulator of immune cell function and activation. Precise activation states of macrophages and other **innate immune cells** are linked to various cellular metabolic conditions, so cell metabolic adaptations aid in macrophage phenotype and plasticity. Metabolic alterations of innate immune cells are essential to inherent immune memory. This means that specific stimuli can promote unspecific memory in innate immune cells, signified by their increased inflammatory functions. The innate immune cells have a more robust inflammatory response when rechallenged. Cellular metabolism regulates the functions of mature **myeloid cells** as well as **myelopoiesis**. Metabolic adaptations of natural immune cell precursors are vital for differentiation and lineage determinations related to myelopoiesis in normal and stressful conditions.

Immunometabolic processes, such as altered metabolism of various immune cells, are essential components of the tumor microenvironment and influence tumor growth. Immunometabolism has also been implicated in type 1 diabetes and multiple sclerosis. Specific alterations may help the loss of immunological tolerance and the emergence of autoreactive immune cells in immune cell metabolism. Immunometabolic modulators can be used therapeutically for various metabolic and inflammatory conditions.

TEST YOUR KNOWLEDGE

1. Why are cytokines important for immunity?
2. How do IFNs affect viral replication?
3. What is immunometabolism?

REGULATED CELL DEATH

Regulated cell death is essential for tissue homeostasis and to restore biological balance during stressful conditions. There are various forms of regulated cell death. The five most important forms are apoptosis, pyroptosis, autophagy-dependent cell death, necroptosis, and ferroptosis. These have different features and pathways yet remain somewhat interactive. There is also **accidental cell death** in which cells die because of uncontrolled biological processes.

The entirely physiological form of regulated cell death is also called **programmed cell death**. Neurodegenerative diseases such as Alzheimer disease, Parkinson disease, amyotrophic lateral sclerosis, multiple sclerosis, and Huntington disease cause progressive nervous system degeneration and widespread neuronal cell death. Regulated cell death is related to these neurodegenerative diseases.

Apoptosis is the process of programmed cell death. During early development, it helps to eliminate unneeded cells. In adults, apoptosis is used to remove cells that have been damaged beyond repair. Apoptosis also has a role in the prevention of cancer. When apoptosis is somehow prevented, this can lead to uncontrolled division of cells and the development of a tumor.

Pyroptosis is a form of cell death triggered by proinflammatory signals. It is linked to inflammation. This type of cell death mainly occurs in macrophages and can be triggered by bacterial or pathogen infections.

Necroptosis is another regulated cell death mode that mimics apoptosis and necrosis features.

Ferroptosis is an intracellular iron-dependent type of cell death that is highly distinct. It plays a pivotal role in tumor suppression and may provide new opportunities for cancer therapies. Ferroptosis is also correlated with cancer therapy resistance, and inducing ferroptosis has been shown to reverse drug resistance.

TEST YOUR KNOWLEDGE

1. What are the five most essential forms of regulated cell death?
2. How do normal and excessive apoptosis occur?
3. What are the three primary subtypes of autophagy?

THE INNATE (NONSPECIFIC) DEFENSE SYSTEM

The innate (nonspecific) defense system is always prepared to protect against foreign substances and responds within minutes. Its first line of defense is made up of intact skin and mucosae. The second line of defense is used once the first line has been breached. It uses internal factors to inhibit pathogens' spread, including antimicrobial proteins, **phagocytes**, and other cells. The hallmark of the second line of defense is inflammation.

Surface Barriers

The surface barriers are the first line of immune defense, including the skin and mucous membranes and their secretions. While the epidermis is unbroken, its strongly keratinized epithelial membrane is an excellent physical barrier to most microorganisms. **Keratin resists** weak acids, bases, bacterial enzymes, and toxins. Intact mucous membranes provide similar mechanical barriers inside the body. They line all cavities that open to the exterior of the body. These include the respiratory, digestive, urinary, and reproductive tracts. The protective chemicals produced by the skin and mucous membranes include the following:

- Acid-bacterial growth is inhibited by the acidity of the skin, vagina, and stomach—collectively known as the **acid mantle**.
- *Defensins:* these broad-spectrum antimicrobial peptides are secreted in small amounts; output increases significantly due to inflammation; the **defensins** help control bacterial and fungal colonization in exposed areas using mechanisms such as disruption of microbial membranes.
- *Enzymes* such as *lysozyme* (in the saliva, respiratory mucus, and lacrimal fluid of the eyes) destroy bacteria; in the stomach, protein-digesting enzymes kill many microorganisms.
- *Mucin:* this substance, dissolved in water, forms thick and sticky mucus, which lines digestive and respiratory passageways; it traps many microorganisms; the **mucin** of the watery saliva traps microorganisms, washing them out of the mouth, into the stomach, where they are digested.
- *Other chemicals:* within the skin, some lipids in the **sebum**, and **dermcidin** in the eccrine sweat are toxic to bacteria.

The mucosae of the respiratory tract have structural alterations that oppose invaders. Tiny mucus-coated hairs of the nose trap inhaled particles, as cilia on the mucosa of the upper respiratory tract push mucus-containing dust and bacteria toward the mouth. This prevents it from entering the lower respiratory passages. Surface barriers such as these are sometimes breached by injuries, such as shaving or brushing the teeth. If this occurs and microorganisms invade more profound tissues, the internal innate defenses act.

Internal Defenses

The internal defenses include many nonspecific cellular and chemical mechanisms, some of which are discussed later. The inflammatory response utilizes macrophages, mast cells, different WBCs, and many chemicals to kill pathogens and aid in tissue repair. Potentially harmful substances are recognized and bound to by these cells. The receptors that recognize various bacteria, viruses, fungi, and parasites are called *pattern recognition receptors*. Pathogens that enter the skin or mucosae and reach the underlying connective tissue are attacked by *phagocytes*.

While neutrophils become phagocytic when encountering infectious material in body tissues, the deadliest phagocytes are the *macrophages*. *Free macrophages* move through tissue spaces, searching for cellular debris or foreign molecules. *Fixed macrophages*, including the stellate macrophages, remain in particular organs. The process of *phagocytosis* is the engulfing of debris or invaders. It begins as receptors on the phagocyte's cytoplasmic extensions bind to the particle and pull it inside. The particle is then enclosed in a membrane-lined vesicle, creating a **phagosome** that fuses with a *lysosome*, forming a **phagolysosome**.

Complement

A complement is a group of 20 or more plasma proteins circulating in the blood in normal conditions. During this time, they are inactive. They are numbered C1 through C9, and there are several others that function as regulatory proteins and other factors. The complement system provides a primary way to destroy foreign substances within the body. When activated, inflammatory chemicals are released. They intensify nearly all aspects of the inflammatory process. Activation also lyses and kills certain bacteria and other types of cells. Though it is a nonspecific defense, the complement system enhances the effectiveness of innate and adaptive defenses. There are three ways in which the complement system can be activated, as follows:

- **The classical pathway** uses antibodies, which are water-soluble protein molecules produced by the adaptive immune system to fight off invaders; when they bind to pathogens, they can also bind to components of the complement system; this double binding begins activation of complement.
- **The lectin pathway** uses lectins, which are water-soluble protein molecules produced by the innate immune system, to recognize invaders; when they bind certain sugars on the surface of microorganisms, they can then bind and activate the complement system.
- **The alternative pathway** is triggered when spontaneously activated complement protein C3 and other factors interact on the surface of microorganisms; the microorganisms do not have the complement activation inhibitors that host cells have.

Complement activation by these three pathways involves a cascade, with proteins activated in an ordered sequence. Each step catalyzes the next. The three pathways converge at C3 and split into C3a and C3b, initiating a common terminal way. This pathway increases inflammation, promotes phagocytosis, and can cause lysis of cells.

Cell lysis starts when C3b binds to the target cell's surface, triggering the insertion of a group of complement proteins called membrane attack complex into the cell's membrane. A hole is formed and stabilized in the membrane, allowing a large influx of water, which lyses the target cell. The C3b molecules also function as **opsonins**, which coat the microorganisms, creating "handles" that macrophage and neutrophil receptors can stick to. They can then engulf the particle more quickly. C3a and other molecules formed as complements are activated to increase the inflammatory response via mast cells and basophils stimulation, releasing histamine and attracting more neutrophils and other inflammatory cells.

TEST YOUR KNOWLEDGE

1. Which protective chemicals act as surface barriers?
2. What do the internal defenses include?
3. What are the three ways in which the complement system can be activated?

Fever

While inflammation is a localized response to infection, the body sometimes responds to a microbial invasion on a more widespread level with a *fever*. This is a systemic response. When leukocytes and macrophages are exposed to foreign substances, they release **pyrogens**, which act on the body's temperature control mechanisms in the **hypothalamus**. The body temperature is then raised above the normal 98.6 °F (37°C). A fever has beneficial results. It causes the liver and spleen to collect iron and zinc, which is believed to make them less available to support the growth of bacteria. Fevers also increase the metabolic rate of tissue cells, which may increase their repair speed.

Inflammation

Inflammation is a nonspecific response to tissue injury regardless of the type, including physical trauma, extreme heat, irritating chemicals, and infections. Inflammation prevents the spread of damaging agents to additional tissues, disposes of cell debris and pathogens, alerts the adaptive immune system, and starts tissue repair. The four cardinal signs of inflammation are redness, heat, swelling, and pain. There may also be impaired function as a result of inflammation. The inflammatory process begins with a flood of chemicals released into the extracellular fluid by injured or stressed tissue cells and immune cells. Key components include mast cells, histamine, kinins, **prostaglandins**, and cytokines. A complement is activated if pathogens provoke the inflammation, forming inflammatory solid chemicals. Soon, phagocytes flood into the damaged area, led by neutrophils, followed by macrophages. The phagocytes are mobilized via **leukocytosis**, **margination**, **diapedesis**, and **chemotaxis**. Antimicrobial proteins, aside from complement, also include IFNs.

You Should Remember

Inflammation develops due to damage or a stimulus—usually from external factors. Many cells are involved in the inflammatory response (mostly macrophages, mast cells, and lymphocytes). Acute inflammation usually heals quickly. However, the immune system can attack healthy tissue when the immune response continues without control, even after the threat has passed.

THE ADAPTIVE (SPECIFIC) DEFENSE SYSTEM

The human body has a specific defense system called the **adaptive immune system**. It finds and eliminates nearly any pathogen and is considered the third line of defense. The adaptive immune system protects against infectious agents and abnormal body cells. If it is weakened or fails, diseases such as cancer and **acquired immunodeficiency syndrome (AIDS)** can develop. Activation of the adaptive immune system dramatically increases the inflammatory response and results in the utmost activation of the complement system. To react, this system must first "meet" a specific antigen. Over time, antibodies develop into antigens. Early studies found that, for example, if an animal had survived a severe bacterial infection and produced antibodies against it, it would likely survive any recurrent bacterial infection. Also, if that animal's antibody-containing serum was injected into another animal without exposure to the pathogen, the injected animal would be protected.

TEST YOUR KNOWLEDGE

1. What are the beneficial results of a fever?
2. What does inflammation prevent?
3. How does the adaptive immune system react to antigens?

Antigens

Antigens are substances that mobilize the body's adaptive defenses and are the ultimate targets of all adaptive immune responses. The term "antigen" means "antibody generating." Most of them are large, complex natural or synthetic molecules that are foreign to the body. Therefore they are considered to be intruders and referred to as nonself. Antigens may be complete or incomplete. Whole antigens have both immunogenicity and reactivity. Immunogenicity is the ability to stimulate specific lymphocytes (B cells) to multiply. Reactivity is the ability to react with activated lymphocytes and antibodies released by immunogenic reactions.

Most foreign molecules can act as **complete antigens**, including most foreign proteins, large polysaccharides, and lesser amounts of lipids and nucleic acids. Proteins are the strongest of all antigens. Microorganisms and pollen grains, including bacteria, fungi, and viral particles, are immunogenic because their surfaces have many foreign macromolecules. Small molecules such as **nucleotides**, peptides, and hormones are not immunogenic. However, if they join with body proteins, the adaptive immune system can recognize this combination as foreign and attack it. These reactions are known as *hypersensitivities*. When this occurs, the **hapten** is implicated. Haptens are also known as *incomplete antigens*. When not attached to protein carriers, haptens have reactivity but no immunogenicity. Haptens are found in animal dander, poison ivy, cosmetics, detergents, many household and industrial products, and certain drugs (especially penicillin).

Antigenic Determinants

Antigenic determinants are foreign proteins that can stimulate an immune response. They bind to specific antigen receptors on the surface of B cells. Binding between receptors and antigenic determinants only occurs when their structures are complementary. When they are, a good fit is required to activate B-cell production of antibodies. The antibodies produced by the B cells are specifically targeted to the antigenic determinants that bind to the cells' antigen receptors. Therefore antigenic determinants are the regions of antigens recognized by specific antibodies that bind to and remove the antigens from the body.

Many antigens have a variety of unique antigenic determinants on their surfaces. Each can react with a different B-cell antigen receptor. The blood serum of an immunized individual or animal usually contains a mixture of antibodies that can all combine with the same antigen but with different antigenic determinants on the surfaces of the antigen. Antibodies that bind to the same antigenic determinant often have differing abilities to attach to that antigenic determinant. Two or more different antigens can have one antigenic factor in common. When this occurs, antibodies that target one antigen can react with all other antigens that carry the same antigenic determinant. These antigens are then called **cross-reacting antigens**.

TEST YOUR KNOWLEDGE

1. What are antigenic determinants?
2. What are cross-reacting antigens?

Antigen-Presenting Cells

The adaptive immune system consists of two distinct populations of lymphocytes, along with antigen-presenting cells (APCs). B cells manage **humoral immunity**, while T cells are non-antibody-producing cells that form the cellular part of adaptive immunity. APCs do not respond to specific antigens but serve supportive functions. T cells cannot recognize their antigens without the help of APCs. B and T cells follow a typical development pattern and shared life cycle stages. The growth, maturation, and activation of B and T cells involve five fundamental steps, which are explained below.

- *Origin* – lymphocytes originate in the red bone marrow from hematopoietic stem cells
- Maturation – lymphocytes (T cells) undergo a complex selection process
- *Self-tolerance* – each lymphocyte must be somewhat unresponsive to self-antigens to avoid attacking body cells; growth of lymphocytes takes

2 to 3 days, occurring in the red bone marrow for B cells and in the thymus for T cells
- *Seeding secondary lymphoid organs and circulation* – **Immunocompetent** B and T cells are called naïve because they have not yet been exposed to antigens; they come from the primary lymphoid organs to colonize the secondary lymphoid organs, where they will probably encounter antigens
- *Proliferation and differentiation* – after being activated, the lymphocyte quickly multiplies to form many identical cells with the same antigen specificity; these similar cells, all derived from the same **ancestor cells**, are called *clones*; most become *effector cells*, which fight off infections, but a few become memory cells

Humoral Immunity

Antibodies provide humoral immunity. They circulate freely and bind primarily to extracellular targets such as bacteria, toxins, and viruses. Antibodies are located in various body areas, including the skin, lungs, tears, saliva, and even breast milk. They temporarily inactivate and "mark" them for destruction by complement or phagocytes. The immune response does not involve antibodies. Instead, cell-mediated immunity is the activation of phagocytes, antigen-specific cytotoxic T lymphocytes, and releasing various cytokines in response to an antigen. **Cellular immunity** has cellular targets: cells infected with pathogens, cancer cells, and cells from foreign tissue grafts. The lymphocytes may act directly or indirectly. Direct action means killing the infected cells, while indirect action means working via the release of chemicals that enhance the inflammatory response, activate macrophages, or regulate the adaptive immune response. Many lymphocytes coordinate humoral as well as cellular immunity.

Activation and Differentiation of B Cells

An immunocompetent, naïve B lymphocyte is activated when matching antigens bind to its surface receptors and then cross-link adjacent receptors. Antigen binding is soon followed by receptor-mediated endocytosis of the cross-linked complexes. This clonal selection is followed by proliferation and differentiation into effector cells. Most clonal cells differentiate into plasma cells, the antibody-secreting effector cells of the humoral response. Plasma cells develop the intricate internal components, mainly the rough endoplasmic reticulum, required to secrete antibodies at a rate of about 2000 molecules per second. This continues for 4 to 5 days, and the plasma cells die. The secreted antibodies have the same antigen-binding properties as the receptor molecules on the parent B cell's surface. They circulate in the blood or lymph nodes, binding to free antigens and marking them for death via other innate or adaptive mechanisms. Clone cells do not become plasma cells; they become memory cells with longer lives. They can create a nearly immediate humoral response when reencountering the same antigen in the future.

Immunological Memory

Cellular proliferation and differentiation comprise the *primary immune response*, occurring on first exposure to a specific antigen. The answer takes 3 to 6 days after the encounter, related to the time needed for the B cells specific for that antigen to increase over about 12 generations and for offspring to differentiate into plasma cells. After this, plasma antibody levels increase, peak within approximately 10 days, and then decline. When reexposure to the same antigen occurs, regardless of how often, a *secondary immune response* happens, which is faster, longer, and more effective because the immune system has been primed to the antigen. Sensitized memory cells have already been alerted, providing **immunological memory**.

Over hours, new plasma cells are generated. Within 2 to 3 days, the **antibody titer** reaches much higher levels than with the primary response. Secondary response antibodies bind more tightly, and their blood levels stay elevated for weeks to months. With appropriate chemical signaling, plasma cells continue functioning longer than in the primary responses. Memory cells remain longer, mostly retaining the capacity to produce secondary humoral responses throughout life. Generally, the same events occur in the cellular immune response. A primary reply sets up many effector T cells and generates memory cells that can mount secondary responses.

TEST YOUR KNOWLEDGE

1. What is humoral immunity provided by?
2. When is an immunocompetent, naïve B lymphocyte activated?
3. What are the descriptions of the primary and secondary immune responses?

Active and Passive Humoral Immunity

Active humoral immunity occurs when B cells encounter antigens and produce antibodies against them. Active immunity is either naturally or artificially acquired. It is natural when a bacterial or viral infection develops, often with symptoms. It is artificial when a *vaccine* is given. Most vaccines contain dead or attenuated pathogens (alive but significantly weakened) or their components. There are two components of vaccines, as follows:

- Their weakened antigens provide immunogenic and reactive functional antigenic determinants.
- They do not cause most of the symptoms and morbidity of a disease that would usually occur during a primary response.

Active and passive immunity, which comprise humoral immunity

You Should Remember

The term *booster* refers to an extra dose of a vaccine after the primary amount. Booster vaccines intensify the immune response at later encounters with the same antigen. They can be given weeks, months, or years later.

Passive humoral immunity has different antibody sources and amounts of protection. Ready-made antibodies are introduced into the body. Antigens do not challenge the B cells, and immunological memory does not occur. The provided protection ends when the antibodies are naturally degraded. Passive immunity is provided naturally to a fetus or infant when maternal antibodies cross the placenta or are ingested via breast milk. For a few months after birth, the infant is protected from all antigens to which the mother was previously exposed. Passive immunity can also be provided artificially by giving exogenous antibodies, such as *gamma globulin*, collected from the plasma of an immune donor. These antibodies help prevent hepatitis A (via antiserum) and treat poisonous bites (via antivenom), botulism, rabies, and tetanus (via antitoxin). Otherwise, some quickly fatal diseases would cause death before establishing active immunity. Donated antibodies provide immediate protection but only have a short effect over 2 to 3 weeks.

Antibodies

Antibodies, called **immunoglobulins** (Igs), comprise the gamma globulin portion of plasma proteins. They are formed in response to many antigens but can be grouped into five Ig classes. Each antibody has four looping polypeptide chains linked by disulfide bonds. The four combined chains form a molecule known as an antibody **monomer** that has two identical halves. The molecule is Y shaped.

The two heavy chains (H chains) are identical to each other. The other two light chains (L chains) are identical but about half as long as the H chains. The heavy chains have a hinge region near their middles. The loops on each chain come from disulfide bonds. Each chain that forms an antibody has a **variable region** (V region) at one end and a **constant region** (C region) at the other end. Antibodies that respond to various antigens have significantly different V regions, while their C regions remain nearly the same in all antibodies of one class. In each monomer arm, the V regions of the heavy and light chains combine, forming an **antigen-binding site** that fits a certain antigenic determinant. Therefore each antibody monomer has two of these antigen-binding regions. The C regions include the stems of antibodies. Some antibodies activate complement, while others circulate in the blood or are found chiefly in secretions. Some are also able to cross the placental barrier.

The five major classes of immunoglobulins are IgM, IgA, IgD, IgG, and IgE, based on the C regions of their heavy chains (Figure 1.2). The antibodies have different characteristics, biological roles, and locations in each class. IgM is much larger and has heavier molecules in the plasma than the other antibodies. It is made up of five Y-shaped monomers linked to form a pentamer. IgA occurs in monomer and dimer (two linked monomers) forms. IgD, IgG, and IgE are all monomers with the same basic Y-shaped structure. B cells primarily switch from manufacturing different classes of antibodies as they become plasma cells. Therefore two or more antibody classes with the same antigen specificity are produced. The first antibody released in the primary response is IgM. Later, plasma cells start secreting IgG. In secondary responses, nearly all of the Ig protein is IgG. There also can be a switch from IgM to IgA or IgE. The Ig classes are further described as follows:

- *IgM (pentamer):* the initial Ig class secreted by plasma cells during the primary response; the presence of IgM in plasma usually means a current pathogenic infection is present and causing IgM formation; complement is readily activated; IgM exists in pentamer (five united monomers) form, but also as a monomer; the pentamer circulates in blood plasma, while the monomer acts as an antigen receptor on the B-cell surface; many antigen-binding sites make IgM a potent agglutinating agent.

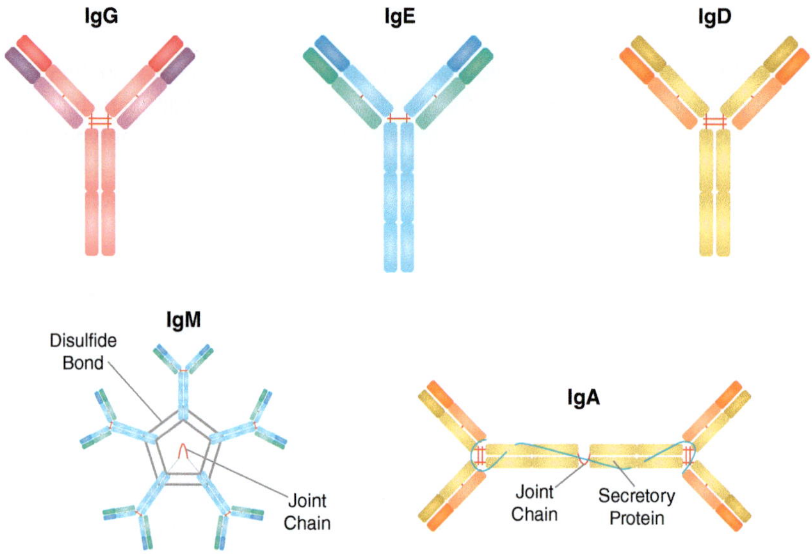

FIGURE 1.2 The five major classes of immunoglobulins.

- *IgA (dimer):* referred to as *secretory IgA*, is found in breast milk, saliva, sweat, and intestinal juice; secretory IgA helps keep pathogens from attaching to epithelial cell surfaces that include the mucous membranes and epidermis.
- *IgD (monomer):* present on B-cell surfaces, functioning (like IgM) as a B-cell antigen receptor.
- *IgG (monomer):* the most abundant antibody in the plasma, making up 75% to 85% of circulating antibodies, it is the primary antibody of secondary and late direct responses; IgG readily activates complement; it protects against bacteria, viruses, and toxins in circulating blood and lymph; it also crosses the placenta and results in passive immunity in the fetus
- *IgE (monomer):* the "stem end" binds to mast cells or basophils; an antigen binding to the "receptor end" triggers these cells to release chemicals such as histamine, mediating inflammation and an allergic reaction; IgE is secreted by plasma cells in the skin, mucosae of the GI and respiratory tracts, and tonsils; there are only traces of IgE in the blood plasma; levels increase during severe allergic attacks or chronic parasitic infections of the GI tract.

Antibodies cannot destroy antigens but can inactivate them and tag them for destruction. There is always a formation of **antigen-antibody complexes**, also called immune complexes. Antibodies use the following defensive mechanisms:

- **Neutralization:** the most basic type; it occurs when antibodies block specific sites on viruses or bacterial exotoxins; the virus or exotoxin cannot bind to tissue cell receptors; phagocytes then destroy the antigen-antibody complexes.
- **Agglutination:** since antibodies have multiple antigen-binding sites, they can bind to the same determinant on several antigens simultaneously; the complexes can be cross-linked into large frameworks; when cell-bound antigens are cross-linked, agglutination (clumping) of the foreign cells occurs; IgM has 10 antigen-binding sites, making it a powerful agglutinating agent.
- **Precipitation:** soluble molecules are cross-linked into large complexes that settle out of solution; precipitated antigen molecules are much more likely to be captured by phagocytes and engulfed in comparison to freely moving antigens.
- **Complement activation:** this is the primary antibody defense against cellular antigens; when several antibodies bind closely on the same cell, complement-binding sites on the stem regions line up, and complement is activated; membrane attack complexes may insert into the antigen cell surfaces, causing lysis; as the inflammatory response and phagocytosis are amplified, a positive feedback cycle brings in more defensive elements.

Monoclonal antibodies are preparations of pure antibodies, specific for one antigenic determinant, produced by descendants of one cell. Commercial monoclonal antibodies are essential for research, clinical tests, and treatments. Monoclonal antibodies help diagnose pregnancy, sexually transmitted infections, hepatitis, rabies, and some cancers. The tests are more specific, sensitive, and rapid than other tests. Monoclonal antibodies are also used for **leukemia** and **lymphoma**, which are easily accessible to injected antibodies. They can deliver anticancer drugs to cancerous tissues and can also be used to treat some autoimmune diseases. Monoclonal antibodies are administered either subcutaneously or as an intravenous infusion. The FDA strongly recommends IV infusion except when IV infusion is not available or would lead to a delay in treatment.

TEST YOUR KNOWLEDGE

1. When are active and passive humoral immunity?
2. What are the basic descriptions of the five types of immunoglobulins?
3. What are the four defense mechanisms used by antibodies?

Antibody Targets and Functions

Each antibody has a unique target (antigen) in an invading organism. The antigen helps the antibody to identify the organism. This is true because the antibody and antigen have a similar structure at the tips of their Y structures. Each antibody has a single antigen key. When the antibody activates, it tags or neutralizes its target. Regarding the biological functions of antibodies, the following are present:

- Specific binding of the corresponding antigen
- Activation of complement
- Binding of Fc receptors (with opsonization promoting phagocytosis, then mediated allergic reactions, and antibody-dependent cellular cytotoxicity [the ADCC effect])
- Through the placenta
- Immune regulation

Cellular Immunity

Cellular immunity is based on T lymphocytes directing adaptive immunity or attacking cellular targets. A cellular immune response is provoked when antigens are presented to T lymphocytes. Some activated T cells kill cells infected by viruses or bacteria, abnormal cancers, or transplantation. Other T cells release chemicals that regulate the immune response. T cells are much more complex than B cells in classification and function. The two major types of

T cells are based on the two structurally similar *cell differentiation glycoproteins* displayed by mature T cells. The CD4 and CD8 glycoproteins are surface receptors distinct from T cell antigen receptors. They affect interactions between T cells and other cells. Once activated, CD4 and CD8 cells differentiate into three major types of effector cells. They are as follows:

- CD4 cells: These usually become helper T cells (T_H cells), which aid in activating B cells, other T cells, and macrophages; they also direct the adaptive immune response.
- CD8 cells: these become cytotoxic T (T_C) cells, which destroy cells that contain anything foreign.
- Regulatory T cells: formed by some CD4 cells, these T_{Reg} cells moderate the immune response.

Activated CD4 and CD8 cells can become memory T cells as well. Helper, cytotoxic, and regulatory effector cells are only related to activated T cells. Naïve T cells are called CD4 or CD8 cells.

TEST YOUR KNOWLEDGE

1. What features are present regarding the biological functions of antibodies?
2. What is cellular immunity based on?
3. What are the three significant types of effector cells?

Major Histocompatibility Complex

The T cells cannot "see" free or naturally occurring antigens. The cells can recognize and respond to processed fragments of protein antigens displayed on the surfaces of APCs and other body cells. APCs are required to activate naïve T cells and the normal functioning of effector T cells. There are two classes of major histocompatibility complex (MHC) proteins, which are summarized in Table 1.1.

Class I MHC proteins are on the surface of nearly all body cells except RBCs. Each protein has a groove holding an antigen. **Endogenous antigens** are always self-antigens for healthy cells, usually pieces of digested cellular proteins. In infected cells, endogenous antigens may include fragments of antigens synthesized within the infected cell. In cancerous cells, endogenous antigens may consist of altered proteins due to the cancer.

The *class II MHC proteins* are less numerous and are usually found only on the surfaces of cells presenting antigens to CD4 cells. These include the dendritic cells, macrophages, and B cells. These proteins are also synthesized at the endoplasmic reticulum and bind to peptide fragments. However, the peptides they bind are longer amino acids and come from **exogenous antigens** from outside the cell that have been engulfed by the cell displaying them.

TABLE 1.1 Summarizing major histocompatibility complex proteins as part of cellular immunity.

Class I MHC proteins	Class II MHC proteins
Displayed by all nucleated cells	Displayed by APCs (dendritic cells, macrophages, B cells)
Recognized by naïve CD8 cells and T_C cells	Recognized by naïve CD4 cells and T_H cells
Foreign antigens on MHC are endogenous (intracellular pathogens or proteins made by cancer cells, with dendritic cells being an exception)	Foreign antigens on MHC are exogenous (phagocytized extracellular pathogens)
Cells displaying foreign antigens on MHC send one of two messages: if the cell is an APC, the message describes it as belonging to self, with a captured foreign invader that looks a certain way, and any cells resembling this will be killed; if the cell is not an APC, the message describes it as belonging to self, and having been invaded or becoming cancerous—this instructs that it should be killed	Cells displaying foreign antigens on MHC are described as belonging to self, having captured a foreign invader that looks a certain way and requesting that a defense be mounted against it

APC, Antigen-presenting cells; *MHC*, major histocompatibility complex, T_C cells, cytotoxic T cells; T_H cells, helper T cells.

TEST YOUR KNOWLEDGE

1. What are the two classes of MHC proteins?
2. Where are class I MHC proteins located, and what are their primary functions?
3. Where are class II MHC proteins located?

Activation and Differentiation of T Cells

Activated T cells may become effector cells or memory cells. T_H cells are essential in adaptive immunity, as they mobilize the humoral and cellular components. Once activated, these T_H cells help activate B and T cells and cause these cells to proliferate. Their cytokines provide the chemical that recruits other immune cells. Destruction of the T_H cells results in severe disease, as is seen in AIDS. T_H cells directly interact with B cells that display antigen fragments bound to class II MHC receptors. When a T_H cell binds to a B cell, the T_H cell releases cytokines that encourage B cells into more rapid division. They also signal the start of antibody formation. B cells keep dividing as long as the stimulation continues. Some B cells activate only by binding to *T cell–independent antigens*, but responses are usually weak and short-lived. Most antigens are *T cell–dependent antigens* that require T cell assistance to activate the B cells to which they bind.

CD8 cells usually need help from T_H cells to activate into destructive T_C cells. The T_H cells cause dendritic cells to express, on their surfaces, costimulatory molecules needed to activate CD8 cells. T_H cells amplify innate immune system responses, such as activating macrophages to become more efficient "killers." The immune response strengthens so that the antigens can be overwhelmed.

Activated CD8 cells, or T_C cells, directly attack and kill other cells. They circulate in and out of the blood and lymph and through the lymphoid organs, searching for cells displaying antigens they can recognize. They primarily target virus-infected cells but also attack tissue cells infected by some intracellular bacteria or parasites, cancer cells, and foreign cells present because of blood transfusions or organ transplants. Initially, a T_C cell must attach to a target cell by binding to a self-nonself complex. After recognizing their targets, T_C cells utilize **perforin** and **granzymes**. They also bind to a specific membrane receptor on the target cell that stimulates the target cell to undergo apoptosis.

Role of Specific T Cells

Depending on the APC that a naïve cell comes across, it can become an *effector T cell*, which has a relatively short lifespan and carries out the functions of immune responses. They can be cytotoxic, helper, or regulatory T cells. T_C cells ($CD8^+$ cells) primarily kill toxic or target cells. Upon recognition, they remove virally infected cells, bacteria, and tumor fragments, such as cancer cells, via apoptosis. T helper cells ($CD4^+$ cells) are similar to cytotoxic cells but have more functions. They are required for most adaptive immune responses and become activated when presented with antigens. They can also differentiate into cell subtypes. Regulatory T cells stop autoimmune responses once the threat has been eliminated. They have no further purpose once T_H cells and T_C cells bind to pathogens and rid them from the body. Regulatory T cells stop them from taking up space or accidentally attacking healthy cells until they are affected by apoptosis. Memory T cells can respond to antigens upon reintroduction, helping the body build **immunological tolerance**. They form after an infection and can expand into many effector T cells once exposed to familiar antigens. Memory T cells are unique because they remember pathogens and infectious cells more quickly than others. They are the reason that vaccines can create immunities within the body.

IMMUNE DEFICIENCIES

Immune deficiencies are disorders that impair the immune system's ability to defend the body against foreign or abnormal cells that invade or attack it.

Examples of foreign or abnormal cells are bacteria, viruses, fungi, parasites, and cancer cells. Immunodeficiency disorders are either congenital or acquired. A genetic or primary disease is one you were born with. A developed, or secondary, condition is one you get later in life. Acquired disorders are more common than congenital disorders.

Primary Immunodeficiency

With *primary immunodeficiency*, the immune system does not function normally. Affected individuals are more likely to contract infections and become very ill. There are over 400 types of primary immunodeficiency, varying in severity. Often, with a milder form, a person may find out they have the condition in adulthood. In other cases, it causes health problems in infancy. All states in the United States include testing for the subtype called **severe combined immunodeficiency** as part of newborn screening.

Signs and symptoms of primary immunodeficiency include more frequent or repeated ear, sinus, or skin infections; pneumonia; bronchitis; meningitis; and **thrush**. Conditions tend to last longer than normal individuals and may be difficult to treat—not responding to medications. Infections are often more severe and require hospitalization, such as **sepsis** or abscesses of internal organs. **Opportunistic infections** are common. Patients often lack weight gain or, in infants, failure to thrive. Chronic diarrhea and certain blood disorders are seen. People with primary immunodeficiency are more likely to have certain cancers. In some cases, primary immunodeficiency is caused by a genetic disorder that involves other health problems, such as **DiGeorge syndrome (DGS)**.

Early diagnosis of DGS can help prevent or delay health problems. Untreated, the condition can cause organ damage and death. For individuals with primary immunodeficiency, it is always important to regularly wash their hands, maintain good oral hygiene, and have physical activity, a healthy diet, and sufficient sleep. Any exposure to sick individuals or crowds should be avoided. Patients often cannot have live vaccines (rotavirus, chickenpox, oral polio, measles/mumps/rubella). Treatments for primary immunodeficiency include antibiotics, immunoglobulin replacement therapy, IFN-gamma therapy, growth factors, stem cell transplants, and gene therapy.

You Should Remember

DGS is a congenital disorder with a broad phenotype, which results predominantly from the defect of chromosome 22. Features of DGS include cardiac anomalies, recurrent infections, abnormal facial expressions, thymic hypoplasia or aplasia, cleft palate, developmental delay, and hypocalcemia.

TEST YOUR KNOWLEDGE

1. What is the function of regulatory T cells?
2. What are immune deficiencies?
3. What are the signs and symptoms of primary immunodeficiency?

Secondary Immunodeficiency

Secondary immunodeficiency (SID) occurs when another treatment or illness weakens the immune system. It occurs when the immune system is compromised due to an environmental factor. SIDs are clinically manifested by an increased frequency or complications of common infections and occasionally by opportunistic infections. The SIDs have a broad spectrum of presentation, depending on the magnitude of the offending external condition and the host's susceptibility.

SIDs are far more common than primary immunodeficiencies. They are clinically manifested by an increased frequency or unusual complications of common infections and sometimes by opportunistic infections. The best-known SID is **AIDS**, primarily because of its prevalence and its high mortality rate without treatment. Even so, the most common SID worldwide is severe malnutrition, affecting innate and adaptive immunity.

AIDS interferes with the activity of T_H cells to impair the immune system. It is caused by the human immunodeficiency virus (HIV), transmitted primarily through blood, semen, and vaginal secretions. HIV usually enters the body through blood-contaminated needles or during sexual intercourse. HIV can also be transmitted from a mother to her fetus via the placenta. The virus targets CD4 cells via their surface proteins. After entering these cells, HIV uses the **reverse transcriptase** viral enzyme to produce DNA from its viral RNA. The DNA copy (*provirus*) inserts itself into the target DNA, directing the cell to create new copies of viral RNA and proteins, allowing the virus to multiply and infect other cells. Therefore HIV destroys the T_H cells, depressing adaptive immunity. The HIV reverse transcriptase enzyme often produces errors, causing the relatively high mutation rate of HIV, plus its ability to develop drug resistance. There is no cure for AIDS, but many antiviral drugs, often combined, can treat it. Unfortunately, this can fail when the virus becomes resistant.

You Should Remember

The most common cause is malnutrition, affecting many global communities with restricted food access. Protein-calorie deficiency and micronutrient deficiencies alter immune responses, and vitamin D deficiency causes a failure of immune activation. Other diseases that may be implicated include metabolic disorders and genetic multisystemic syndromes. Immune defects seen in SID are usually heterogeneous, and the prognosis is based on the severity of the immune deficiency.

TEST YOUR KNOWLEDGE

1. When does SID occur?
2. What is the best-known SID?
3. How does AIDS impair the immune system?

KEY TERMS

Accidental cell death
Acid mantle
Acquired immunodeficiency syndrome
Active humoral immunity
Adaptive immune system
Adenoid
Agglutination
Alveolar macrophages
Allogeneic cells
Ancestor cells
Antibody titer
Antibodies
Antigen-antibody complexes
Antigen-binding site
Antigenic determinants
Antigens
Antigen-presenting cells
Apoptosis
Astrocytes
Auditory tubes
Basophils
Bone marrow
Cellular immunity
Chemokinesis
Chemotaxis
Complement activation
Complement
Complete antigens
Constant region
Cross-reacting antigens
Cytokines
Cytotoxic T cells
Defensins
Dendritic cells
Dermcidin
Diapedesis
DiGeorge syndrome
Diffuse lymphoid tissue
Dust cells
Endogenous antigens
Eosinophils
Exogenous antigens
Ferroptosis
Fibroblasts
Genital warts
Granzymes
Hapten
Haptotaxis
Homeostasis
Humoral immunity
Hypothalamus
Immune deficiencies
Immunoglobulins
Immunological memory
Immunological tolerance
Immunometabolism
Innate immune cells
Innate immunity
Intracellular degradation
Interferons
Interleukins
Keratin
Kupffer cells
Lamina propria
Leukocytosis
Leukemia
Lingual tonsil
Lipolysis
Lymph nodes
Lymphocytes
Lymphoma
Lymphoid follicles
Macrophages
Margination
Memory T cells
Microglia
Monoclonal antibodies
Monocytes
Monomer
Mucin
Multiple sclerosis
Myeloid cells
Myelopoiesis
Necroptosis
Neutralization
Neutrophils
Nucleotides
Opportunistic infections
Opsonins
Palatine tonsils
Passive humoral immunity
Perforin
Peyer patches
Phagocytosis
Phagosome
Phagolysosome
Plasma cells
Platelets
Precipitation
Prostaglandins
Pyrogens
Pyroptosis
Regulatory T cells
Reticular cells
Reverse transcriptase
Sebum
Sepsis
Severe combined immunodeficiency
Stem cells
Sternum bone
Thrush
Thymus
Tubal tonsils
Variable region

FURTHER READING

1. Abbas, A.K., Lichtman, A.H., Pillai, S., 2023. Basic Immunology: Functions and Disorders of the Immune System, 7th Edition. Elsevier.
2. Agmon-Levin, N., Shoenfeld, Y., Tomjerovic, L., 2015. Vaccines and Autoimmunity. Wiley Blackwell.
3. Chang, C., Lu, Q., 2020. Epigenetics in Allergy and Autoimmunity (Advances in Experimental Medicine and Biology Book 1253). Springer.
4. Dettmer, P., 2021. Immune: A Journey into the Mysterious System that Keeps You Alive. Random House.
5. Faass, N., Saputo, L., 2011. Boosting Immunity: Creating Wellness Naturally. New World Library.
6. Faustman, D., 2018. The Value of BCG and TNF in Autoimmunity, 2nd Edition. Academic Press.
7. Glaser, R., Kiecolt-Glaser, J.K., 2014. Handbook of Human Stress and Immunity. Academic Press.
8. Haseltine, W.A., Gurch, J., 2022. Natural Immunity and COVID-19: What It Is and How It Can Save Your Life. Access Health Press.
9. Mummery, C.L., van de Stolpe, A., Roelen, B., Clevers, H., 2021. Stem Cells: Scientific Facts and Fiction, 3rd Edition. Academic Press.
10. Parham, Peter, 2021. The Immune System, 5th Edition. W.W. Norton & Company.
11. Parmar, G., 2022. Arming the Immune System: The Incredible Power of Natural Immunity & The Fever Response. Parmar.
12. Perricone, C., Shoenfeld, Y., 2019. Mosaic of Autoimmunity: The Novel Factors of Autoimmune Diseases. Academic Press.
13. Shoenfeld, Y., Mahroum, N., Watad, A., 2020. Infection and Autoimmunity, 3rd Edition. Academic Press.
14. Sompayrac, L., 2019. How the Immune System Works, 6th Edition. Wiley Blackwell.
15. University Press, 2021. Immune System: A Brief History. University Press.
16. Zouali, M., 2005. Molecular Autoimmunity. Springer.

Chapter 2

Integrative Immunology

Chapter Outline

Learning Objectives

1. Describe immunologic tolerance.
2. Differentiate the peripheral and central tolerance.
3. Explain the role of Fc receptors in immune responses.
4. Describe the mucosa-associated lymphoid tissue.
5. Explain mechanisms for the secretion of polymeric IgA and IgM antibodies.
6. Describe neuroinflammatory disorders.
7. Explain the structure of a virus.
8. Compare the characteristics of chlamydiae and rickettsiae.
9. Describe the classifications of bacteria.
10. Explain deep fungal infections and give five examples.

OVERVIEW

The immune system protects us from infection through various lines of defense. If the immune system is not functioning as it should, it can result in diseases such as autoimmunity, allergy, and cancer. The immune system

Vaccinology and Immunizations. http://doi.org/10.1016/B978-0-443-23915-1.00002-0

has two lines of defense: innate immunity and adaptive immunity. Innate immunity is the first immunological, nonspecific (antigen-independent) mechanism for fighting against an intruding pathogen. It is a rapid immune response that occurs minutes or hours after aggression and has no immunologic memory. On the other hand, adaptive immunity is antigen dependent and antigen specific; it has memory capacity, which enables the host to mount a more rapid and efficient immune response upon subsequent exposure to the antigen. There is a great deal of synergy between the adaptive immune system and its innate counterpart, and defects in either system can provoke illness or disease, such as autoimmune diseases, immunodeficiency disorders, and hypersensitivity reactions. Immunological tolerance is the process by which immune cells are made unresponsive to self-antigens to prevent damage to healthy tissues. It contains an immune response to antigens produced by the body itself or recognized from a prior encounter. Various microorganisms may act as a pathogen to which the immune system responds and provides immunity.

IMMUNOLOGIC TOLERANCE

Immunologic tolerance, also known as *immune tolerance*, is the state of an active, highly regulated unresponsiveness of the immune system to self-antigens or against a particular antigen that can induce an immune response in the body. Immunological tolerance is broadly categorized as central and peripheral mechanisms that provide and maintain **self-tolerance**. Central tolerance is achieved through negative selection by newly developing lymphocytes in primary lymphoid organs tolerant to self-antigens. Peripheral tolerance describes the mechanisms that prevent autoreactive lymphocytes from initiating potentially harmful immune responses against the body's antigens, food, and commensal organisms through anergy, deletion, or development of induced regulatory T cells.

Immunologic tolerance describes a diverse range of host processes that prevent potentially harmful immune responses within that host. This is achieved by avoidance of adaptive immunity, such as the forms of immune privilege seen in maternal acceptance of the fetus, in cancer, and diverse body tissues, or through fine control of adaptive immunity in lymphocytes throughout their lifetime. Understanding mechanisms underlying tolerance promises opportunities to therapeutically reprogram the immune system to treat autoimmune diseases and allergies, ensure improved acceptance of transplants, and provide better vaccines against microbes and cancers.

The tolerance of the immune system is essential in maintaining immune homeostasis. Immune tolerance is carried out through central and peripheral immune tolerance. The T-regulatory cells, directed from the thymus, regulate the central tolerance. However, the T-regulatory cells must hold the peripheral tolerance peripherally after central tolerance.

Central Immune Tolerance

Central immune tolerance is performed in the host body's thymus and bone marrow parts. During the development of an embryo and neonate stages, the immature T cells and B cells obtain tolerance against self-antigens by the selection processes, which may be positive or negative at the maturation time. During the process, the self-antigen receptors possessing cells are eliminated. T cells that do not recognize either major histocompatibility complex I (MHC-I) or MHC-II molecules degenerate through apoptosis, known as "positive selection." The high-affinity binding of T cells to MHC I and II is also directed to programmed cell death and is known as "negative selection." A similar negative selection process has been observed during B-cell development in the bone marrow. The B cells possessing autoreactive antibodies on their surface are induced to programmed cell death. The process can be named clonal deletion. The immune system is assimilated to differentiate the self and nonself by deleting the autoreactive T and B cells before fully maturing into functional immune cells by these central tolerance phenomena.

Peripheral Immune Tolerance

Peripheral immune tolerance refers to immunological tolerance developed after autoreactive T and B cells mature and enter the periphery. It enables the immune system to recognize and tolerate self-antigens or nonharmful foreign antigens in the body. Peripheral immune tolerance mainly occurs in adults. Its mechanism prevents the immune system from overreacting to environmental factors. Thus peripheral tolerance processes exist wherein self-reactive T cells become functionally unresponsive (anergy) or are deleted after encountering self-antigens outside the thymus.

You Should Remember

Central tolerance is a state of immune tolerance induced initially in the thymus and bone marrow. At the same time, peripheral tolerance is a state of immune tolerance induced initially in the lymph nodes and other tissues.

TEST YOUR KNOWLEDGE

1. What are the differences between central and peripheral immune tolerance?
2. How is immune tolerance carried out?
3. Where is central immune tolerance performed?

THE ROLE OF FC RECEPTORS

The receptors for the Fc of immunoglobulins, **Fc receptors** (FcRs), link the humoral and cellular branches of the immune system, and they have essential functions in the activation and downmodulation of immune responses. Balanced signaling through activating and inhibiting FcRs regulates various cells' activity in the immune system.

Immune responses to self-antigens in various tissues cause autoimmune diseases. **Rheumatoid arthritis**, for example, involves joint inflammation and destruction caused by autoimmune antibody responses to unknown synovial antigens. By contrast, patients with type 1 diabetes develop insulitis due to T-cell infiltration and destruction of the pancreatic islets. Autoimmune reactions are thought to have the same basis as adaptive immune responses to foreign antigens, in which **antigen-specific T cells** are activated by antigen-presenting cells.

Even before identifying cell surface receptors for the Fc of antibodies, it was well-known that passively administered antibodies can activate or suppress immune responses. Therefore antibody- or Fc-mediated activation and suppression have been studied since the 1960s, which led to identifying FcRs in B cells. During the past decade, we have learned much more about FcRs at the molecular level and have shown that they are not simply cell surface molecules that bind immunoglobulins—they can initiate various biological functions.

You Should Remember

FcRs control the humoral and innate immune responses, essential for appropriate responses to infections and the prevention of chronic inflammation or autoimmune diseases. Following their cross-linking by immune complexes, FcRs play various roles, such as modulation of the immune response by released cytokines or phagocytosis.

THE MUCOSAL IMMUNE SYSTEM

The immune system may be viewed as an organ distributed throughout the body to provide host defense against pathogens wherever these may enter or spread. Within the immune system, a series of anatomically distinct compartments can be distinguished, each of which is specially adapted to generate a response to pathogens present in a particular set of body tissues. Part of the immune system responds to antigens that have entered the tissues or spread into the blood. Another compartment located near the surfaces where most pathogens invade is the **mucosa-associated lymphoid tissue**. Two further distinct compartments are the body cavities (peritoneum and pleura) and the skin.

Two key features define these compartments. The first is that immune responses induced within one chamber are confined mainly in expression to that particular compartment. The second is that lymphocytes are restricted to specific cases by expressing homing receptors bound by ligands, known as addressins, that are expressed explicitly within the tissues of the compartment. The mucosal surfaces of the body are particularly vulnerable to infection. They are thin and permeable barriers to the body's interior because of their physiological activities in gas exchange in the lungs, food absorption in the intestinal tract, sensory activities (eyes, nose, mouth, and throat), and reproduction (uterus and vagina). The necessity for permeability of the surface lining these sites creates an apparent vulnerability to infection. Unsurprisingly, most infectious agents invade the human body through these routes.

A second important point to remember when considering the immunobiology of mucosal surfaces is that the intestine acts as a portal of entry to a vast array of foreign antigens in food. The immune system has evolved mechanisms to avoid a vigorous immune response to food antigens on the one hand and, on the other, to detect and kill pathogenic organisms gaining entry through the intestine. These are beneficial to their host in many ways. They protect against pathogenic bacteria by occupying the ecological niches for bacteria in the large intestines. They also serve a nutritional role in their host by synthesizing vitamin K and B_{12}. However, in certain circumstances, they may cause infectious diseases.

The other principal sites within the intestinal mucosal immune system for the induction of immune responses are the Peyer patches of the small intestine, the appendix, and solitary lymphoid follicles of the intestine. Peyer patches are a significant site for the induction of immune responses in the small intestine and have a distinctive structure, forming domelike structures extending into the lumen of the intestine.

There are unique mechanisms for the secretion of **polymeric** IgA and IgM antibodies into the intestine lumen. Polymeric IgA and IgM are synthesized throughout the gut by plasma cells in the lamina propria. They are transported into the intestine by immature epithelial cells located at the base of the **intestinal crypts**. These express the polymeric immunoglobulin receptor on their basolateral surfaces. This receptor binds polymeric IgA or IgM and transports the antibody by **transcytosis** to the luminal surface of the intestine. Upon reaching the luminal surface of the **enterocyte**, the antibody is released into the secretions by proteolytic cleavage of the extracellular domain of the polymeric IgA receptor. Secreted IgA and IgM bind to the mucus layer overlying the gut epithelium, where they can bind to and neutralize gut pathogens and their toxic products.

The feeding of foreign antigens typically leads to specific and active unresponsiveness, a phenomenon known as **oral tolerance**. Thus no antibody response follows feeding a foreign protein such as **ovalbumin**. However, injecting it subcutaneously can induce a strong antibody response to this protein, especially if an adjuvant is also given. However, the feeding of ovalbumin is followed by a prolonged period during which the administration of ovalbumin by injection, even in the presence of an adjuvant, elicits no antibody response.

We each harbor more than 400 species of **commensal bacteria** present in the most significant numbers in the colon and ileum. Although these bacteria collectively weigh approximately 1 kg and outnumber us by about 1014 to 1, we usually cohabitate with our intestinal bacterial flora in a happy **symbiotic relationship**.

One protective activity of our normal intestinal tract flora is competition against pathogenic bacteria for space and nutrients, preventing their intestinal colonization. This activity is dramatically illustrated by one of the adverse effects of antibiotics. Taking an antibiotic kills large numbers of commensal gastrointestinal tract (GIT) bacteria and thereby offers an **ecological niche** to bacteria that would not otherwise be able to compete successfully with the typical flora and grow in the gut. One example of a bacterium that grows in the antibiotic-treated GIT and can cause a severe infection is *Clostridium difficile*; this produces two toxins that can cause severe bloody diarrhea associated with mucosal injury.

There are some circumstances in which the normal bacterial inhabitants of the intestinal tract cause disease, for example, following the breakdown of the integrity of the mucosa lining the intestine. This may occur following poor blood flow in the intestine or following **endotoxemia**. In these circumstances, innocuous gut bacteria, such as nonpathogenic *Escherichia coli*, can cross the mucosa, invade the bloodstream, and cause fatal systemic infection. This illustrates the vital importance of the barrier to infection by the body's mucosal surfaces. The normal intestinal tract flora also becomes a significant cause of systemic disease in patients with immunodeficiency. This illustrates the role of the adaptive immune system in the host's defense against the flora of the intestine but also shows that this response does not result in the elimination of bacteria from the lumen of the gut but rather a state resembling symbiosis.

You Should Remember

Probiotics are live microorganisms intended to have health benefits when consumed or applied to the body. They can be found in yogurt, other fermented foods, dietary supplements, and beauty products.

TEST YOUR KNOWLEDGE

1. What do immune responses to self-antigens in various tissues cause?
2. Why are the mucosal surfaces of the body particularly vulnerable to infection?
3. What principle sites are utilized for the induction of immune responses?

NEUROIMMUNOLOGY

Neuroimmunology, as a separate discipline, has its roots in neurology, neuroscience, and immunology. While neuroimmunologists initially focused on classical neuroinflammatory disorders such as multiple sclerosis and CNS infections, there is strong evidence to suggest that the immune response contributes to genetic white matter disorders, epilepsy, neurodegenerative diseases, neuropsychiatric disorders, peripheral nervous system, and neurooncological conditions, as well as aging.

Technological advances have greatly aided our knowledge of how the immune system influences the nervous system during development and aging and how such responses contribute to disease, regeneration, and repair. Molecular biological studies may push many areas of neuroimmunology. Understanding neuroimmunology will open up new avenues for therapeutic approaches to manipulate neuroinflammation.

One of the greatest misconceptions that impeded progress in neuroimmunology was the idea that the **blood-brain barrier** and the perceived immunological privilege of the brain prevent cross-talk between the CNS and immune systems.

Probing neuroinflammatory diseases has been aided with improved higher-resolution MRI, single-photon emission computed tomography and PET ligands, and **optical coherence tomography** to visualize the progression of disease in patients and, for some modes, the contribution of inflammation.

While current therapies aim to modulate neuroinflammation arising during the disease, future approaches should aim at disease prevention. The etiological agents are known for some conditions. As a result, vaccination strategies are essential for disease prevention. In other cases, the specific genes or environmental agents triggering disease require clarification. Prophylactic approaches for genetic disorders could exploit genetic modification during development, while cell therapy strategies may aid the regeneration of the damaged nervous system. Exploitation of infectious agents may also be beneficial.

Rapid and specific diagnosis and adequate ways to monitor the disease course and response to therapy are crucial for disease prevention. Thus advancements in **biomarker** research will be critical to faster diagnosis and more efficient monitoring in clinical trials, speeding up drug development, and reducing costs. Biomarkers of neuroimmunological diseases may include markers of blood-brain barrier disruption, **demyelination**, oxidative stress and axonal/neuronal damage, **gliosis**, and repair. Still, they should also focus on features of altered immune function, such as cytokines, chemokines, antibodies, adhesion molecules, and antigen presentation.

CLASSIFICATIONS OF PATHOGENS

Discussing the various pathogen classes is essential to better understanding immune responses to pathogens. Many microorganisms are pathogens and affect the immune system. The microbial pathogens cause human disease and are classified as viruses, chlamydiae, rickettsiae, mycoplasmas, bacteria, fungi, and protozoa.

Viruses

Viruses differ significantly from all the other microbes, as they consist of only nucleic acid surrounded by a protein coat (**capsid**) and contain only one instead of two types of nucleic acid. Once inside human cells, the viruses remove the standard nuclear control of the cells to take over cellular metabolism to synthesize new virions.

Some viruses also have an envelope. Viruses cannot reproduce without a host. Therefore the obligate intracellular parasites require their host to replicate them and facilitate their spread to others. Some common diseases caused by viruses include the flu, the common cold, and COVID-19. Mortality commonly occurs when viruses jump species (such as Ebola or human immunodeficiency virus [HIV]) when the virus undergoes a significant antigenic change (influenza viruses) or when host immunity is compromised. HIV represents one of the most dramatic human examples of an exotic virus that kills its host. However, HIV kills slowly, providing the time needed to spread to new hosts and an effective strategy for persistence in the species. In most situations, defense against viruses involves multiple immune components, and the impact of a single mechanism varies significantly according to the method by which individual viruses enter, replicate, and spread within the host.

Several common human viral pathogens enter through the GIT, including rotavirus, enteric adenoviruses, and hepatitis A virus. These are usually spread via person-to-person contact or contaminated food and water. Respiratory infections caused by influenza viruses, rhinoviruses, coronaviruses, measles viruses, varicella-zoster viruses, and respiratory syncytial viruses are often spread by aerosol transmission and person-to-person contact. Many herpes viruses target the skin or the mucosae, such as herpes simplex virus and varicella-zoster virus. Herpes simplex virus, in particular, can infect oral and genital mucosa, the eye, and the skin through minor cuts and abrasions. Cytomegalovirus targets the mucosa. Cytomegalovirus can also spread from mother to baby or, rarely, via blood transfusions. Human papillomavirus targets skin and mucosa, causes warts, and may cause cervical cancer. Viruses like West Nile and Semliki Forest viruses may also enter through the skin via insect vectors. HIV, hepatitis C virus, and hepatitis B virus are commonly spread via sexual contact. They can also infect humans via direct entry into the bloodstream via transfusions or contaminated needles.

TEST YOUR KNOWLEDGE

1. Besides multiple sclerosis and CNS infections, what other disorders may the immune response contribute to?
2. What may biomarkers of immunological diseases include?
3. How do viruses differ from all other microbes?

Chlamydiae

Chlamydiae are among the most common human infectious agents and produce much disability, although little acute mortality. They are gram-negative obligate intracellular bacteria that are pathogenic for humans. The chlamydiae consist of three species, *C. trachomatis, C. psittaci*, and *C. pneumoniae*. Trachoma occurs worldwide and is prevalent in Africa and Asia. *C. trachomatis* is usually inoculated into the eye by contaminated fingers or fomites or, in neonates, by passage through an infected birth canal. Genital infections are spread venereally, and respiratory infections are usually by inhalation. Psittacosis transmitted by *C. psittaci* is acquired from infected birds.

Rickettsiae

The **rickettsiae** are a diverse collection of obligately intracellular gram-negative bacteria found in ticks, lice, fleas, mites, and **chiggers**. *Rickettsia* species cause **Rocky Mountain spotted fever** (RMSF), rickettsialpox, and Rickettsia typhi. Patients present with febrile exanthems and visceral involvement; symptoms may include nausea, vomiting, abdominal pain, encephalitis, hypotension, acute renal failure, and respiratory distress.

RMSF is an infection caused by the bite of an infected tick. It affects over 2000 people annually in the United States and usually occurs from April until September. It can occur anytime during the year when the weather is warm. RMSF was first recognized in the Rocky Mountain states but may occur throughout the United States. The most common areas where the disease occurs are in the southeastern and south-central United States. The condition is not spread from person to person. A classic case of RMSF involves a rash that appears 2–4 days after the onset of fever as small, flat, pink macules on the wrists, forearms, and ankles and spreads to the trunk and sometimes the palms and soles (Figure 2.1). RMSF is among the most severe of human infectious

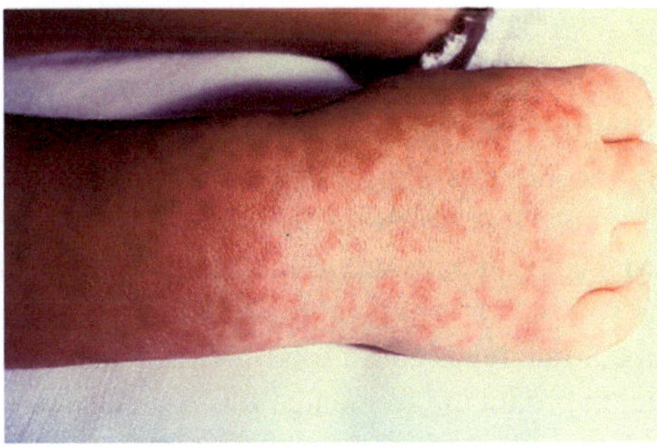

FIGURE 2.1 The classic rash of Rocky Mountain spotted fever.

diseases, with a mortality of 20%–25% unless treated with an appropriate antibiotic. The severity and mortality are higher for males, elderly persons, and Black males with glucose-6-phosphate dehydrogenase deficiency.

Rickettsialpox is a mite-borne and predominately urban **zoonosis** that cycles among house mice. Confirmed or suspected cases of rickettsialpox have been reported from at least 14 countries worldwide, making this disease one of the few spotted fever–group **rickettsioses** with a cosmopolitan distribution.

Rickettsia typhi is associated with rats and fleas, mainly the oriental rat flea, although other ecologic cycles have been implicated. Fleas are infected by transovarial transmission or by feeding an animal with rickettsiae circulating in the blood. Rickettsiae are shed from fleas in the feces, from which humans acquire the infection through the skin, respiratory tract, or conjunctiva.

TEST YOUR KNOWLEDGE

1. What are the three species of *Chlamydiae*?
2. What do the species of *Rickettsia* cause?
3. How does the classic rash of RMSF appear?

Mycoplasmas

Mycoplasmas are the smallest and simplest self-replicating bacteria. The mycoplasma cell contains the minimum organelles essential for growth and replication: a **plasma membrane**, **ribosomes**, and a **genome** consisting of a double-stranded circular DNA molecule. Unlike all other prokaryotes, the mycoplasmas have no cell walls. All mycoplasmas cultivated and identified thus far are parasites of humans, animals, plants, or arthropods. The primary habitats of human and animal mycoplasmas are the mucous surfaces of the respiratory and urogenital tracts and the joints in some animals. Although some mycoplasmas belong to the normal flora, many species are pathogens, causing various diseases that tend to run a chronic course.

Bacteria

Bacteria are tiny single-celled organisms and **prokaryotes**. They are found in every **habitat** on Earth: soil, rock, oceans, and even arctic snow. Some live in or on other organisms, including plants, animals, and humans. There are approximately 10 times as many bacterial cells as human cells in the human body. A lot of these bacterial cells are found lining the digestive system. Some bacteria live in the soil or on dead plant matter, playing an essential role in the cycling of nutrients. Some types cause food spoilage and crop damage, but others are instrumental in producing fermented foods such as yogurt and soy sauce. Bacteria are microbes with a more straightforward cell structure than many other organisms. Their nucleus contains genetic information and is contained in a single loop of DNA. Some bacteria have an extra circle of genetic material called a **plasmid**, rather than a nucleus. The plasmid often contains genes that give the bacterium some advantage over other bacteria. For example, it may have a gene that makes the bacterium resistant to a particular antibiotic.

Bacteria are classified into five groups according to their basic shapes: spherical (cocci), rod (bacilli), spiral (spirilla), comma (vibrios), or corkscrew (spirochaetes). They can exist as single cells, in pairs, chains, or clusters.

Most bacteria reproduce by **binary fission**. In this process, the bacterium, a single cell, divides into two identical daughter cells. Binary fission begins when the DNA of the bacterium divides into two. The bacterial cell then elongates and splits into two daughter cells, each with identical DNA to the parent cell. Each daughter cell is a clone of the parent cell. Bacterial infections are common diseases that can affect all body systems. Some of them may release toxins into the body.

Fungi

Fungi are **eukaryotic** microorganisms. They can occur as yeasts, molds, or mushrooms. Some fungi are capable of causing superficial, cutaneous, subcutaneous, and systemic diseases. **Yeasts** are microscopic fungi of solitary cells that reproduce by **budding**. They digest food externally and absorb nutrients directly through their cell walls. Most fungi reproduce by spores and have a body composed of microscopic tubular cells called **hyphae**. Fungi are like animals; they obtain carbon and anergy from other organisms. Some fungi obtain nutrients from a living host (plant or animal). Others get their nutrients from dead plants or animals. Some fungi infect a resident host but kill host cells to obtain their nutrients, which is called necrotrophy.

In humans, there are several fungal infections called **mycoses**. Dermatophytes cause the most common. The fungi colonize dead **keratinized tissue**, including skin and toenails. They cause superficial infections such as unsightly **ringworm**, which is challenging to treat but rarely severe. Some fungi are members of the resident **microflora** in healthy people but become pathogenic in people with predisposing conditions. For example, *Candida* species cause annoying yeast infections in the mucosal tissues of many healthy people but can also cause diseases collectively called **candidiasis** in babies and immunocompromised individuals. Another group of fungi is inhaled as spores, initiating lung infection.

Fungal infections usually affect the skin, hair, nails, or mucous membranes, but they can also infect the lungs or other parts of the body. Fungal infections are more common in places on the body that trap moisture or have much friction. People are at higher risk for disease, especially severe ones, if they have poor circulation or diabetes or a weakened immune system from cancer or cancer treatment, immunosuppressant medications, and HIV/AIDS. Subcutaneous fungal infections are more common in tropical and subtropical areas. Examples include **sporotrichosis**, **chromoblastomycosis**, and **eumycetoma**.

Deep fungal infections are found in the lungs, blood, urinary tract, or brain. The most common deep fungal infections include:

- **Histoplasma** is the fungus that causes histoplasmosis and can infect your lungs, brain, or other body parts. It is commonly found in the Ohio and Mississippi River valleys.
- **Cryptococcus** causes cryptococcosis. The disease usually infects the lungs but sometimes can infect the brain and spinal cord.
- **Blastomyces** species are the fungi that cause blastomycosis, commonly infecting the bones, skin, and lungs. Rarely, it can also infect the brain and spinal cord.
- The mold of *Aspergillus* causes aspergillosis and can cause several lung infections, including allergic bronchopulmonary aspergillosis and chronic pulmonary aspergillosis. It may infect other body parts or form a fungus ball (**aspergilloma**).
- **Pneumocystis pneumonia** is caused by the fungus *Pneumocystis jirovecii*, which can infect the lungs.
- **Coccidioidomycosis** is a disease caused by a fungus called Coccidioides that grows in the soil and dirt in some areas of California and Arizona. It is also referred to as **valley fever**, which affects the lungs.

TEST YOUR KNOWLEDGE

1. What are the primary habitats of mycoplasmas?
2. What are the five classifications of bacteria?
3. What are examples of fungal infections in humans?

Protozoa

Protozoa are single-celled organisms. They come in many different shapes and sizes, ranging from an amoeba, which can change its shape, to a paramecium, with its fixed shape and complex structure. They live in moist habitats, including freshwater, marine environments, and soil. Infections range from asymptomatic to life-threatening, depending on the parasite's species and strain and the host's resistance.

Most of the parasitic diseases in humans are attributed to protozoa. These diseases induce sickness in humans when they turn into human parasites. Protozoal infections in humans, such as malaria, **amoebic dysentery**, and **African sleeping sickness**, cause the most prevalent and fatal diseases.

IMMUNE RESPONSES TO PATHOGENS

The innate immune responses are the first line of defense against invading pathogens. They are also required to initiate specific adaptive immune responses. Innate immune responses rely on the body's ability to recognize conserved features of pathogens not in the uninfected host. Because the adaptive system comprises small numbers of cells with specificity for any individual pathogen, toxin, or allergen, the responding cells must proliferate after encountering the antigen to attain sufficient numbers to mount an effective response against the microbe or the poison. Thus the adaptive response generally expresses itself temporally after the innate response in the host defense. A vital feature of the adaptive response is that it produces long-lived cells that persist in a dormant state but can reexpress effector functions rapidly after another encounter with their specific antigen. This allows the adaptive response to manifest immune memory. Therefore this permits it to contribute prominently to a more effective host response against particular pathogens or toxins.

The immune system employs many potent effector mechanisms that can destroy a broad range of microbial cells and clear a wide range of toxic and allergenic substances. Therefore the immune response must avoid unleashing these destructive mechanisms against the human host's tissues. The ability of the immune response to prevent damaging self-tissues is referred to as self-tolerance. Failure of self-tolerance underlies the broad class of autoimmune diseases. Mechanisms to avoid reaction against self-antigens are expressed in many parts of the innate and adaptive immune response.

Because an essential aspect of the T-cell arm of the immune system is to recognize host cells infected by viruses, intracellular bacteria, or other intracellular parasites, T cells have evolved an elegant mechanism that recognizes foreign antigens together with self-antigens as a molecular complex.

Myeloid stem cells give rise to several forms of granulocytes, **megakaryocytes**, platelets, and erythrocytes. Cells of the granulocyte lineage that play prominent immune functions include neutrophils, monocytes, macrophages, eosinophils, basophils, and mast cells. The immune functions of the classical granulocytes have been inferred from the immunologically active molecules. For example, neutrophils produce large quantities of reactive oxygen species that are cytotoxic to bacterial pathogens. They also have enzymes that appear to participate in tissue remodeling and repair following injury. Neutrophils accumulate in large quantities at sites of bacterial infection and tissue injury. They possess prominent phagocytic capabilities that permit them to sequester microbes and particulate antigens internally, which can be destroyed and degraded. Thus it is clear that they play a significant role in the clearance of microbial pathogens and the repair of tissue injury. More recently, however, neutrophils have been recognized to produce substantial amounts of cytokines tumor necrosis factor and interleukin-12. This supports an additional immunoregulatory role of neutrophils.

Like neutrophils, monocytes are also highly phagocytic for microbes and particles marked for clearance by binding Ig and complement. They appear to be mobilized shortly after the recruitment of neutrophils and persist for long periods at sites of chronic inflammation and infection. In addition to participating in acute inflammatory responses, they are prominent in **granulomatous** processes throughout the body. Eosinophils are readily recognized by their prominent cytoplasmic granules that contain toxic molecules and enzymes that are particularly active against **helminths** and other parasites.

Basophils and mast cells are morphologically similar cells that represent distinct lineages. By the cell surface expression of high-affinity receptors for IgE, they are critical initiators of immediate hypersensitivity responses and the host response to helminthic parasites, releasing histamine and heparin from their granules. Recent studies have demonstrated that in addition to their role in immediate hypersensitivity responses, mast cells also play prominent roles in the host response to bacterial infection.

The monocyte also plays critical roles in the adaptive immune response by taking up microbial antigens, processing them by proteolysis to peptide fragments, and presenting them in forms that activate T responses. Additional cells in this lineage include **Langerhans cells** in the epidermis, Kupffer cells in the liver, and microglial cells in the CNS.

TEST YOUR KNOWLEDGE

1. Which protozoal infections cause the most fatal and prevalent human diseases?
2. What do innate immune responses rely on?
3. What is the ability of the immune response to prevent damaging self-tissues referred to as?

KEY TERMS

African sleeping sickness
Amoebic dysentery
Antigen-specific T cells
Aspergilloma
Biomarker
Binary fission
Blastomyces
Blood-brain barrier
Budding
Candidiasis
Capsid
Central immune tolerance
Chiggers
Chlamydiae
Chromoblastomycosis
Coccidioidomycosis
Commensal bacteria
Cryptococcus
Demyelination
Ecological niche
Endotoxemia
Enterocyte
Eukaryotic
Eumycetoma
Fc receptors
Gliosis
Genome
Granulomatous
Habitat
Helminths
Histoplasma
Hyphae
Immunologic tolerance
Intestinal crypts
Keratinized tissue
Langerhans cells
Megakaryocytes
Microflora
Mucosa-associated lymphoid tissue
Mycoplasmas
Mycoses
Neuroimmunology
Optical coherence tomography
Oral tolerance
Ovalbumin
Peripheral immune tolerance
Plasma membrane
Plasmid
Pneumocystis pneumonia
Polymeric
Prokaryotes
Ribosomes
Rickettsialpox
Rickettsia typhi

Ringworm
Rocky Mountain spotted fever
Rheumatoid arthritis
Self-tolerance
Sporotrichosis
Symbiotic relationship
Transcytosis
Valley fever
Yeasts

CASE STUDIES

Case Study 1

A 9-year-old girl was brought by her parents to the local hospital with complaints of a frontal headache, fever, abdominal pain, and severe myalgia. She also had a maculopapular rash over much of her body. The patient soon developed hypotension, oliguria, hepatic dysfunction, and coagulopathy. She was transferred to the intensive care unit and placed on a ventilator. Treatment with gamma immunoglobulin was started due to the possibility of Kawasaki disease. After testing, Kawasaki disease was ruled out, and diagnoses that were considered included rickettsiosis, staphylococcemia, leptospirosis, ehrlichiosis, and meningococcemia. Intravenous ciprofloxacin was applied. Within 4 days, the bacterial cultures that had been taken returned negative. The young patient died within a few hours afterward. During the autopsy, detailed studies were undertaken, and it was found that the patient had died from severe RMSF complications.

Critical Thinking Questions

1. What is the description of RMSF, and how prevalent is it?
2. What are the classic manifestations of RMSF?
3. How severe can RMSF be?

Case Study 2

A 25-year-old male was hospitalized because a necrotic skin lesion on his back did not respond to treatment. He had recently visited from a vacation in Honduras. Within 10 days, he developed generalized weakness, night sweats, chills, and a persistent headache. He also admitted to losing much of his appetite. The patient described a feeling of heaviness behind his sternum. Medical imaging confirmed abdominal and inguinal adenopathy. Doxycycline had been used for a suspected rickettsial infection, which resolved the lesion, while the other symptoms persisted. Histopathology isolated a fungus in culture, and the final diagnosis was histoplasmosis.

Critical Thinking Questions

1. What do fungal infections usually affect, and where in the body are they most common?
2. Which groups of people are at a higher risk of disease due to fungal infections?
3. Which fungus causes histoplasmosis?

FURTHER READING

1. Bansal, S.S., 2022. Immune Cells, Inflammation, and Cardiovascular Diseases (Methods in Signal Transduction Series). CRC Press.
2. Bennett, A., 2023. Human Diseases and Bacterial Pathogens. American Medical Publishers.
3. Bielekova, B., Birnbaum, G., Lisak, R.P., 2019. Neuroimmunology (Contemporary Neurology Series). Oxford University Press.
4. Cheeseman, H.R., Fulder, S., Mizrahi, A., Sheinman, N., 2013. Potentiating Health and the Crisis of the Immune System: Integrative Approaches to the Prevention and Treatment of Modern Diseases. Springer.
5. Dietert, R.R., Luebke, R.W., 2012. Immunotoxicity, Immune Dysfunction, and Chronic Disease (Molecular and Integrative Toxicology). Humana Press.
6. Hameed, S., Fatima, Z., 2019. Pathogenicity and Drug Resistance of Human Pathogens: Mechanisms and Novel Approaches. Springer.
7. Hangartner, L., Burton, D.R., 2020. Vaccination Strategies Against Highly Variable Pathogens (Current Topics in Microbiology and Immunology Book 428). Springer.
8. Hemsworth, R., 2023. Ticks and Tick-Borne Pathogens. American Medical Publishers.
9. Horwitz, R., Muller, D., 2010. Integrative Rheumatology (Integrative Medicine Library). Oxford University Press.
10. Jacobs, P., 2023. Human Fungal Pathogens. American Medical Publishers.
11. Kierzenbaum, F., 2013. Parasitic Infections and the Immune System. Academic Press.
12. Kudva, I.T., Cornick, N.A., Plummer, P.J., Zhang, Q., Nicholson, T.L., Bannantine, J.P., Bellaire, B.H., 2016. Virulence Mechanisms of Bacterial Pathogens, 5th Edition. ASM Press.
13. Mak, T.W., Saunders, M.E., Jett, B.D., 2014. Primer to the Immune Response, 2nd Edition. Academic Press – Cell.
14. McGuire, R.A., Coelho, P.R.P., 2011. Parasites, Pathogens, and Progress: Diseases and Economic Development. The MIT Press.
15. Nelson, R., 2023. Fc Receptors and their Antibodies: Role in Disease and Immunotherapy. Foster Academics.
16. Platt, J., 2018. Immunological Tolerance and Accommodation. Academic Press.
17. Smith, D., Ryan, M.J., Buddie, A.G., 2023. Managing Microorganisms. CABI.
18. Wisneski, L., 2017. The Scientific Basis of Integrative Health, 3rd Edition. Routledge.

Unit II

Vaccinology

Chapter 3

History of Vaccines

Chapter Outline

Learning Objectives

After study of this chapter, readers should be able to:

1. Identify the various types of viral hepatitis.
2. Discuss the signs and symptoms of rabies in humans.
3. Describe the most significant achievement in international public health concerning smallpox.
4. Identify the different types of diphtheria.
5. Describe yellow fever and how it is transmitted to humans.
6. Describe the historical events related to meningococcal disease.

Vaccinology and Immunizations. http://doi.org/10.1016/B978-0-443-23915-1.00003-2

7. Explain the history of Spanish influenza.
8. Describe the manifestations of acute respiratory distress syndrome.
9. Explain the link between human papillomavirus and illness.
10. Explain the COVID-19 pandemic.

OVERVIEW

Although inoculation practices started more than 500 years ago, Edward Jenner first described the term "vaccine" in the 18th century. The history of vaccines did not begin with his smallpox vaccine and will not end with the recent vaccines against the novel coronavirus that caused the COVID-19 pandemic. The history of vaccines started before the first vaccine, with an immunizing procedure called "inoculation" by some and "variolation" by others. Inoculation with materials from smallpox lesions to trigger immunity against smallpox dates to ancient China, and the first account of the procedure was written in 1549. An English physician, Dr. Jenner, created the world's first successful vaccine. He found out that people infected with cowpox were immune to smallpox. In 1796, he inoculated 8-year-old James Phipps with matter collected from a cowpox sore on the hand of a milkmaid. Smallpox vaccination with the vaccinia virus is the most famous example of a highly effective vaccine. The typical vaccine development timeline takes 5 to 10 years, and sometimes longer, to assess whether a vaccine is safe and efficacious in clinical trials, complete the regulatory approval processes, and manufacture enough vaccine doses for widespread distribution.

POLIOMYELITIS

Poliomyelitis (polio) is a disabling and life-threatening disease. It is caused by the *poliovirus*, which spreads between individuals. It can invade the spinal cord, causing **paralysis** (Figure 3.1).

Polio has existed since prehistoric times, and Egyptian images show children walking with canes and "withered" limbs, characteristic of the disease. The first known clinical description of polio did not occur, however, until 1789, when British physician Michael Underwood described it. Polio was formally recognized as a condition in 1840 by German physician Jakob Heine. In the late 19th and early 20th centuries, regular epidemics resulted in polio becoming the most feared global disease. In 1916, a large outbreak in New York City killed more than 2000 people. The worst recorded attack, in 1952, killed over 3000 Americans. Survivors often face lifelong consequences. Limb deformities result in the need for leg braces, crutches, or wheelchairs. Some people required breathing devices such as the iron lung, an early artificial respirator invented for polio treatment. By the mid–20th century, poliovirus killed or paralyzed more than 500,000 people annually throughout the world. There was an urgent need for a vaccine.

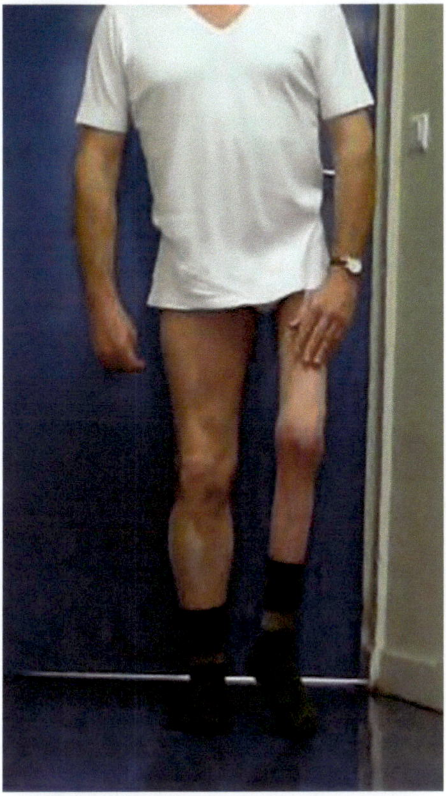

FIGURE 3.1 A patient with poliomyelitis.

In 1949, the poliovirus was cultivated in human tissue at Boston Children's Hospital, resulting in a 1954 Nobel Prize for the participating scientists. Soon, Dr. Jonas Salk created the first successful vaccine (Figure 3.2). He tested his experimental "killed-virus" vaccine on himself and his family and then on volunteer children in the United States, Canada, and Finland. His inactivated poliovirus (IPV) vaccine was released in 1955, and by 1957, annual cases decreased from 58,000 to 5600. By 1961, only 161 patients remained. Six pharmaceutical companies were licensed to produce IPV. Physician and microbiologist Albert Sabin developed the oral poliovirus (OPV), which was approved in 1960 (Figure 3.3). It was live attenuated, using the virus in a weakened form, and could be given orally, such as in the form of drops placed on a sugar cube.

There was initially low interest in this new vaccine in the United States. However, the ease of administering the OPV made it originally famous in other countries such as Hungary, Czechoslovakia, and Cuba. By 1994, polio had been eliminated from the Americas, and by 2000, it had been eradicated in

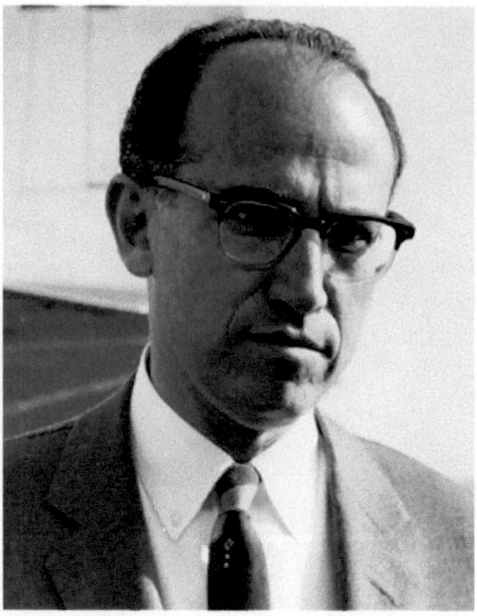

FIGURE 3.2 Dr. Jonas Salk.

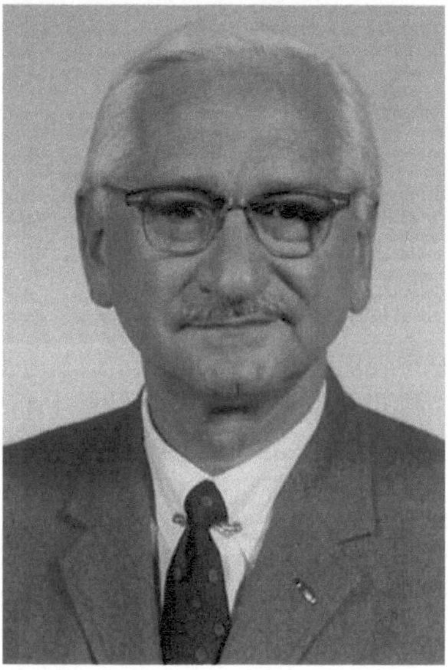

FIGURE 3.3 Dr. Albert Sabin.

the Western Pacific. By 2006, polio remained endemic in only four countries. The 21st century saw additional advances, with cases reduced by over 99% worldwide in less than two decades. Southeast Asia was polio free by 2014, and Africa achieved this in 2020. As of 2021, just two "wild poliovirus" cases were recorded (one each in Afghanistan and Pakistan).

You Should Remember

While the IPV was successful, it did not prevent it from spreading between children. The OPV interrupted the chain of transmission, meaning that it was able to stop polio outbreaks from occurring.

TEST YOUR KNOWLEDGE

1. When did the worst recorded outbreak of polio occur?
2. When were the Salk and Sabin vaccines first used publicly?
3. When was polio eradicated from the Americas?

TUBERCULOSIS

Tuberculosis (TB) is caused by the bacterium known as *Mycobacterium tuberculosis*, which usually attacks the lungs. However, TB bacteria can attack any body part—primarily the kidneys, spine, and brain. Not all infected patients become ill.

TB in humans can be traced back to 9000 years ago to a location near Israel, where the remains of a mother and child were still found to contain the TB bacteria. Throughout the 1600s to the 1800s in Europe, TB caused 25% of all deaths. In the 1700s, TB was referred to as the *white plague* because it caused infected people to become extremely pale. It was commonly called *consumption* in the 1800s because of how it caused weight loss and the appearance of "wasting away."

The term "TB" was coined in 1834 by Johann Schonlein, though it is estimated that the bacteria may have existed for up to 3 million years. Dr. Robert Koch announced his discovery of *M. tuberculosis* in 1882. At this time, TB killed one in every seven people in the United States and Europe. Today, the subtypes of TB identify its locations within the body (pulmonary or extrapulmonary). The disease is also classified as drug susceptible, drug resistant, multidrug resistant, and extensively drug resistant.

Extrapulmonary TB includes genitourinary, meningeal, peritoneal, pericardial, and cutaneous forms. *Miliary TB* is a potentially fatal form of disseminated disease due to the hematogenous spread of tubercle bacilli to the lungs and other organs. It causes millet seed–sized tuberculous foci to form, each 1 to 2 mm in size. There is simultaneous involvement of two or more noncontiguous organ sites of the body or infection of the blood, bone marrow, or liver. The classical hallmark is **mottling**, seen in chest radiographs. *Genitourinary TB* usually involves the urinary tract or genital organs from the hematogenous spread of chronic latent pulmonary TB.

Diagnosis is often delayed because the signs and symptoms are often masked by another disease (usually a urinary tract infection). *Meningeal TB*, also called *tuberculous meningitis*, is caused by the seeding of the meninges with the bacilli of *M. tuberculosis*. It is characterized by membrane inflammation (meninges) around the brain or spinal cord. *Peritoneal TB* is a form of abdominal TB that often presents as an insidious progression of abdominal pain in 50% to 100% of cases and distention due to ascites in 40% to 73% of cases. It causes weight loss, fever, and, sometimes, night sweats. *Pericardial TB* causes coughing, dyspnea, chest pain, night sweats, orthopnea, weight loss, and edema of the ankles. The most frequent signs include cardiomegaly, pericardial rub, fever, and tachycardia. *Cutaneous TB* causes friable, painful, red-to-yellow papules and nodules that measure 1 to 3 cm in diameter. The condition can lead to painful ulcers with fibrinous bases in the skin surrounding body orifices. Edema and inflammation are seen in the perilesional tissue.

You Should Remember

By the beginning of the 19th century, TB, or "consumption," had killed one out of every seven people. Famous people who died from TB included author Jane Austen, author George Orwell, first lady Eleanor Roosevelt, actress Vivien Leigh, author Emily Bronte, US president James Monroe, clergyman Cardinal Richelieu, historical figure Pocahontas, and gunfighter Doc Holliday.

TEST YOUR KNOWLEDGE

1. In the 1800s, how lethal was TB?
2. What is miliary TB?
3. What causes meningeal TB?

VIRAL HEPATITIS

Hepatitis is liver inflammation that results in abnormal function of the organ. A virus often causes it, and there are five types of viral hepatitis, which include hepatitis A, B, C, D, and E. The most common types are hepatitis A, hepatitis B, and hepatitis C.

The oldest evidence of hepatitis (specifically, hepatitis B) was found in a tooth of a male who lived around 5000 BCE. Outbreaks of jaundice (probably hepatitis A) were reported in the 17th and 18th centuries, often during military campaigns. Hepatitis A was formerly called **infectious hepatitis** and was first differentiated from hepatitis B in the 1940s. In the 1970s, identifying the virus and developing serologic tests helped differentiate hepatitis A from other types. The most significant number of cases in 1 year was 59,606 in 1971. The hepatitis A virus was first isolated in 1979. Hepatitis A vaccines were first licensed in the United States in 1995, providing long-term protection. From 1996 through 2011, hepatitis A cases decreased by more than 95%. Before 2004, hepatitis A was the most frequently reported subtype in the United States. In 2016, hepatitis A reemerged in the United States due to widespread outbreaks among drug users and people experiencing homelessness.

Hepatitis B was formerly called **serum hepatitis**. The first recorded cases are believed to be those following the administration of the **smallpox** vaccine, which was given to shipyard workers in Germany in 1883. In the early and middle 20th century, serum hepatitis was seen repeatedly after using contaminated needles and syringes. In 1943, the role of blood as a vehicle for hepatitis B virus (HBV) transmission was clearly described, and the hepatitis B surface antigen was first identified in 1965. The complete hepatitis B virion, the *Dane particle*, was identified in 1970. A plasma-derived hepatitis B vaccine was first licensed in the United States in 1982. Recombinant HBV replaced the plasma-derived vaccine in 1986, and the plasma-derived type is no longer used in the United States. In 2018, 3322 cases of acute hepatitis B were reported to the CDC, with an overall incidence of one point per 100,000 population. The rate of reported acute HBV infections declined by about 90% since recommendations for vaccination were first issued.

Hepatitis C was first discovered in the 1980s when a different virus (not hepatitis A or hepatitis B) was found to be causing liver damage. It was identified as the hepatitis C virus in 1989. In 1991, a screening process was developed to detect hepatitis C virus in blood samples. Though there is not yet a hepatitis C vaccine, the best way to prevent the condition is to avoid behaviors that spread the disease, such as injecting drugs using shared needles or having unprotected sex. Testing for hepatitis C is vital because current treatments can cure most people within 8 to 12 weeks.

Hepatitis D is a rare form of viral hepatitis first discovered in 1977 in patients with chronic hepatitis B infection. It is also called **delta hepatitis**. Hepatitis D was initially thought to be an unrecognized HBV antigen. Later, it was found that hepatitis D was part of a new pathogen called the *delta agent*. Hepatitis D virus (HDV) is a hybrid virus because it uses hepatitis B surface antigen as its envelope protein. Therefore it can only infect patients who harbor HBV. For unknown reasons, HBV replication is suppressed when HDV is present. HDV is mainly transmitted via the parenteral route through blood or blood product exposure. It is most prevalent in the Mediterranean, East Africa, the Amazon basin, the Middle East, Central and Northern Asia, and certain Pacific areas. There is no vaccine to prevent HDV, but prevention of HBV also protects against HDV infection.

Hepatitis E was first discovered in 1980 during a waterborne epidemic of acute hepatitis in India. A single-stranded RNA viral genome has been identified and named hepatitis E virus (HEV). Genotypes 1 and 2 only infect humans, while genotypes 3 and 4 primarily infect other mammals. In highly endemic areas, the disease is acquired through the fecal-oral route, mainly from contaminated water supplies. HEV infections in humans also occur because of eating undercooked game meat, raw liver from supermarkets, and natural pork sausages called *Fratelli* in Corsica, an island owned by France. Blood transfusion–associated HEV infections occur in many countries, and the screening of donors for HEV RNA is under consideration. HEV is very severe in pregnant females and has a high mortality rate. There is no approved vaccine for hepatitis E in the United States, but a recombinant vaccine was approved for use in China in 2012.

You Should Remember

Hepatitis B causes severe and lifelong health problems. About 25% of chronic infections progress to liver cancer. It also causes liver damage, cirrhosis, liver failure, and death. Vaccination within 24 hours of birth, followed by two to three additional doses, provides life-long protection against hepatitis B infection. The vaccine is estimated to prevent 38 million deaths over the lifetimes of persons born between 2000 and 2030 in 98 low- and middle-income countries.

TEST YOUR KNOWLEDGE

1. How is hepatitis E transmitted?
2. When did the hepatitis A and hepatitis B vaccines first become available?
3. What is the best way to prevent hepatitis C?

MALARIA

Malaria is a life-threatening disease spread to humans by *Anopheles* mosquitoes and is most preventable in tropical countries. Only *Anopheles* mosquitoes can transmit malaria, and they must have been infected through a previous blood meal taken from an infected person. Malaria is not a contagious disease because it is not spread person-to-person. The disease causes fever, chills, headache, fatigue, confusion, seizures, and difficulty breathing. Young children, pregnant females, travelers, and immunocompromised people are at the highest risk of severe disease.

The history of malaria began with documentation of similar disease symptoms recorded in Chinese documents dating from about 2700 BCE. There was additional documentation in Greece from approximately 850 BCE. Scientific studies became possible after the discovery of the malaria parasite in 1880. By 1884, it was found that a protozoan and not a bacterium caused malaria. *Anopheles* mosquitoes were determined to be the vector in 1897. When an accidental discovery was made in 1891 of a methylene blue eosin stain, searches for malaria parasites were simplified. By 1900, it was known that there were three species of parasites, and by 1918, a fourth species was discovered. The four kinds of malaria parasites that infect humans include *Plasmodium falciparum, P. vivax, P. ovale*, and *P. malaria*.

In 1945, malaria research intensified globally, and the disease soon began to decrease in prevalence. In the United States, there were 15,000 reported cases in 1947 and 2000 in 1950, and by 1951, malaria was considered eliminated. However, malaria remains a major global health problem, with 350 to 500 million infections and about 1 million deaths occurring annually worldwide. The areas of the world most affected today include Central and South America, Africa, Asia, Eastern Europe, and the South Pacific.

RABIES

Rabies is a preventable viral disease usually transmitted through a rabid animal's bite. The rabies virus infects the CNS of mammals, eventually causing **encephalitis**, coma, and death. Most reported rabies cases occur in wild animals such as raccoons, bats, skunks, and foxes, though any mammal can be affected. The rabies virus is transmitted through direct contact with saliva from an infected animal. Humans usually get rabies from the bite of a rabid animal. Less often, transmission occurs from scratches, abrasions, or open wounds exposed to infectious saliva or other material from an infected animal.

After exposure, the virus must travel from the bite site or scratches to the brain before symptoms develop. The **incubation period** in humans is typically between 20 and 90 days, although incubation periods as short as 4 days and more prolonged than 6 years have been documented. This variation is probably related to the site of inoculation, the severity of the wound, and the amount of virus, based on the location of the exposure site, the type of rabies virus, and any existing immunity. Initial symptoms may include weakness, discomfort, fever, headache, prickling, and an itching sensation at the bite site. Signs and symptoms then progress to brain dysfunction, anxiety, confusion, and agitation. Later, there may be **hydrophobia**, delirium, abnormal behaviors, **hallucinations**, and insomnia. The acute period usually ends within 2 to 10 days. Once clinical signs and symptoms appear, the disease is nearly always fatal, and treatment is generally supportive.

The first written record of rabies causing death in humans and dogs was found in Babylon, dating from 2300 BCE. In the 1st century CE, the Roman scholar Celsus suggested that the saliva of a biting animal may transmit rabies. In 18th century America, home remedies to treat rabies included using hairballs called mudstones from the stomachs of cows, goats, and deer. They were believed to have curative powers that pulled the "madness" out of bite wounds. These objects were highly valued and passed down through generations of families. President Abraham Lincoln reportedly transported his son Robert for "Maidstone" treatment in 1849 after a rabid dog bit the boy. The boy survived. The same year, writer Edgar Allan Poe traveled to Baltimore, Maryland, where he was found lying in the street. A lifelong alcoholic, it was assumed that Poe was suffering from **delirium tremens**. When offered water, he had great difficulty swallowing it. Poe slipped in and out of a coma, hallucinated, and showed extreme aggression, and he finally died 4 days later. His body had no bite wounds, but less than one-third of human rabies victims showed evidence of these wounds.

The first actual treatment for rabies occurred in the 1880s because of the work of Louis Pasteur in developing the vaccine. In 1885, a young boy was attacked by a rabid dog. Pasteur inoculated the boy 13 times over 11 days, and the boy completely recovered. Over 20,000 people had received his postexposure prophylactic vaccine by Pasteur's death. Today, the protocol for the rabies vaccine is as follows:

- Four 1-mL doses of the human diploid cell culture vaccine or purified chick embryo cell rabies vaccine should be administered intramuscularly (IM) to previously unvaccinated persons.
- The first dose must be given as soon as possible after rabies exposure.
- Additional dose are given on days 3, 7, and 14.
- For adults, the vaccination is always administered IM into the deltoid muscle.
- For children, the anterolateral aspect of the thigh can also be injected.
- The gluteal area is never used for rabies vaccine injections because observations suggest that this results in lower neutralizing antibody titers.

The first vaccination is given concurrently with the human rabies immune globulin (HRIG) at a site distant from the HRIG. An additional fifth dose of rabies vaccine is given on day 28 to immunocompromised patients. Certain people with a higher risk for rabies exposure, such as those who work with potentially infected animals, are recommended to receive the vaccine to help prevent rabies if an exposure happens. For individuals at higher risk of exposure to the rabies virus:

- Two doses of rabies vaccine are given on days 0 and 7.
- Depending on the level of risk, a booster dose may be delivered within 3 years after the first two doses.

HRIG is infiltrated around the bite(s) site and provides rapid passive immune protection with a half-life of approximately 21 days. It is administered only once, on the first day of the postexposure prophylaxis (PEP) regimen (designated day 0). A maximum of the recommended dosage of HRIG should be given because excessive HRIG can partially suppress the active production of antibodies. If the HRIG was not administered on day 0, it may be administered up to and including day 7 of the PEP regimen. Beyond day 7, HRIG is not indicated, as the patient's antibody response to the vaccine occurs in that time frame.

- The recommended dosage of HRIG is 20 IU per kg of body weight for all ages, including children.
- Infiltrate as much of the HRIG as possible into and around the bite wound.
- Administer the remaining HRIG IM at a site distant from the first vaccination site, generally in the quadriceps or deltoids.
- If there is no wound, such as following a bat-in-the-bedroom exposure, then administer the entire dose of HRIG in the quadriceps or deltoids.

You Should Remember

Following an exposure, previously vaccinated persons are given two 1-mL doses of vaccine IM in the deltoid muscle on days 0 and 3. No HRIG is administered. The CDC states that the standard two-dose vaccination schedule will protect for at least 3 years.

You Should Remember

About 5000 animal rabies cases are reported in the United States annually, with more than 90% occurring in wild animals. There were 89 human rabies deaths in the country from 1960 to 2018. In 2021, five people in the United States died from rabies.

Most were due to bat exposure, though raccoons, skunks, and other wild mammals can also be infected with rabies. In several countries, canine rabies is also a risk.

You Should Remember

Rabies can spread to people from bats after minor, seemingly unimportant or unrecognized bites or scratches. Rabies PEP, including vaccination, is recommended for anyone with a bite or scratch from a bat unless the bat has been captured to be tested for rabies.

TEST YOUR KNOWLEDGE

1. In which animals do most cases of rabies occur?
2. What is typically the incubation period for rabies?
3. How is the rabies immunization protocol administered?

SMALLPOX

Smallpox is an acute contagious disease caused by the variola virus, a member of the **Orthopoxvirus** family. The first symptoms of smallpox usually appear 12 to 14 days after a patient is exposed to the smallpox virus. After the incubation period, sudden flulike symptoms occur. These include fever, headache, muscle aches, severe back pain, and fatigue. A few days later, flat red spots appear on the body. They may start in the mouth and on the tongue and then spread to the skin. The face, arms, and legs are often affected first, followed by the torso, hands, and feet. Within a day or two, many spots become small blisters filled with clear fluid. Later, the blisters fill with pus. These sores are

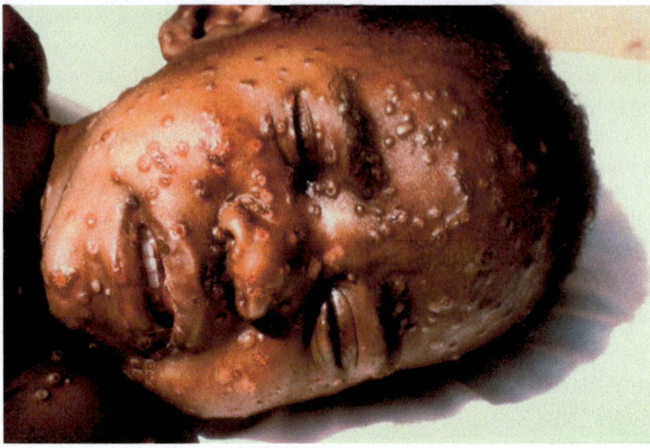

FIGURE 3.4 A patient with smallpox.

called **pustules** (Figure 3.4). Scabs form 8 to 9 days later and eventually fall off, leaving deep, pitted scars.

Smallpox was a severely devastating disease and caused millions of deaths before it was eradicated. The origin of smallpox is unknown. Smallpox-like rashes have been found on Egyptian mummies, suggesting that the disease existed for at least 3000 years. The first written description of a condition with the characteristics of smallpox occurred in China during the 4th century CE. Other early reports appeared in India (7th century) and Asia Minor (10th century).

The global spread of smallpox was due to the growth of civilizations and world exploration. As trade routes increased over many centuries, the disease spread. Highlights from the history of smallpox include the following:

- The 6th century: Smallpox reached Japan due to increased trade with China and Korea.
- The 7th century: Smallpox reached northern Africa, Spain, and Portugal because of the expansion of Arab nations.
- The 11th century: Smallpox reached Europe during the Crusades.
- The 15th century: Smallpox reached western Africa, which Portugal partly occupied.
- The 16th century: Smallpox reached the Caribbean and Central and South America as European settlers and the African slave trade grew.
- The 17th century: Smallpox reached North America, carried by European settlers.
- The 18th century: Smallpox reached Australia, carried by explorers from Great Britain.

Smallpox had an average mortality rate of three out of 10 infected as it developed. It usually caused scarring, which was often severe. An early control method was **variolation**, in which uninfected people were exposed to material from smallpox pustules by scratching the material into their forearms or arms. After variolation, some of the disease's symptoms usually develop, including fever and rash. Fortunately, fewer people died from variolation than when the infection was naturally acquired.

Variolation began in 1796, as English physician Edward Jenner (Figure 3.5) realized that farmworkers who had contracted cowpox were protected from developing smallpox. He correctly guessed that exposure to cowpox could be used to protect against smallpox (Figure 3.6). He took material from a cowpox sore on a farm worker's arm and inoculated the arm of a friend's son. Months

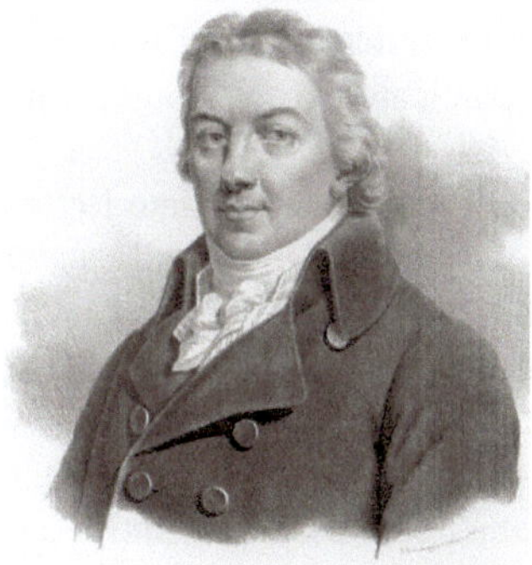

FIGURE 3.5 Dr. Edward Jenner.

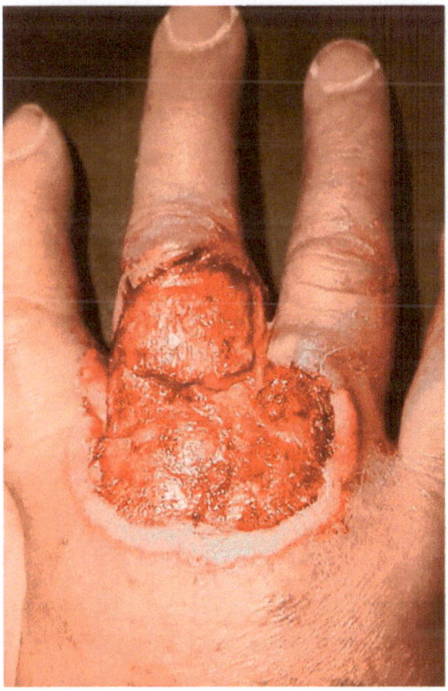

FIGURE 3.6 Cowpox on the hand.

later, the child was exposed to the variola virus several times yet never developed smallpox. After many other experiments, Jenner published "On the Origin of the Vaccine Inoculation," which summarized his work and predicted how smallpox would eventually be eradicated. Vaccination then became widely accepted and slowly replaced variolation. In the 1800s, the virus used to manufacture the smallpox vaccine was changed from cowpox to vaccinia. By 1952, smallpox was eliminated in North America and, by 1953, in Europe.

In 1959, the World Health Organization (WHO) planned to eradicate smallpox globally. Still, the disease remained widespread due to insufficient funding, lack of personnel, poor commitment from many countries, and a shortage of vaccines. In 1967, laboratories in many countries with large smallpox outbreaks produced better freeze-dried vaccines. Additional improvements included the bifurcated needle, case **surveillance** systems, and mass vaccination programs. By 1971, smallpox was eradicated from South America, followed by Asia (1975) and Africa (1977).

The last cases of smallpox occurred in the late 1970s. A girl from Bangladesh was the last person in the world to have naturally acquired a variola major and survived. A male from Somalia was the last person in the world to have naturally contracted smallpox caused by variola minor, and he survived but later died of malaria. The last person to die of smallpox was a female in England in 1978. Today, only two locations officially store and handle the variola virus, supervised by the WHO: the Centers for Disease Control and Prevention (CDC) and the State Research Center of Virology and Biotechnology (VECTOR Institute) in Koltsovo, Russia.

You Should Remember

Nearly two centuries after Edward Jenner isolated the causative virus, smallpox was declared eradicated globally in 1980. It is widely considered to be the most significant achievement in international public health.

TEST YOUR KNOWLEDGE

1. How did Edward Jenner treat smallpox?
2. When was smallpox declared eradicated?
3. When did the last cases of smallpox occur?

ANTHRAX

Anthrax is a severe infectious disease. It is caused by a gram-positive, rod-shaped bacterium known as *Bacillus anthracis*, which occurs naturally in soil and often affects animals worldwide. There are four types of anthrax: cutaneous (affecting the skin), inhalation (involving the lungs), gastrointestinal (affecting the digestive system), and injection anthrax (affecting the skin or other body parts).

Anthrax is believed to have originated in Egypt and Mesopotamia somewhere around 700 BCE. Cutaneous anthrax was first described clinically in 1752. In 1877, TB pioneer Robert Koch studied the causative bacterium, discovering its spore-forming abilities. He isolated the bacterium and injected it into animals for testing, which allowed him to determine the life cycle of the bacterium. In 1881, Louis Pasteur created a vaccine, injecting animals with weakened anthrax bacteria (Figure 3.7). After two rounds of this vaccine, he injected the animals with live anthrax bacteria, and all the prevaccinated animals survived. The first deliberate use of anthrax occurred in World War I (1914 to 1918) when the German army used it to infect livestock and animal feed traded to the Allied Nations by neutral partners. Anthrax immunization will be discussed in Chapter 10.

By the early 1900s, anthrax cases were documented in the United States, Great Britain, and Germany. In 1932, Japan began producing anthrax as a weapon, attacking at least 11 Chinese cities with it. In 1937, Max Sterne created the anthrax live spore vaccine for animals, which is still used today in many countries. Though penicillin was discovered in 1928, it was first used in 1944 to treat anthrax and became the drug of choice. In 1950, the first human anthrax vaccine was created, which was 92.5% effective in preventing cutaneous anthrax. In 1970, an updated human anthrax vaccine was released, which is essentially the same vaccine used today.

In 1979, there was an unusual anthrax outbreak in Sverdlovsk, USSR, with 96 human cases (most of which were gastrointestinal). In 2001, letters filled

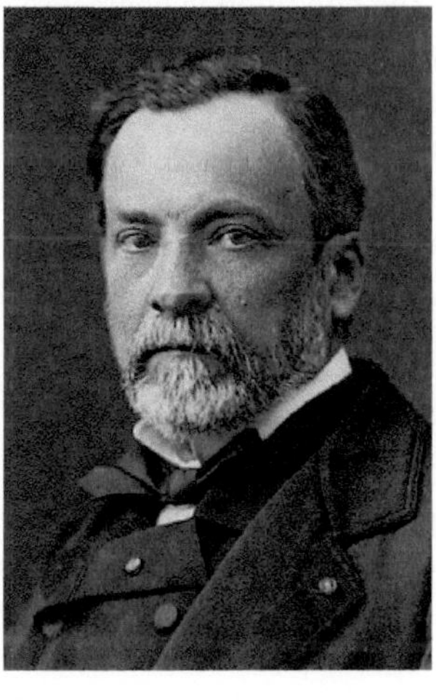

FIGURE 3.7 Dr. Louis Pasteur.

with a white powder containing anthrax spores were mailed to US Senate offices and news media agencies. Twenty-two people became ill from anthrax, of which five people died. It was found that all the dead individuals had inhaled anthrax, which is the most severe form of the disease. In 2010, a small anthrax outbreak occurred in the United Kingdom and Germany. All the patients were illicit drug users who had injected heroin before having symptoms. The signs and symptoms did not resemble typical cutaneous anthrax. Physicians determined it was a new subtype and named it *injection anthrax*. It was believed that anthrax spores had somehow gotten into the heroin that was injected.

You Should Remember

The natural form of anthrax infects cows and other animals with hooves. Anthrax rarely infects humans, and human anthrax cases are rare in the United States but occur more commonly in developing countries. Very infrequently, anthrax spores have been released intentionally as a fine powder to cause harm.

TEST YOUR KNOWLEDGE

1. What are the four types of anthrax?
2. When was the first human anthrax vaccine created?
3. What is the most severe form of anthrax?

TETANUS

Tetanus is an acute disease caused by an **exotoxin** produced by the bacterium *Clostridium tetani*. The condition is characterized by generalized rigidity and convulsive spasms of the skeletal muscles. The muscle stiffness usually begins in the jaw, known as *lockjaw*, and the neck before becoming generalized. Tetanus is often fatal. The bacterium usually enters the body through a wound. The incubation period is usually about 8 days, from 1 to 21 days. There are three general forms of tetanus. *Generalized tetanus* causes 80% of cases and usually presents with a descending pattern, first affecting the jaw, followed by the neck, throat, and abdominal muscles. *Localized tetanus* is uncommon, with persistent contractions of muscles in the same anatomic area as the injury. *Cephalic tetanus* is rare, occasionally occurring along with otitis media. Another form, *neonatal tetanus*, only occurs in newborns, usually through infection of the unhealed umbilical stump.

Tetanus was first described clinically in approximately 500 BCE. However, it was not until 1884 that tetanus was first produced in animal test subjects by injecting them with pus from a human patient who had died. The same year, tetanus was also induced in test animals by injecting them with infected soil samples. The causative organism was isolated from a human in 1889 by Kitasato Shibasaburō, who showed that it caused disease when injected into animals. The toxin could be neutralized, however, by specific antibodies. In 1897, Edmond Nocard proved the protective effect of passively transferred antitoxin. During World War I, **passive human immunization** was used for treatment and prevention. A method for inactivating the tetanus toxin with formaldehyde was developed early in the 1920s, leading to the tetanus toxoid development in 1924. It was first used extensively during World War II.

MUMPS

Mumps is a viral infection that previously was most common in children and adolescents, leading to inflammation in salivary glands and organs that could result in chronic problems. Hippocrates described **Parotitis** and orchitis in the 5th century BCE in Greece. During World War I, mumps was the third highest cause of hospitalization of soldiers (after influenza and gonorrhea). In 1934, it was proven that mumps could be transmitted from infected patients to rhesus monkeys and that a filterable agent in the saliva caused the condition. The agent was shown to be a virus in 1935. Until the 1967 mumps vaccine, the state was one of the most common causes of **aseptic meningitis** and sensorineural hearing loss in children in the United States. The two-dose vaccination program led to a greater than 99% reduction in annual mumps cases.

MEASLES

Measles is also known as rubeola and is a highly contagious viral disease. Before the measles vaccine was introduced, significant epidemics occurred every 2 to 3 years, with 2.6 million deaths occurring annually. One of the first documented accounts of measles was in Persia (Iran) in the 9th century. In 1757, a Scottish physician showed that an infectious agent in the blood caused measles. In 1912, the disease became nationally notifiable in the United States. An average of 6000 related deaths were reported annually in the next 10 years. Before the development of a vaccine, nearly all children contracted measles before the age of 15. An estimated 3 to 4 million Americans were infected annually, with about 400 to 500 annual deaths.

In 1954, the measles virus was isolated in the blood of a 13-year-old patient. In 1963, the Edmonston-B strain of the measles virus was transformed into a vaccine. In 1968, an improved, weaker vaccine known as the Edmonston-Enders (formerly Moraten) strain was licensed and is the only measles vaccine still in use in the United States. Today, it is usually combined into the measles, mumps, and rubella (MMR) vaccines. In 1981, the reported cases were 80% less than in the previous year. A 1989 outbreak occurred in vaccinated school-age children, resulting in a second MMR dose being recommended for children. Measles was declared eliminated from the United States in 2000.

RUBELLA

Rubella (German measles or three-day measles) is a contagious viral infection. It was initially considered a variant of measles or scarlet fever, but this has been proven incorrect. Rubella was first described as a unique disease in 1814 in Germany. One hundred years later, in 1914, Alfred F. Hess used his studies of monkeys to propose a viral etiology. After a widespread epidemic in 1940, an Australian ophthalmologist reported the occurrence of congenital cataracts occurring in infants born following maternal rubella. This is known as **congenital rubella syndrome**. The rubella virus was first isolated in 1962, and the first rubella vaccines were licensed in 1969. The MMR vaccine was approved for use in the United States in 1971. In 2005, a combination measles, mumps, rubella, and varicella vaccine was licensed.

TEST YOUR KNOWLEDGE

1. What is the most common complication of mumps?
2. How lethal was measles in previous history?
3. What is congenital rubella syndrome?

PERTUSSIS

Outbreaks of **pertussis** (whooping cough) were first described in 1578 in Paris, France. The organism was first isolated in 1906. In the 20th century, whooping cough was one of the most common childhood diseases and a significant cause of childhood mortality in the United States. Before the vaccine became available in the 1940s, over 200,000 cases were reported annually. After the widespread use of the vaccine started, the incidence of whooping cough decreased by more than 75% compared to the prevaccine era. However, pertussis is still a significant health problem worldwide. According to the WHO, there are still an estimated 24.1 million cases and about 160,700 deaths from whooping cough per year.

TYPHOID

Typhoid, also called typhoid fever, is a life-threatening infection caused by *Salmonella enterica* serovar Typhi. It is usually spread through contaminated food or water. Patients carry the bacteria in the bloodstream and intestinal tract.

Jamestown, Virginia, had a severe typhoid outbreak, killing over 6000 settlers between 1607 and 1624. More than 80,000 soldiers died as a result of typhoid or dysentery during the American Civil War. The Spanish-American War also led to typhoid infections. Mary Mallon (*Typhoid Mary*) was the most widely known carrier of typhoid fever (Figure 3.8). She was the first person in the United States to be identified as a carrier, but she never developed any disease symptoms. She worked as a cook, preparing food for many people. She is

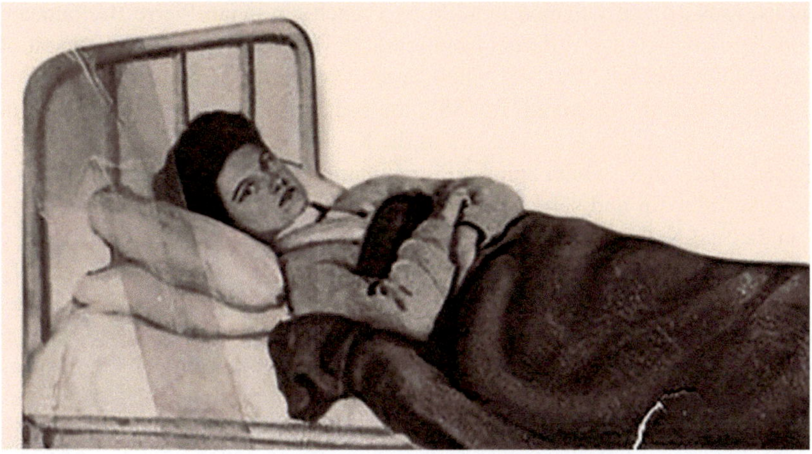

FIGURE 3.8 Mary Mallon, commonly referred to as "Typhoid Mary."

believed to have infected 51 people; three of these infections were fatal. Mary Mallon was quarantined twice because of carrying the disease and died the second time in quarantine.

In 1838, while treating a typhoid outbreak in England, Dr. William Budd noted that the bacterium could be transmitted to healthy people by consuming contaminated water. He suggested quarantines to help control future episodes. Karl Joseph Eberth first described the bacterium in 1880. The first effective vaccine was developed by Almroth Edward Wright and was introduced for military use in 1896. This vaccine was further developed over the following years in London, England. Throughout the 20th century, the incidence of typhoid has steadily declined due to the introduction of vaccinations and improved public sanitation and hygiene. The chlorination of drinking water significantly impacted the number of people affected by typhoid. Today, it is considered a rare condition in developed countries, with an incidence rate of about five cases per million people yearly.

DIPHTHERIA

Diphtheria is a severe bacterial infection caused by *Corynebacterium diphtheriae*, which produces a toxin. It can result in dyspnea, arrhythmia, and death. The disease is spread between people from coughing or sneezing. The condition can also be spread by touching infected open sores or ulcers. Those at increased risk for contracting diphtheria include people in the same household or healthcare individuals with close contact with a patient.

The history of diphtheria began in 1613 with an epidemic in Spain. In 1735, an epidemic swept through New England, wiping out entire families. The case-fatality rate was nearly 40%. Treatments could have been more effective. The disease was officially named in 1826 by French physician Pierre Bretonneau, who distinguished it as different from scarlet fever based on the development of its pseudomembrane. Tracheotomies were often performed, allowing patients to breathe as they recovered. In 1883, the bacterium was identified by Edwin Klebs. This bacterium is also known as the Klebs-Löffler bacillus. It has a club-shaped appearance, which helps differentiate it from other microbes. In 1890, the first antitoxin and serum therapy were developed, and Emil von Behring won the first Nobel Prize in medicine for his work.

In 1894, New York City regulated the antitoxin, which had previously come chiefly from two suppliers in Germany. In 1901, 13 children in St. Louis, Missouri, died from contaminated diphtheria antitoxin, leading to federal regulation of biological products. The worst year for cases of diphtheria was 1921, with 206,000 recorded in the United States, resulting in 15,520 deaths (a case-fatality ratio of 7.5%). World War II sparked additional outbreaks. In 1943, there were 1 million cases in Europe, with 50,000 deaths. In 1954, the concentration of diphtheria toxoid in the adult tetanus and diphtheria booster was reduced, which lowered the concentration of toxoid-induced adverse reactions (fever, swelling, body aches, fatigue, headaches, and chills). In 1974, the WHO included the diphtheria, tetanus, and pertussis vaccine in its Expanded Programme on Immunization for developing countries. In 1994, declining diphtheria immunization among children and reductions in adult immunity led to an epidemic in the former Soviet Union, with 39,703 recorded cases.

You Should Remember

Respiratory diphtheria has almost disappeared in the United States. Since 2004, the CDC has recorded no cases at all. In less than 75 years, both forms of diphtheria have been virtually eliminated in the United States. Diphtheria was once the leading cause of childhood deaths.

TEST YOUR KNOWLEDGE

1. How is diphtheria spread?
2. When did the history of diphtheria begin?
3. What was the worst year for diphtheria in the United States?

YELLOW FEVER

Yellow fever is an acute viral hemorrhagic disease transmitted by infected mosquitoes. It is referred to as "yellow" because patients often develop jaundice. Yellow fever was a feared lethal disease that was first documented in 1547. Before 1900, its etiology and mode of transmission were not understood. At the turn of the 20th century, Walter Reed and his colleagues identified these factors based on an 1881 theory by Carlos Finlay of Cuba. The causative virus originated in Africa and was brought to the Western hemisphere during the slave trade period. The first epidemic occurred in the Yucatan in 1648. Over the next 200 years, outbreaks occurred in tropical America, North American coastal cities, and Europe. By the end of the 19th century, every soldier in the Spanish-American war who died in battle was outnumbered by 13 by those who died from yellow fever.

After Walter Reed's discovery, a Cuban campaign against the urban mosquito **vector** was able to eliminate yellow fever in 1902, followed by the same result in Panama in 1906. It took more than 25 years before the causative virus was isolated. Testing of a viral subculture known as 17D revealed that the virus had become attenuated but could still induce a protective immune response. The 17D subculture would serve as the basis of the vaccine still in use today. A second live attenuated vaccine was developed from a different strain in 1927.

In the 1940s, mass campaigns were done using the 17D vaccine in South America, and vaccination with the *French neurotropic vaccine* was made compulsory in French territories in Africa. Also, in the 1960s, epidemics occurred in Africa and the Americas, causing thousands of cases in West Africa, where vaccine coverage had significantly been reduced, and in Ethiopia, where the disease had not previously been reported. Yellow fever virus is antigenically related to other group B arboviruses, now called *flaviviruses*, because "flavus" means yellow in Latin. Vertical transmission of the virus in mosquitoes was confirmed in the 1970s. In 1982, concern about the high rate of postvaccinal encephalitis following the use of the French neurotropic vaccine resulted in the vaccine being abandoned.

In the late 1980s, serological studies revealed that just one in seven people infected with yellow fever became ill. Also during this time, another major expansion of activity occurred in Africa, with an estimated 120,000 cases and 24,000 deaths in Nigeria alone; since 1988, the WHO and the Pan American Health Organization have promoted the yellow fever vaccine in routine immunization programs. In the 1990s, the 17D vaccine was harnessed as a live vector for genes of other flaviviruses. This resulted in new vaccines being tested to prevent **dengue**, **Japanese encephalitis**, and **West Nile virus infection**. Though much has been learned about yellow fever over the past century, much more is still to be discovered concerning its natural transmission cycle, recently fatal adverse events from the 17D vaccine, and upswings in enzootic transmission.

VARICELLA

Varicella is a highly contagious disease caused by the varicella-zoster virus. It is also called chickenpox. The earliest reports of the vesicular rashes now recognized as those caused by varicella-zoster date back to ancient civilizations. However, it was not until 1888 that a relationship between the virus and chickenpox was suggested. This relationship was proven in the 1950s. A live attenuated varicella vaccine was developed in Japan in the 1970s. The complete DNA sequence of varicella-zoster virus was established in 1986. The Japanese vaccine was licensed for general use in Japan and Korea in 1988 and in the United States in 1995 for people aged 12 months or older. In 2005, a combination measles, mumps, rubella, and varicella vaccine was licensed in the United States for children between 12 months and 12 years of age.

CHOLERA

Cholera is an acute diarrheal infection caused by ingesting food or water contaminated with the bacterium known as *Vibrio cholerae*. Cholera remains a global threat to public health. The highly **virulent** disease can cause severe, acute, watery diarrhea. After ingesting contaminated food or water, the disease takes 12 hours to 5 days to cause symptoms. Children and adults can be affected; the disease can be fatal within hours without treatment. However, most infected people do not develop any symptoms even though the bacteria are present in their feces for up to 10 days following infection. The bacteria can be shed back into the environment to infect other people. In those patients who do have symptoms, most have only mild to moderate symptoms. A minority of patients develop acute watery diarrhea with severe dehydration that can lead to death.

In the 19th century, cholera spread worldwide, initiating in the Ganges delta in India. Six pandemics killed millions of people globally. The current (seventh) pandemic began in South Asia in 1961, reaching Africa in 1971 and the Americas in 1991. Cholera is now endemic in many countries. Only two serogroups of the bacteria (labeled O1 and O139) cause outbreaks. The O1 serogroup caused all recent episodes. The O139 serogroup was first identified in Bangladesh in 1992 and caused previous attacks, but today, it is only identified sporadically and has never been identified outside of Asia. The illness is the same when caused by either serogroup.

Cholera may be endemic or epidemic. A *cholera-endemic* area is one where confirmed cases were detected over the last 3 years, with evidence of local transmission. An outbreak can be seasonal or sporadic, representing more than expected cases. A *cholera-epidemic* area occurs in endemic countries and those in which cholera is uncommon. In a country where cholera is unique, an outbreak is defined by at least one confirmed case, with evidence of local transmission in an area where cholera does not usually occur.

Cholera transmission is linked tightly to insufficient access to clean water and sanitation. At-risk areas include slums and camps for refugees or internally displaced people. Clean water and sanitation requirements still need to be met in these locations. The consequences of this humanitarian crisis can increase risks for cholera transmission if the bacterium is present or introduced. The number of cholera cases reported to the WHO has remained high. During 2020, there were 323,369 cases, and 857 deaths were confirmed in over 24 countries. The discrepancy between these amounts and the estimated disease burden is because many instances are not recorded due to limited surveillance and the fear of the disease's impact on trade and tourism.

Preventing and controlling cholera requires combined surveillance, good water sources, sanitation and hygiene, social mobilization, treatments, and oral cholera vaccines. Surveillance must be part of an integrated disease surveillance system, including feedback at local levels and information sharing at the global level. Cholera is detected based on clinical suspicion of profuse diarrhea and is confirmed by identifying the bacteria in stool samples. Detection is assisted via rapid diagnostic tests in which one or more positive samples trigger an alert. The results are confirmed by culture or polymerase chain reaction. Under international health regulations, public health events involving cholera must be assessed against the criteria provided to determine if there is a need for official notification so that an outbreak does not result.

Most cholera patients can be treated by promptly administering an oral rehydration solution. Adults may require up to 6L of the solution to treat moderate dehydration on the first day. Severely dehydrated patients risk shock and need rapid intravenous (IV) fluid administration. They are also given appropriate antibiotics to reduce the duration of diarrhea, volume of rehydration fluids needed, and amount and duration of bacterial excretion via the stool. Rapid access to treatment is essential during cholera outbreaks. Oral rehydration must be available in communities, along with larger treatment centers that can provide IV fluids and 24-hour care. With these treatments, fatalities should be below 1%. Zinc is a necessary adjunctive therapy for children under age 5. It also reduces the diarrhea duration and can prevent future episodes of other causes of acute watery diarrhea. Breastfeeding is also promoted because immune factors against cholera are present in breast milk. Antibiotics shorten the course and diminish the severity of the illness, but they are not as important as rehydration. Persons who develop severe diarrhea and vomiting in countries where cholera occurs should seek medical attention promptly.

To prevent contracting cholera, there must be adoption of protective hygiene measures. These include handwashing with soap, safe preparation and storage of food, and safe disposal of feces. For cholera patients who die from the disease, funeral practices must be performed that include methods of preventing infection in other people. Communities must become engaged via better communication about potential risks, awareness of symptoms, preventive precautions, and how to report cases and seek immediate treatment. Several oral vaccines against cholera can be given to prevent cholera infection (Chapter 12).

You Should Remember

The WHO and Global Task Force on Cholera Control, working together, have launched a strategy for cholera control called Ending Cholera: A Global Roadmap to 2030. This aims to reduce cholera deaths by 90% and eliminate the disease in as many as 20 countries by 2030.

TEST YOUR KNOWLEDGE

1. How is cholera spread?
2. What is the difference between cholera-endemic and cholera-epidemic areas?
3. What are some strategies to prevent cholera?

PNEUMOCOCCAL DISEASE

Pneumococcal disease is an infection caused by the bacterium known as *Streptococcus pneumoniae*, which can cause pneumonia, bacteremia, or meningitis. In children, pneumococcal disease is the most common cause of serious infections. Pneumococcal pneumonia is the most common type of bacterial pneumonia. Pneumococcal meningitis is the leading cause of bacterial meningitis among children and adults in the United States. Severe pneumococcal infections are more common in children under age 2 and adults over age 65, persons with certain diseases (sickle cell disease, HIV infection), and those with poorly functioning or removed spleens. The most likely infected include those with African-American heritage, Alaska Natives, and Native Americans.

S. pneumoniae was first isolated by Louis Pasteur in 1881 from the saliva of a patient with rabies. Pneumococcal pneumonia was confused with other types of pneumonia until the development of the **gram stain** in 1884. More than 80 serotypes of pneumococci came to be described by the year 1940. By the late 1960s, efforts were underway to develop a polyvalent pneumococcal vaccine. The first vaccine licensed in the United States became available in 1977. The first conjugate pneumococcal vaccine was approved in the United States in 2000.

MENINGOCOCCAL DISEASE

Meningococcal disease is a rare and severe illness caused by the bacterium called ***Neisseria meningitidis***. It can cause meningitis or bacteremia. Between 10% and 14% of those infected die from the disease. About 20% of surviving patients have permanent disabilities such as deafness, brain damage, loss of limbs, or seizures.

N. meningitidis was first discovered in 1887 from the cerebrospinal fluid analysis of a patient infected with meningitis. During widespread epidemics of meningococcal meningitis at the start of the 20th century, German and US physicians produced immune serum and antiserum that contained specific antibodies from animals injected with meningitis-causing bacteria. This protected against meningitis and also had a therapeutic effect. Direct injection of horse antiserum into humans (via the CSF) became the primary therapy for meningococcal meningitis and was the first effective treatment, saving many lives during WWI. In the 1930s, meningitis vaccines that were safe, stable, and effective against pneumococcal meningitis were produced for the first time. In 1935, sulfonamides became the treatment of choice because they were less expensive and risky than antiserum. By 1941, penicillin became the first antibiotic that was commonly used.

During WWII, several epidemics, mainly among military personnel, occurred. Treatment with penicillin proved highly successful. By the 1960s, the causative bacterium had developed increased resistance to sulfonamides. Therefore vaccines against meningococcal meningitis were designed for use. There is still no single vaccine that can protect against all forms of meningitis. However, the various available vaccines have reduced bacterial meningitis globally by 25%, and 90% of this reduction is attributable to vaccination. Between 1996 and 1997, 250,000 people across the "meningitis belt" in Africa were affected by meningococcal "A" meningitis, resulting in 25,000 deaths. Various world organizations worked together to produce an affordable vaccine for Africa. Since the vaccine's introduction in 2010, more than 250,000 people have been vaccinated across the meningitis belt, and the disease has virtually disappeared.

TEST YOUR KNOWLEDGE

1. What percentage of people die from meningococcal disease?
2. What are the possible permanent disabilities associated with meningococcal disease?
3. How much have the various meningococcal vaccines reduced meningococcal disease globally?

SPANISH INFLUENZA

The *Spanish influenza* (*Spanish flu*) epidemic of 1918 infected approximately 33% of the global population. There were no effective treatments and no significant efforts to prevent its spread. The flu was caused by an H1N1 virus that started in some birds. It was a new influenza A virus that spread quickly throughout the world. Very few people had some amount of immunity to the disease. From 1918 to 1919, this flu infected an estimated 500 million people worldwide. About 50 million cases were fatal, and about 675,000 deaths occurred in the United States. The Spanish flu was extremely deadly to infants under age 5 and those over 65. However, it also killed many healthy adults between 20 and 40.

Symptoms of the Spanish flu included high fever, dry cough, headache, body aches, sore throat, chills, **rhinorrhea**, loss of appetite, and fatigue. As a result, many people died from pneumonia or other respiratory illnesses. Some were even killed on the same day that they became ill. No diagnostic tests were available then, and healthcare providers had to rely on reported signs and symptoms. No medications were effective in treating complications of the Spanish flu. There were also no mechanical ventilators or intensive care units at the time. Preventive measures in 1918 and 1919 included the following:

- Quarantine
- Closing public facilities such as schools and gymnasiums
- Washing hands thoroughly and frequently
- Wearing protective masks and gloves
- Avoiding touching items belonging to other people
- Avoiding spitting on the ground in public

Though the Spanish flu may have started in the United States or France, Spain was neutral during World War I and did not censor its news. Therefore Spanish news sources reported about the disease outbreak occurring worldwide. Other countries censored their news and avoided reports about the disease. The flu was deadly because of the lack of effective treatments, cramped living arrangements (especially in the military), a lack of healthcare providers due to them being involved in the war, and the ability of the virus to replicate and infect the lungs. The Spanish flu was similar to the COVID-19 virus because it was spread by breathing in infected respiratory droplets and caused **acute respiratory distress syndrome** (ARDS). Once ARDS developed, the fatality rate was 100% for the Spanish flu.

One of the first recorded cases of the Spanish flu was on March 11, 1918, at Fort Riley, Kansas, a military encampment. Overcrowding and poor sanitation resulted in 522 soldiers being admitted to the camp hospital with the same signs and symptoms of severe influenza. Soon after, the US Army reported similar outbreaks in Virginia, South Carolina, Georgia, Florida, Alabama, and California. Navy ships also reported attacks. By May 1918, the attacks began to subside in the United States. However, soldiers from Fort Riley had incubated the virus while traveling to fight in France. Once they arrived, the virus infected fighting forces from all countries involved in the battles. Individual names were given to the disease by each of the nations, which included the following:

- United States: 3-day fever or purple death
- France: purulent bronchitis
- Italy: sand fly fever
- Germany: Blitzkatarrh or Flanders fever

Aside from the relatively general flu symptoms, the disease ravaged its victims' lungs. Some patients died of respiratory failure within hours. Autopsies revealed that the lungs were stiff, red, and fluid. Microscopic views showed that the alveoli were filled with fluid—the patients drowned. Slow suffocation would begin when a patient developed reddish-brown spots on the face. Within hours, the patient would appear cyanotic. While nurses were performing **triage** for patients, they would look first at their feet—if they were black, the affected patient was considered beyond help and taken to a particular area to die. Unlike other types of influenza, many healthy males and females (especially pregnant females) died, leaving behind orphaned children.

By the summer of 1918, the Spanish flu had spread to Norway, China, the Philippines, India, New Zealand, Puerto Rico, the Caribbean, Mexico, and Hawaii. Eventually, it returned to the United States, with second and third "waves" of the flu occurring in the cold-weather months of 1918. This time, many civilians were infected. It disproportionately affected Native Alaskans and hit certain cities harder than others, with 33,000 deaths in New York City and about 13,000 in Philadelphia. Many towns ran out of coffins, and some had to convert streetcars into hearses to carry the bodies. Sometimes dead people were left in their homes for days due to cities being overwhelmed. Everyday life was shut down in many locations, and businesses were closed. Though, generally, the pandemic ended in the summer of 1919, a minor fourth wave appeared in the spring of 1920 in isolated areas of New York City. The pandemic ended because infected individuals either died or developed immunity.

You Should Remember

The Spanish flu was the deadliest pandemic that has ever occurred. Its "second wave" was much more dangerous than the first, believed to be related to virus mutations. The second wave was thought to have spread widely because many soldiers were being moved worldwide as part of World War I. More US soldiers died from the Spanish flu than died in battle.

TEST YOUR KNOWLEDGE

1. What are the signs and symptoms of typhoid?
2. What were the preventive measures used for the Spanish flu?
3. How was the Spanish flu similar to COVID-19?

WEST NILE VIRUS INFECTION

Mosquitoes spread West Nile virus infection to humans after having bitten an infected bird. The virus can infect humans, birds, mosquitoes, horses, and other mammals. The disease primarily occurs during the summer and fall. While most infected patients do not become ill, about 20% may develop a fever, headache, fatigue, rash, vomiting, diarrhea, and body aches. Patients with mild West Nile virus infection do well after supportive care treatment. For those with severe disease, the outlook is more uncertain. West Nile encephalitis or meningitis may lead to brain damage and death. Risks can be reduced by using insect repellent and wearing long-sleeved shirts and long pants to prevent mosquito bites. There are no available vaccines or medications to treat this virus.

West Nile virus was first identified in 1937 in Uganda in eastern Africa. In 1957 in Israel, the virus became recognized as a cause of severe **meningoencephalitis** in older adults. It was first discovered in the United States in the summer of 1999 in New York and quickly spread across the country. Illinois has had the most cases and deaths from West Nile virus, but between 1999 and 2022, western states such as California and Colorado had the highest case counts. Researchers believe the virus is spread when a mosquito (*Culex pipiens*) bites an infected bird and then bites a person.

You Should Remember

Severe illness can occur in people of any age. However, people over 60 are at greater risk for severe disease if infected (one in 50 people). People with certain medical conditions such as cancer, diabetes, hypertension, and kidney disease, and those who have received organ transplants, are also at greater risk.

TEST YOUR KNOWLEDGE

1. Which war is associated with ARDS?
2. What are the signs and symptoms of West Nile virus infection?
3. Where was the West Nile virus first identified?

HUMAN PAPILLOMAVIRUS INFECTION

Human papillomavirus (HPV) infection is the most common sexually transmitted infection in the United States. There are more than 200 types of HPV that have been identified. Among those, 85 genotypes have been characterized. The link between HPV and cervical cancer was discovered in the 1980s by Harald zur Hausen, which led to the 2008 Nobel Prize in Physiology or Medicine. There were about 43 million HPV infections in 2018, mostly in people in their late teenage years and early 20s. There are many different types of HPV. Some cause health conditions such as **genital warts** and cancers (Figure 3.9). However, HPV

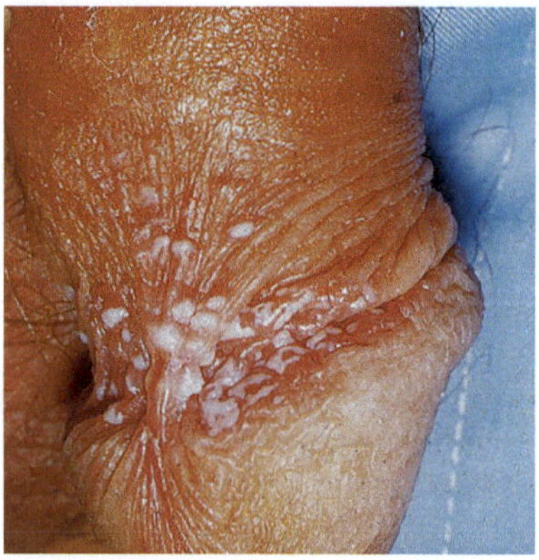

FIGURE 3.9 Genital warts.

vaccines can prevent these conditions from developing. HPV can be spread through all sexual intercourse and even close skin-to-skin touching.

The relationship between cervical cancer and sexual intercourse was suspected for more than 100 years before being established in the 1960s. In the early 1980s, cervical cancer cells were shown to contain HPV DNA. Epidemiologic studies showing a strong association between HPV and cervical cancer were published in the 1990s. HPV has since been identified as a cause of other mucosal cancers. A quadrivalent vaccine to prevent infection with four types of HPV was licensed in the United States in 2006. A bivalent vaccine was approved in 2009, and a nine-valent vaccine was licensed in 2014.

You Should Remember

Most males who get HPV never have symptoms. The infection usually goes away by itself. But if HPV does not go away, it can cause genital warts or certain kinds of cancer. Patients must talk to their healthcare provider about anything new or unusual affecting the genitals, scrotum, anus, mouth, or throat.

TEST YOUR KNOWLEDGE

1. Which populations are most at risk of severe pneumococcal infections?
2. What is the most common sexually transmitted infection in the United States?
3. Which cancer is most commonly linked to HPV?

ACUTE RESPIRATORY DISTRESS SYNDROME

ARDS is a life-threatening condition characterized by poor oxygenation and noncompliant lungs. The disorder is associated with capillary endothelial injury and diffuse alveolar damage. Once ARDS develops, patients usually have varying degrees of pulmonary artery vasoconstriction and may develop pulmonary hypertension. ARDS can develop at any age.

ARDS was first described in 1967. Though it originated in the United States, ARDS was closely associated with the Vietnam War. During the war, American Army Medical Corps physicians identified patients who initially responded to respiratory resuscitation but became distressed. Persistent **hypoxia** would not react to oxygen masks. Plain chest X-rays suggested **pulmonary edema** associated with left ventricular failure, which was unlikely in combat soldiers. It was quickly learned that ARDS was signified by noncardiogenic pulmonary edema and is life-threatening.

In 1994, ARDS was given a new definition, with patients subdivided into *formal ARDS* and a second form known as *acute lung injury*. In 2011, European and American physicians came up with the *Berlin definition* in which patients are divided into mild, moderate, or severe ARDS based on the degree of hypoxia present. Each stage is associated with increased mortality. Survival has improved significantly since the early 1990s, primarily because of newer lung-protective strategies. Today, ARDS is most commonly associated with elective surgeries. Ultrasound is also helpful in determining the presence of ARDS.

ROTAVIRUS INFECTION

Rotavirus infection is a highly contagious virus that causes severe watery diarrhea. The virus mainly affects infants and young children, who may become dehydrated. Early signs and symptoms are fever and vomiting, followed by 3 to 7 days of watery diarrhea. The infection can cause abdominal pain as well. The infection can be fatal. It is essential to protect infants and young children with the rotavirus vaccine.

In 1973, Dr. Ruth Bishop and her colleagues observed a virus particle in the intestinal tissue of children with diarrhea via electron micrography. The virus was named "rotavirus" because it is similar in appearance to that of a wheel. By 1980, rotavirus was recognized as the most common cause of severe gastroenteritis in American infants and young children. Before the vaccine, most children were infected by the age of 5 years. There were up to 500,000 deaths among children annually worldwide. The first rotavirus vaccine was licensed in the United States in 1998 but was withdrawn the next year because it caused bowel **intussusception**. Second-generation vaccines became available in the United States in 2006 and 2008.

EBOLA INFECTION

Ebola, or *Ebola virus infection*, is a deadly condition with occasional outbreaks that mainly occur in Africa. It usually affects humans and nonhuman primates and is caused by the Ebola virus. Scientists do not know where the virus comes from but believe it is animal-borne, with bats or nonhuman primates being the most likely source. The virus first spreads through contact with infected blood, body fluids, and tissues. It causes fever, aches, pains, fatigue, sore throat, loss of appetite, gastrointestinal symptoms, bleeding, and **ecchymosis**.

Ebola was identified in 1976 because of nearly simultaneous outbreaks in the Democratic Republic of the Congo and Sudan. Since 1994, episodes have been frequently observed mostly near tropical rainforests in Central and West Africa. Between 2014 and 2016, West Africa saw more than 28,000 reported cases, and other countries also reported increased cases (Italy, Mali, Nigeria, Senegal, Spain, the United Kingdom, and the United States). Between 2017 and 2022, the countries with the most significant outbreaks have been the Democratic Republic of the Congo, Guinea, and Uganda.

COVID-19 PANDEMIC

COVID-19, also known as *coronavirus disease 2019*, is highly infectious and is caused by the SARS-CoV-2 virus. Though most infected people have mild to moderate respiratory illness, some become seriously ill and die. Those at the highest risk of severe COVID-19 include older people, those who are obese, and those with underlying chronic medical conditions such as cardiovascular disease, diabetes mellitus, chronic respiratory disease, or cancer. The virus can spread via small liquid particles through coughing, sneezing, speaking, or breathing.

COVID-19 began in December 2019 when patients in Wuhan, China, started experiencing symptoms of a pneumonia-like illness that did not respond well to standard treatments. The first death from the disease occurred in January 2020 in China. The disease then spread to Thailand, Japan, the Republic of Korea, and the United States. By February 2020, there were 1013 worldwide deaths. Italy next became a "hotspot" for the virus, and the first US death occurred on February 29, 2020. On March 11, the WHO declared the COVID-19 pandemic after more than 118,000 cases in 114 countries and 4291 deaths.

Schools and businesses began to be shut down in many countries. People were instructed to stay home as much as possible as a quarantine measure. Vaccine trials in human subjects started on March 17, 2020. Mask mandates and other safety precautions became commonplace. By April 4, more than 1 million cases were confirmed worldwide, with a 10-fold increase in less than 1 month. On April 10, the United States became the country with the most reported cases and deaths. Millions of people had to file for unemployment because of being unable to go to work. On May 8, the US Food and Drug Administration authorized the first COVID-19 test with the option of using home-collected saliva samples. On May 28, the recorded death toll in the United States surpassed 100,000. On August 17, COVID-19 became the third leading cause of death in the United States, behind cardiovascular disease and cancer.

On August 24, the first documented case of COVID-19 reinfection was confirmed in Hong Kong, and the first reinfection in the United States was established on August 28. On September 22, the reported US death toll surpassed 200,000; on the 28th, the global death toll reached 1 million. On December 11, 2020, the FDA issued an *emergency use authorization* (EUA) for the Pfizer-BioNTech COVID-19 vaccine. The US death toll surpassed 300,000 on December 14—the same day a nurse in New York became the first American (outside of clinical trials) to receive a COVID-19 vaccine. On December 18, the FDA issued an EUA for the Moderna COVID-19 vaccine. By December 24, more than 1 million COVID-19 vaccine doses had been administered in the United States. Variants of the virus began to appear.

On January 18, 2021, the US death toll surpassed 400,000. On January 26, the number of recorded cases worldwide exceeded 100 million. On February 21, the US death toll reached 500,000. On February 27, the FDA approved the

EUA for Johnson & Johnson's single-dose COVID-19 vaccine for adults—the other two mRNA vaccines required two doses. On March 13, over 100 million vaccines had been administered in the United States. On April 21, more than 200 million vaccine doses were issued in the United States. On December 15, 2021, the recorded US death toll surpassed 800,000—1 of every 100 people aged 65 or older had died due to COVID-19 infection.

On January 3, 2022, the United States reported almost 1 million new infections, the highest daily total of any country worldwide. By January 24, the "Omicron" variant had accounted for nearly 99% of all current US cases. On February 4, the US death rate surpassed 900,000. On March 5, over 10 billion people received a COVID-19 vaccine worldwide, and public mask mandates started to be withdrawn. Even so, on March 10, worldwide deaths surpassed 6 million, and the number of cases reached 450 million. On May 5, the WHO estimated about 15 million deaths globally between January 2020 and December 2021. On May 12, 2022, the number of recorded deaths in the United States reached 1 million. On June 1, the United States announced a total of 84,145,569 COVID-19 infections. For adult vaccination against COVID-19, see Chapter 10.

You Should Remember

Symptoms of COVID-19 develop within 2 to 14 days of exposure to the virus. A person infected with SARS-CoV-2 is contagious for up to 2 days before symptoms appear. They remain infectious to others for 10 to 20 days, depending upon their immune system and the severity of the illness.

You Should Remember

Some people infected with COVID-19 have mild illness, and others have no symptoms. In some cases, however, COVID-19 can lead to lung damage, myocarditis, stroke, hearing loss, kidney failure, respiratory failure, and death.

TEST YOUR KNOWLEDGE

1. How does Ebola infection spread?
2. Which people have the highest risk of death from COVID-19?
3. When and where did COVID-19 originate?

KEY TERMS

Acute respiratory distress syndrome
Anthrax
Aseptic meningitis
Cholera
Congenital rubella syndrome
Delirium tremens
Delta hepatitis
Dengue

Diphtheria
Ebola
Ecchymosis
Encephalitis
Exotoxin
Genital warts
Gram stain
Hallucinations
Human papillomavirus infection
Hydrophobia
Hypoxia
Incubation period
Infectious hepatitis
Intussusception
Japanese encephalitis
Malaria
Measles
Meningoencephalitis
Mottling
Mumps
Neisseria meningitidis
Orthopoxvirus
Paralysis
Parotitis
Passive human immunization
Pertussis
Pneumococcal disease
Poliomyelitis
Pulmonary edema
Pustules
Rabies
Rhinorrhea
Rotavirus infection
Rubella
Serum hepatitis
Smallpox
Surveillance
Tetanus
Triage
Varicella
Variolation
Virulent
West Nile virus infection

Case Study 1

A 6-year-old boy was bitten by a bat while playing outside. He told his parents, but no PEP was sought because there were no visible bite marks, and his parents were unaware that bats could transmit rabies. Later, the boy was hospitalized for altered mental status, seizures, fever, and hypersalivation. A diagnosis of rabies was made. Experimental therapies were tried, but the boy died 22 days after his symptoms had begun.

Critical Thinking Questions

1. How is the rabies virus transmitted?
2. How long is the incubation period for rabies?
3. When did the first actual treatment for rabies occur?

Case Study 2

A 29-year-old female presented to a local clinic with anorexia and malaise. When questioned, she admits to being sexually promiscuous, with several partners over the past 9 months. Physical examination reveals she has mild yellowing of the sclera and liver tenderness upon palpation. Acute viral hepatitis is considered. Her complete blood count is average. Viral serology is ordered, and the patient is found to have hepatitis B.

Critical Thinking Questions

1. When did the first recorded cases of hepatitis B occur?
2. When did the hepatitis B vaccines come about?
3. How has vaccination affected the number of cases of acute HBV infections?

Case Study 3

A 64-year-old male went to the emergency department because of coughing and shortness of breath. He was worried additionally because there was blood in his sputum over the past 3 days. He had been waking up at night drenched in sweat for a few weeks. The patient states that he never tested positive for TB and was last screened a few years ago. He had gone to the emergency department the previous week, was diagnosed with community-acquired pneumonia, and was sent home with a prescription for azithromycin.

Critical Thinking Questions

1. What is the cause of TB?
2. Which organs of the body can TB affect?
3. What is miliary TB?

Case Study 4

A 69-year-old female with a history of pulmonary TB was brought to the emergency department complaining of sharp left-sided chest pain, myalgia, fever, chills, and a productive cough. Lung examination revealed crackles on the upper left lung fields, extending to the left midlung. The patient tested positive for COVID-19. Blood cultures showed gram-positive cocci in chains and pairs on preliminary gram stain, later identified as *S. pneumoniae*. Antibiotics were started, and repeated blood cultures showed no growth. Eventually, worsening hypoxemia required the patient to be placed on noninvasive positive pressure ventilation, but this failed, so mechanical ventilation was started. Weeks later, the patient developed unstable atrial flutter and required chest tube placement. She also developed severe emphysema and multiple complicating infections. She went into asystolic cardiac arrest and could not be revived.

Critical Thinking Questions

1. What is pneumococcal disease?
2. In which age groups are severe pneumococcal infections more common?
3. When was the first pneumococcal vaccine licensed for use in the United States?

Case Study 5

A 39-year-old male presented to the emergency department with pain and a darkening of the fifth toe of his left foot. An ultrasound reveals no significant stenosis. Because his symptoms have been linked to COVID-19, the patient is tested for the disease and found to be positive. It was determined that his toe discoloration was due to a microvascular embolic event. The patient had previously received phlebotomy treatments secondary to an elevated hematocrit. He is given IV fluids, and his hemoglobin and hematocrit both improve. A heparin drip is started, and the patient has 3 months of anticoagulation therapy because coagulopathy has been reported in up to half of all patients with severe COVID-19.

Critical Thinking Questions

1. Which people are at the highest risk for developing severe COVID-19 disease?
2. When did the history of COVID-19 begin?
3. How long did it take before more than 1 million cases of COVID-19 were confirmed worldwide?

FURTHER READING

1. Blaxill, M., Olmsted, D., 2015. Vaccines 2.0: The Careful Parent's Guide to Making Safe Vaccination Choices for Your Family. Skyhorse.
2. Conis, E., 2014. Vaccine Nation: America's Changing Relationship with Immunization. University of Chicago Press.
3. Conniff, R., 2023. Ending Epidemics: A History of Escape From Contagion. MIT Press.
4. Cowan, T., Fallon Morell, S., 2018. Vaccines, Autoimmunity, and the Changing Nature of Childhood Illness. Chelsea Green Publishing.
5. Davidson, T., 2017. Vaccines: History, Science, and Issues (The Story of a Drug). Greenwood.
6. Humphries, S., Bystrianyk, R., 2013. Dissolving Illusions: Disease, Vaccines, and the Forgotten History. CreateSpace Independent Publishing Platform.
7. Kinch, M., Foster, M., 2020. Between Hope and Fear: A History of Vaccines and Human Immunity. Dreamscape Media.
8. Lam, A., 2023. The Masters of Medicine: Our Greatest Triumphs in the Race to Cure Humanity's Deadliest Diseases. BenBella Books.
9. Loomis, J., 2020. Epidemics: The Impact of Germs and Their Power Over Humanity. Turner.
10. Miller, J., Tureci, O., Sahin, U., 2022. The Vaccine: Inside the Race to Conquer the COVID-19 Pandemic. St. Martin's Press.
11. Offit, P.A., Dixon, T., 2022. Vaccinated: From Cowpox to mRNA, the Remarkable Story of Vaccines. Harper.
12. Oldstone, M.B.A., 2020. Viruses, Plagues, and History: Past, Present, and Future. Oxford University Press.
13. Plotkin, S.A., 2011. History of Vaccine Development. Springer.
14. Polinsky, P.V., Ginevra, D., 2022. Vaccines: A Graphic History (Medical Breakthroughs). Graphic Universe.
15. Rees, A.R., 2022. A New History of Vaccines for Infectious Diseases: Immunization – Chance and Necessity. Academic Press.
16. Schama, S., 2023. Foreign Bodies: Pandemics, Vaccines, and the Health of Nations. Ecco.
17. Schwartz, H.E., 2023. Vaccine Breakthroughs (Edge of Medicine). Mayo Clinic Press.
18. Tizard, I.R., 2023. A History of Vaccines and their Opponents. Academic Press.
19. Veronese, K., 2022. Making Medicine: Surprising Stories From the History of Drug Discovery. Prometheus.
20. Wadman, M., Linari, N., 2017. The Vaccine Race: Science, Politics, and the Human Costs of Defeating Disease. Penguin.
21. Youngdahl, K., Hammond, B., Sipics, M., Cicchini, D., Hicks, R., 2013. The History of Vaccines. College of Physicians of Philadelphia.
22. Zaitchik, A., 2023. Owning the Sun: A People's History of Monopoly Medicine from Aspirin to COVID-19 Vaccines. Counterpoint.

Chapter 4

Vaccine Preparation and Classifications

Chapter Outline

Learning Objectives

After study of this chapter, readers should be able to:

1. Describe vaccine safety research accomplishments.
2. Explain the vaccine development process.
3. Discuss the general stages of vaccine development.
4. Describe the official federal government agency that approves vaccines.
5. Identify the "blinding" phases of vaccine trials.
6. Explain the classifications of vaccines.
7. Identify some examples of live attenuated vaccines.
8. Describe some examples of inactivated vaccines.
9. Explain the polysaccharide vaccines.
10. Discuss the messenger RNA vaccines.

Vaccinology and Immunizations. http://doi.org/10.1016/B978-0-443-23915-1.00004-4

OVERVIEW

Vaccines have a long history of successfully protecting people and communities against infectious diseases. Vaccination has improved the quality of life for many, and severe conditions such as smallpox have been eliminated. As vaccine technology advances, researchers can develop better and safer vaccines. There are several different types of vaccines, including inactivated, live attenuated, messenger RNA (mRNA), subunit, recombinant, polysaccharide, conjugate, and toxoid. Protection from a live attenuated vaccine typically outlasts the protection provided by a killed or inactivated vaccine. Both subunit and conjugate vaccines contain only pieces of the pathogens they protect against. Subunit vaccines use only part of a target pathogen to provoke a response from the immune system. This can be done by isolating a specific protein from a pathogen and presenting it as an antigen. Conjugate vaccines are similar to recombinant vaccines made using two different components. Conjugate vaccines, however, are made using pieces from the coats of bacteria. These coats are chemically linked to a carrier protein, and the combination is used as a vaccine. Proper preparation is critical for maintaining the integrity of the vaccine during the transfer from the vial to the syringe. Always use aseptic techniques and follow infection prevention guidelines when preparing vaccines. The aseptic technique involves handling, organizing, and storing medications and injection equipment/supplies (e.g., syringes and needles) to prevent microbial contamination and infection.

RESEARCH AND DISCOVERY OF VACCINES

The concept of immunization is an ancient idea. Edward Jenner was an 18th-century scientist considered to be the founder of vaccinology. However, before his time, immunization was recorded in 17th-century China when Buddhist monks drank snake venom to create immunity to snake bites. The concept of variolation (deliberate infection) occurred even earlier in history. For example, smallpox survivors in 430 BCE were called upon to nurse other individuals with the disease. The history of vaccines is discussed in greater detail in Chapter 3.

The United States's traditional vaccine safety system ensures vaccines are as safe as possible. As science improves and new information becomes available, this system will continue to improve. Vaccine safety research accomplishes the following:

- Ensure that the benefits of vaccines approved in the United States outweigh the risks.
- Define which groups should not receive certain vaccines.
- Describe adverse events and side effects reported after vaccination.
- Evaluate whether reported side effects and adverse events can be directly linked to a vaccine.

In collaboration with public health departments, the CDC evaluates vaccine effectiveness through observational studies that employ many methods. They use information collected through surveillance platforms, electronic health records, and prospective studies. Vaccine effectiveness studies utilize sources of vaccine history data to minimize bias. These include medical records, state and jurisdiction vaccine registries, and vaccination cards. Factors influencing vaccine effectiveness include age and underlying medical conditions such as diabetes mellitus, cancer, and history of prior infection.

Collecting information and adjusting for epidemiologic factors allow the CDC to minimize bias in measuring vaccine effectiveness. This effectiveness may differ in specific populations, such as older individuals or those with immunocompromising conditions. Therefore effectiveness estimates are often presented by age group, by immunocompromising conditions, or among people at increased risk for severe COVID-19, such as long-term care facility residents. Vaccine effectiveness can also differ by the chosen vaccine products, the total number of doses received, and how long it has been since the most recent vaccine dose was received.

Aside from time-dependent weakening, vaccine effectiveness is generally not expected to change meaningfully without new **immune escape variants** or recommendations for new vaccine products or doses. The timing of updates from specific data platforms is based on sample size limitations, especially in a setting of low disease incidence.

TEST YOUR KNOWLEDGE

1. What does vaccine safety research accomplish?
2. What do vaccine effectiveness studies utilize?
3. How does the CDC minimize bias in measuring vaccine effectiveness?

INITIAL VACCINE PREPARATION FOR DEVELOPMENT

Vaccine development usually begins in a university, medical center, or small biotech company research laboratory. Grants from the government or private foundations most often fund scientists in these laboratories. These scientists often spend years researching the effectiveness of their ideas, developing reagents and tests to measure their success, and, finally, using animals for testing. Sometimes products are tested on small animals such as mice, rats, or rabbits and then on larger animals such as monkeys.

During this time, several different groups of scientists may be working toward the same goal: to develop a vaccine against a particular virus or bacteria. Others evaluate the progress of these scientists through presentations at meetings and peer-reviewed papers in journals. Scientists working at pharmaceutical companies often attend such conferences and review journals to see which ideas appear to be working. If any of the work seems promising, pharmaceutical scientists may approach those working on it about expanding their research geared toward product development. This may take 5–10 years. Most university scientists have yet to develop ideas that are turned into products. Most enjoy the success of adding to the general body of scientific knowledge. Most vaccines have been used for decades, with millions receiving them safely every year. Like other medications, each vaccine must undergo extensive and rigorous testing to ensure it is safe before being introduced into a vaccine program.

Each vaccine under development must first undergo evaluations to determine which antigen should be used to invoke an immune response. This preclinical phase is done without human testing. An experimental vaccine is first tested in animals to evaluate its safety and potential to prevent disease.

TEST YOUR KNOWLEDGE

1. Where does vaccine development begin?
2. How do others evaluate the progress of vaccine development?
3. How long does it usually take for vaccine development?

VACCINE TRIALS AND INFECTIOUS DISEASES

If a tested vaccine triggers an immune response, it is tested in three phases in human clinical trials. The general stages of vaccine development are as follows:

- Research and discovery: 10 to 15 years.
- Proof of concept: the period is quite varied; vaccine effectiveness measures how well vaccination protects humans against infections, symptomatic illnesses, hospitalization, and death.
- Testing: usually contains four-phase trials, during which an **investigational new drug** application is submitted to the FDA. It includes data from animal studies, information on manufacturing technology, and the vaccine's quality, which is essential because it affects how well the vaccine will work to provide long- and short-term protection.
- Manufacturing: requires varying amounts of time.
- Approving: requires a **biological license application** submitted to the FDA, including preclinical and clinical data, manufacturing process details, and manufacturing facility information.
- Recommending the vaccine for use: this is done by the Advisory Committee on Immunization Practices (ACIP), which consists of medical and public health experts who develop recommendations for vaccine use. The ACIP only does this for vaccines approved by the FDA. The group considers the safety and effectiveness of the vaccine for people of certain ages, how severe the vaccine-preventable disease is, and how many people would get the disease if there was no vaccine. Once the ACIP recommends a vaccine,

the CDC decides to approve the recommendation. Once this occurs, the approval becomes the official CDC public health guidance for safe vaccine use in the United States. The approved proposal can make the vaccine part of the official US childhood and adult immunization schedules.

- Monitoring safety after approval: the CDC and FDA use different systems. They include the following:
  - The Vaccine Adverse Event Reporting System is an early warning system that helps monitor problems following vaccination. Anyone can report suspected vaccine reactions and issues to the Vaccine Adverse Event Reporting System.
  - The Vaccine Safety Datalink (VSD) is a collaboration between the CDC and health organizations, allowing for ongoing monitoring and proactive searches of data related to the vaccine.
  - The CDC's Clinical Immunization Safety Assessment (CISA) project is a partnership between the CDC and medical centers to conduct clinical research on vaccine-related health risks for certain groups of people.

You Should Remember

The biological license application also contains prescribing information on vaccine usage, dosage, and route of administration. Sometimes the prescribing information must be updated, which is then reviewed by the FDA. This leads to the FDA's decision on whether to approve the vaccine.

Sometimes the Vaccines and Related Biological Products Advisory Committee (VRBPAC) provides input on scientific data about the vaccine's safety, effectiveness, and use. The VRBPAC consists of independent scientific and public health experts. They discuss the vaccine in a public forum. Once the vaccine is approved, the manufacturer can make larger batches to distribute to the public. The FDA monitors vaccine production procedures and regularly inspects the manufacturing facility. This will continue for as long as the manufacturer holds a vaccine license.

The FDA monitors the quality of the vaccine by requiring the manufacturer to submit samples of each vaccine lot for testing. These tests regularly report on their safety, purity, and potency. Regarding purity, the vaccine can only contain the necessary ingredients. Regarding potency it must produce the desired immune response. If the vaccine is consistent across the various lots, the FDA can confirm that it is reliable and safe for use by the public.

TEST YOUR KNOWLEDGE

1. What are the general stages of vaccine development?
2. What does a biological license application include?
3. What does the FDA test to monitor vaccine manufacturing processes?

Phase I Trials

The vaccine is given to a few volunteers (20 to 100) to determine its safety, confirm that it generates an immune response, and find the proper dosage. Generally, in this phase, vaccines are tested on young, healthy adult volunteers. Information is gathered on the vaccine's safety, side effects, and how well the vaccine works to cause an immune response.

Phase II Trials

The vaccine is then given to 100 to 300 volunteers to assess further its safety and ability to generate an immune response. Participants have the same characteristics (such as age, gender, or physical health) as those for whom the vaccine is intended. There are usually multiple trials to evaluate various age groups and different vaccine formulations. A group that did not get the vaccine is generally included as a control group to determine whether the changes in the vaccinated group are attributed to the vaccine or have happened by chance.

Phase III Trials

The vaccine is next given to 1000 to 3000 volunteers and compared to a similar group of people who did not get the vaccine but received a control product to determine if it is effective against the disease it is designed to protect against and to study its safety in a much larger group of people. A control product is also known as a *placebo*, a substance with no therapeutic effect used in the *control group* of subjects. Most of the time, phase III trials are conducted across multiple countries and sites within a country to ensure that the findings of the vaccine performance will apply to many different populations.

During phase II and III trials, the volunteers and scientists conducting the study are kept from knowing which volunteers had received the vaccine being tested or the control product. This is called "blinding." It is necessary to ensure that neither the volunteers nor the scientists are influenced in their assessment of safety or effectiveness. After the trial and all the results are finalized, the volunteers and trial scientists are informed who received the vaccine and the control product.

You Should Remember

During phase III clinical trials, the FDA inspects the manufacturing facility where the vaccine will be made to ensure that it has everything needed for reliable, consistent, large-scale manufacturing. Batches known as "lots" are made, which undergo a series of tests to ensure vaccine consistency. Manufacturers must submit data from these tests to the FDA to support successful manufacturing processes, even after the vaccine has been approved.

Phase IV Trials

When the results of all clinical trials are available, a series of steps are required, including reviews of efficacy and safety, for regulatory and public health policy approvals. Officials in each country closely review study data and decide whether to authorize the vaccine. A vaccine must be proven safe and effective across a broad population before it is approved and introduced into a national immunization program. The bar for vaccine safety and efficacy is exceptionally high because vaccines are given to people who are otherwise healthy and specifically free from the illness. Once the FDA licenses a vaccine for the general population, it may suggest this fourth clinical trial phase with thousands of participants. Phase IV is a formal, continuing study that evaluates the vaccine's safety and effectiveness over extended periods (Figure 4.1).

Further monitoring takes place over time after the vaccine is introduced. There are systems to monitor the safety and effectiveness of all vaccines. This allows scientists to keep track of vaccine impact and safety even when used on many people over a long time frame. These data are used to adjust policies for vaccine use to optimize their impact and allow the vaccine to be safely tracked throughout its use. Once a vaccine is used, it must be continuously monitored to remain safe for continued widespread use.

TEST YOUR KNOWLEDGE

1. What do phase II trials assess?
2. Where are phase III trials usually conducted?
3. What do phase IV trials evaluate?

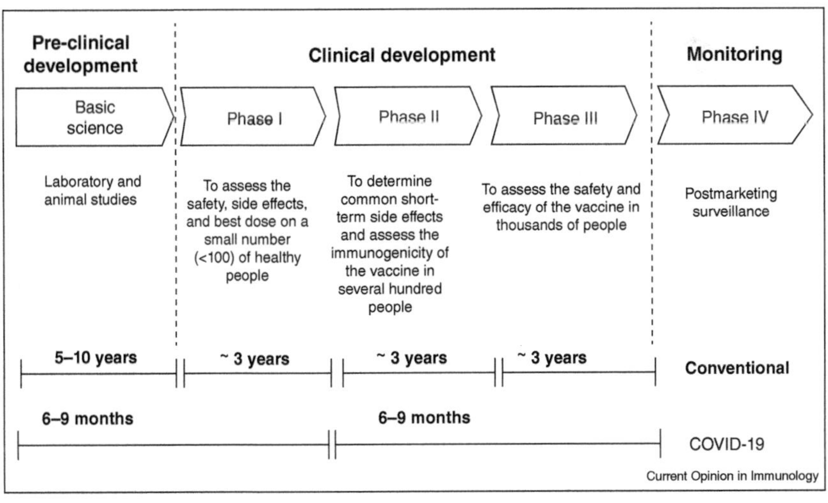

FIGURE 4.1 A depiction of the scope of vaccine trial phases.

CLASSIFICATIONS OF VACCINES

There are several classifications of vaccines, with the most commonly used including live attenuated and inactivated vaccines. Other types include subunit, mRNA, recombinant, toxoid, and vector vaccines.

Live Attenuated Vaccines

Live attenuated vaccines contain live pathogens from a bacterium or a virus that have been "attenuated," which means weakened. Live attenuated vaccines are produced by selecting strains of a bacteria or virus that continue to make a robust enough immune response but do not cause disease. Because these vaccines contain a live pathogen, the immune system reacts very well to them and usually remembers them for a long time. Additional doses, known as booster shots, are only sometimes needed. Live attenuated vaccines include those for influenza (intranasal), measles/mumps/rubella, typhoid (oral), rotavirus, varicella, and yellow fever.

Inactivated Vaccines

Inactivated vaccines take a live pathogen and inactivate (kill) it. When the vaccine is injected into humans, the inactivated pathogen is strong enough to create an immune response. However, it cannot cause the related disease. Multiple doses are often needed to build up immunity and offer complete protection. Some vaccines are manufactured from the inactivated whole virus (hepatitis A, polio, and rabies). Others are made from subunits of the bacterium or virus, such as acellular pertussis, hepatitis B, HPV, and influenza vaccines. Other vaccines are made from the toxoids of the bacterium, such as diphtheria and tetanus. The inactivated product is modified or purified even more to obtain the desired component for vaccines made from fractions of a virus or bacterium. These products do not replicate in the body and cannot cause disease.

Subunit Vaccines

Subunit vaccines are made from a piece of a pathogen, not the entire organism. They do not contain any live pathogens. Some necessary subunit vaccines include polysaccharide, conjugate, and protein-based vaccines.

- **Polysaccharide vaccines** target an immune response to pathogenic bacteria encased in a sugar layer. Therefore they assist in manufacturing protective responses against the surface of the bacteria, allowing the body to kill the bacteria. Therefore these vaccines do not work and are not used in children under age 2.
- **Conjugate vaccines** are the same in that they have a polysaccharide component, but that sugar is stuck to a protein, meaning that the immune system

will respond to the sugar on the bacteria better. They also help the body remember the bacteria better. If a future infection develops, the immune response will be more robust.

- **Protein-based vaccines** allow for a protective response against a protein on the surface of a virus, a protein on the surface of a bacterium, or a secreted toxin. The immune response opposes the protein components of the bacterium or virus, not the sugar coating. Specific proteins on the surface of bacteria or viruses help them cause disease. Therefore inducing an immune response against them can help the body fight against the infection or the toxic effects of the toxin.
- **Subunit vaccines** can be produced from the original pathogen or **recombinantly**. *Recombinant vaccines* use another organism to make the vaccine antigen.

You Should Remember

Live attenuated vaccines are derived from "wild" bacteria or viruses. They are usually weakened by repeated culturing. For example, the measles virus was isolated from a child with the disease in 1954. Nearly 10 years of serial passage using tissue culture media were needed to transform the wild virus into the attenuated vaccine virus.

You Should Remember

Inactivated vaccines are not live, cannot replicate, and cannot cause disease in any human being. Inactivated antigens are less affected by circulating antibodies than live antigens are. Therefore they can be given when antibodies are present in the blood, such as during infancy or after receiving antibody-containing blood products. The immunity provided by inactivated vaccines is usually not as long-lasting as that provided by live attenuated vaccines.

Messenger RNA Vaccine

One of the newest, most exciting areas in vaccine technology is using **messenger RNA (mRNA) vaccines**. Unlike conventional vaccines, mRNA vaccines can be developed quickly using the pathogen's genetic code. When an mRNA vaccine is delivered, RNA material instructs the body to make a specific protein unique to the virus but does not cause illness. The protein triggers an immune response that includes the generation of antibodies, which recognize the protein. When the person is exposed to that virus in the future, the body now has many antibodies to fight against it. The mRNA vaccine is a powerful technique to create many vaccine doses quickly. The benefit is that the technology is highly adaptable. Researchers can potentially go in and alter the mRNA in the formulation to target a new antigen and then manufacture a lot of high-quality vaccine material relatively quickly. The best examples are the Pfizer-BioNTech and Moderna COVID-19 vaccines.

You Should Remember

Scientists design each bit of mRNA to give cells the directions to make specific proteins. It is wrapped with lipids to protect the mRNA and help deliver it to the cells. While current mRNA vaccines are injected, an infusion may deliver future vaccines. After having one of these vaccines, the body can manufacture the desired protein. However, mRNA does not stay in the body very long and causes no permanent changes or alterations of DNA.

Recombinant Vaccines

Recombinant vaccines are made by recombinant DNA technology. This technology allows for the combination of DNA from two or more sources. The human papillomavirus, influenza, and hepatitis B vaccines are produced by inserting a segment of the respective viral gene into a yeast cell or virus gene. The modified yeast cell or virus has HPV capsid protein, influenza hemagglutinin, or pure **hepatitis B surface antigen**. Serogroup B meningococcal vaccines utilize proteins and outer membrane vesicles generated by recombinant technology.

Toxoid Vaccines

Toxoid vaccines use inactivated toxins to target the toxic activity created by bacteria instead of targeting the bacteria. The goal of toxoid vaccines is to neutralize those toxins with antibodies through vaccination. They effectively prevent toxin-mediated diseases such as diphtheria, pertussis, and tetanus. Booster shots are usually recommended about every 10 years. Toxoids are exotoxins secreted by bacteria. They have weakened toxicity, whereas their immunogenicity is maintained. Therefore they can cause a protective immune response but cannot lead to active toxin-induced disease.

Viral Vector Vaccines

Viral vector vaccines use a harmless virus to deliver the genetic code of an antigen to host cells, allowing the immune system to fight the antigen. They are a *gene delivery system*. Information about the antigen is delivered, triggering the immune response. Viral vector vaccines usually cause a robust immune response. Only one dose is generally needed to develop immunity. Boosters may be required to maintain immunity. Examples include the Ebola and COVID-19 vaccines (the AstraZeneca and Johnson & Johnson products).

You Should Remember

Recombinant vaccines include recombinant protein, DNA, and live vaccines using bacterial or viral vectors. Most vaccines currently being studied rely on highly purified recombinant proteins or subunits of pathogens. Posttranslational modifications offer advantages such as enhanced immunogenicity, more stability and solubility, and more controlled activity of antigenic proteins.

TEST YOUR KNOWLEDGE

1. What are some methods of preventing infectious diseases?
2. How are live attenuated vaccines different from inactivated vaccines?
3. What are the advantages of mRNA vaccines?

KEY TERMS

Biological License Application
Conjugate vaccines
Hepatitis B surface antigen
Immune escape variants
Inactivated vaccines
Investigational new drug
Live attenuated vaccines
Messenger RNA vaccines
Protein-based vaccines
Recombinant vaccines
Subunit vaccines
Toxoid vaccines
Viral vector vaccines

Case Study 1

This case study focuses on an experimental herpes simplex type 2 (HSV-2) vaccine. Though herpes simplex virus type 1 is standard, HSV-2 is usually a more severe disease. Therefore an HSV-2 vaccine was developed by a company previously known as Chiron, now called Novartis Vaccines & Diagnostics. Two phase II studies randomized more than 100 people with no antibodies to HSV-2 in their blood to receive one of three vaccine doses. The studies indicated that the vaccine induced an antibody response similar to individuals with a naturally acquired HSV-2 infection. Two phase III studies followed, involving nearly 2400 individuals with no detectable antibodies for HSV-2. They were observed for 1 year after their final immunization. However, these studies revealed that despite producing an antibody response similar to natural HSV-2 infection, the vaccine recipients acquired an HSV-2 infection at a rate comparable to placebo. Therefore researchers concluded that the vaccine produced only partial, transient protection against HSV-2 disease.

Critical Thinking Questions

1. What are the characteristics of phase II trials?
2. What are the characteristics of phase III trials?
3. What "blinding" process is used in phase II and III trials?

Case Study 2

This case study focuses on a glutamic acid decarboxylase (GAD) vaccine proposed by Diamyd Medical to preserve insulin secretion in patients with recent-onset type 1 diabetes. In a phase II study, 70 patients within 18 months of their type 1 diabetes diagnoses were randomly assigned to receive injections of GAD or placebo. Both groups gradually decreased C-peptide levels, but patients receiving GAD injections showed much less decline than patients receiving placebo. This indicated that vaccination with GAD could preserve the insulin-producing function of the beta cells. In a phase III trial, 334 patients were randomly assigned to receive either four doses of GAD, two doses of GAD followed by two doses of placebo, or four doses of placebo. This trial did not confirm the results of the phase II trial, and it was concluded that treatment with GAD did not significantly reduce the loss of C-peptide or improve any critical clinical outcomes.

Critical Thinking Questions

1. What are the general stages of vaccine development?
2. During the approval process, what is a biological license application?
3. What is the definition of a placebo?

Case Study 3

This case study focuses on a MAGE-A3 vaccine produced by GlaxoSmithKline for treating patients with non–small cell lung cancer (NSCLC) following surgery. MAGE-A3 is a cell surface antigen that is tumor specific. About 33% of NSCLCs express MAGE-A3, which is not seen in normal lung cells, making it a potential target for NSCLC therapies. A phase II study evaluated the vaccine, with postsurgical patients receiving either the actual vaccine or placebo 13 times over 27 months. There was a significant improvement in disease-free and overall survival in vaccine patients. In the follow-up phase III trial, 2272 patients received 13 vaccine or placebo injections. However, this trial did not show that the vaccine increased patients' disease-free survival. Therefore it was decided that this vaccine offered no clinical benefit in patients with NSCLC.

Critical Thinking Questions

1. What does vaccine safety research accomplish?
2. To reach a phase II trial, a new vaccine must first undergo a phase I trial. What does this trial consist of?

Case Study 4

This case study focuses on the V710 vaccine Intercell (now known as Valneva) produced when the company worked alongside Merck. The vaccine was intended to prevent *Staphylococcus* (staph) *aureus* infections. Between 10% and 30% of patients with this bacteria in their blood will die. In a phase II trial, 206 chronic hemodialysis patients at high risk for a staph infection received either V710 or placebo on days 1, 28, and 180. Results indicated that V710 produced an antibody response by day 28, sustained for up to 1 year. A phase III trial followed, utilizing nearly 8000 patients from 26 countries. The patients were scheduled to have cardiothoracic surgery and received either one injection of V710 or a placebo. The study was terminated early because of low efficacy and safety concerns. The V710 vaccine did not prevent staph infection any better than the placebo, and there were more cases of multiorgan failure and death in those who acquired a staph infection in the V710 group compared to the placebo.

Critical Thinking Questions

1. What data sources do vaccine effectiveness studies utilize?
2. In which setting does vaccine development usually begin?

FURTHER READING

1. Abbas, A.K., Lichtman, A.H., Pillai, S., 2023. Basic Immunology: Functions and Disorders of the Immune System, 7th Edition. Elsevier.
2. Ashfield, R., Nnamdi Oli, A., Simone, C., Anagu, L., 2022. Vaccinology and Methods in Vaccine Research (Developments in Immunology Series). Academic Press.
3. Bansal, R., 2021. Antibodies and Their Role in Therapeutics: Monoclonal Antibodies/Immunology/Biotechnology. Roohi Bansal.
4. Begg, N., 2022. The Remarkable Story of Vaccines – Milkmaid to Genome. CRC Press.
5. Bhatt, T.K., Nimesh, S., 2021. The Design and Development of Novel Drugs and Vaccines – Principles and Protocols. Academic Press.
6. Buonaguro, L., Van Der Burg, S., 2022. Cancer Vaccines as Immunotherapy of Cancer. Academic Press.
7. Chandler, M., 2022. Vaccines (Focus on Current Events). Focus Readers.
8. Cowan, T., Fallon Morell, S., 2018. Vaccines, Autoimmunity, and the Changing Nature of Childhood Illness. Chelsea Green Publishing.
9. Flajnik, M., 2022. Paul's Fundamental Immunology, 8th Edition. Wolters Kluwer.
10. Hamadache, O., 2023. The Development of the COVID-19 Vaccine. Hamadache.
11. Kesharwani, P., Greish, K., 2022. Polymeric Micelles for Drug Delivery (Series in Biomaterials). Woodhead Publishing.
12. Kolhe, P., Ohtake, S., 2021. Practical Aspects of Vaccine Development. Academic Press.
13. Levinson, W., 2014. Review of Medical Microbiology and Immunology, 13th Edition. McGraw-Hill/Medical.
14. Martin, S.J., Burton, D.R., Roitt, I.M., Delves, P.J., 2017. Roitt's Essential Immunology (Essentials), 13th Edition. Wiley Blackwell.
15. Miller, N.Z., 2015. Miller's Review of Critical Vaccine Studies: 400 Important Scientific Papers Summarized for Parents and Researchers. New Atlantean Press.
16. Murphy, K.M., Weaver, C., Berg, L., 2022. Janeway's Immunobiology, 10th Edition. W.W. Norton & Company.
17. Plotkin, S.A., 2011. History of Vaccine Development. Springer.

18. Prasad, A.K., 2022. Vaccine Development: From Concept to Clinic (Drug Development and Pharmaceutical Science). Royal Society of Chemistry.
19. Prasad, G., Kumar Manna Mohanta, P., 2020. Textbook of Pharmacovigilance: Concept and Practice, 2nd Edition. BSP.
20. Punt, J., Stanford, S., Jones, P., Owen, J., 2018. Kuby Immunology, 8th Edition. W.H. Freeman.
21. Rhodes, J., 2021. How to Make a Vaccine: An Essential Guide for COVID-19 and Beyond. University of Chicago Press.
22. Rich, R.R., Fleisher, T.A., Schroeder Jr., H.W., Weyand, C.M., Corry, D.B., Puck, J.M., 2022. Clinical Immunology: Principles and Practice, 6th Edition. Elsevier.
23. Sears, R.W., 2011. The Vaccine Book: Making the Right Decision for Your Child (Parenting Library). Sears.
24. Singh, M., Srivastava, I.K., 2011. Development of Vaccines: From Discovery to Clinical Testing. Wiley.
25. Thomas, S., 2022. Vaccine Design – Methods and Protocols, Volume 3: Resources for Vaccine Development, 2nd Edition. Humana Press. (Methods in Molecular Biology Book 2412)
26. Wen, E.P., Ellis, E., Pujar, N.S., 2014. Vaccine Development and Manufacturing (Series in Biotechnology and Bioengineering). Wiley.
27. Wehling, M., 2021. Principles of Translational Science in Medicine: From Bench to Bedside, 3rd Edition. Academic Press.

Chapter 5

The Process of Vaccine Approval

Chapter Outline

Learning Objectives

After study of this chapter, readers should be able to:

1. Describe biotechnology platform–based vaccine development.
2. Explain the general stages of vaccine development.
3. Discuss the role of the Advisory Committee on Immunization Practices.
4. Describe the part of the Center for Biologics Evaluation and Research.
5. Explain the preclinical research and testing for vaccines.
6. Explain the clinical development of vaccines.
7. Identify the organizations that are involved with regulatory approval of vaccines.
8. Describe the emergency use authorization for vaccines.
9. Discuss vaccine shipment and the use of specialized equipment.
10. Explain the FDA Review of Vaccines Labeling Requirements.

Vaccinology and Immunizations. http://doi.org/10.1016/B978-0-443-23915-1.00005-6

OVERVIEW

For more than 80+ known infectious agents pathogenic to humans, there are now more than 30 vaccines against 26 mainly viral and bacterial infections. These greatly minimize subsequent disease and prevent death after exposure to those pathogens. To date, all licensed vaccines cause particular antibodies that attach to the infectious agent and therefore can prevent infection. The FDA's expert investigators inspect manufacturing facilities to carefully examine and evaluate the process of making the vaccine to determine compliance with the FDA's requirements. Manufacturing facilities are inspected before a vaccine can be approved and then on a routine basis following approval. If there is substantial evidence that the vaccine is effective and does no harm, then the FDA approves the vaccine for general public use. If a vaccine is not proven safe, has significant side effects, or does not show efficacy, the vaccine is not distributed to the public.

DEVELOPMENT OF VACCINES IN BIOTECHNOLOGY

Vaccination technology was worked out considerably before any underlying science was understood. In the late 19th century, the observation that people infected or exposed to a disease agent were subsequently immune to it was extended by rigorous experimentation. The fact that the immune response is faster and stronger on reinfection than on first infection, meaning that the host "remembers" that it has once been infected and how to deal with it, became known as immunological memory. The organismic system responsible for the immune response became known as the *immune system.*

Biotechnology platform–based vaccine development involves cultivating a flexible baseline structure that can be customized to create new vaccines for related viruses. Researchers identify the changes when pathogens mutate and apply them to the existing system. When COVID-19 started, there was an urgent need for vaccines that could be made quickly, safely, and cost-effectively; traditional manufacturing approaches were insufficient to meet the demand. Biopharmaceutical companies shifted to novel biotechnology platform–based techniques that could be more rapidly adapted to manufacture COVID-19 vaccines and were more robust, customizable, and flexible than traditional approaches. An examination of this transition by a Penn State–led team concludes that such clever manufacturing techniques could, in the future, be applied to other viruses, potentially allowing vaccine development.

Pfizer/BioNTech and Moderna used one such platform, based on messenger RNA, to develop their vaccines. The mRNA platform had already been designed to serve as the basis of a vaccine for coronaviruses that mutate rapidly, which includes the common cold. SARS-CoV-2, the virus that causes COVID-19, was sequenced within weeks of the pandemic's start. Researchers used this information to modify the existing mRNA platform to develop a vaccine tailored to that version of SARS-CoV-2—a process that took less than a week once they had the genetic data. Johnson & Johnson used a similar approach called a **viral vector**. In contrast, traditional vaccine manufacturing, which involves the culture of disease-causing pathogens and injecting some form of these pathogens, can take 10 to 15 years to develop.

The different white blood cells that orchestrate and execute this complex response circulate freely in the blood, where they are relatively easy to access. For this and other reasons, advances in understanding the immune response in the 20th century were widespread. The exponential increase in scientific knowledge plays out in sophisticated methods that exploit the immune system to meet specific goals.

TEST YOUR KNOWLEDGE

1. What is immunological memory?
2. What does biotechnology platform–based vaccine development involve?
3. Why were biotechnology platform–based techniques used to develop the COVID-19 vaccines?

THE FOOD AND DRUG ADMINISTRATION

Vaccines undergo a very rigorous FDA review concerning their laboratory and clinical data. This is to ensure vaccine safety, efficacy, purity, and strength. Vaccines approved for marketing may also have to undergo further studies to include additional evaluation and often to address questions about safety, effectiveness, or adverse effects. The FDA's Center for Biologics Evaluation and Research (CBER) regulates vaccine use in the United States. The general stages of vaccine development include the following:

- Research and discovery: researchers explore ideas for the potential vaccine, often over 10 to 15 years of laboratory research, usually in private companies, but often in collaboration with university researchers.
- Proof of concept: the ability of the vaccine to cause an immune response is studied in small animals.
  - Adjustments to the vaccine's effectiveness may be needed.
- Testing: the clinical development (trial) stage, during which an investigational new drug application is submitted to the FDA.
  - This includes animal study data, manufacturing technology information, and vaccine quality data.
  - The clinical development stage has three phases and sometimes a fourth phase after the FDA approves it.

- The manufacturing process: during the phase III clinical trials, the FDA studies the manufacturer's strategies that will be used for the vaccine and inspects the manufacturing facilities.
  - Vaccine batches are made in "lots," which undergo many tests to ensure vaccine consistency between the lots.
  - Manufacturers must submit data from these tests continually, even after approval.
- Approval: a biological license application (BLA) is submitted to the FDA, which includes preclinical and clinical data, manufacturing details, and manufacturing facility information.
  - The FDA assesses safety and effectiveness.
  - The BLA also contains prescribing information about usage, dosage, and administration.
  - Sometimes the prescribing information must be updated and reviewed by the FDA.
  - The FDA then decides on the vaccine's approval.
  - In some cases, the FDA's Vaccines and Related Biological Products Advisory Committee (VRBPAC) provides input on the scientific data, larger-scale manufacturing may begin, and there is FDA tracking of vaccine quality after this occurs.
- Recommending the vaccine for use: the Advisory Committee on Immunization Practices (ACIP) develops recommendations on the vaccine's usage, considering safety and effectiveness when given at certain ages, how severe the vaccine-preventable disease is, and how many people would contract the disease without the vaccine.
  - The director of the CDC then decides whether to approve the ACIP recommendation.
  - If so, the recommendation becomes the official CDC public health guidance for safe vaccine usage.
  - In some cases, this may lead to the vaccine becoming part of the US adult and childhood immunization schedules.
- Monitoring safety after approval: the FDA and CDC continue to monitor the vaccine's protection to ensure continued success.
  - This is via the following: the Vaccine Adverse Event Reporting System, the Vaccine Safety Datalink, and the Clinical Immunization Safety Assessment project.

TEST YOUR KNOWLEDGE

1. Why do vaccines undergo a very rigorous FDA review?
2. What does the testing stage of a vaccine involve?
3. What does a BLA include?

VACCINES AND RELATED BIOLOGICAL PRODUCTS ADVISORY COMMITTEE

This committee reviews and evaluates data about the safety, effectiveness, and appropriate use of vaccines and related biological products intended to prevent, treat, or diagnose human diseases. The committee considers the quality and relevance of the FDA's research program that provides scientific support for vaccine regulation and makes appropriate recommendations to the FDA commissioner.

The committee consists of a core group of 15 voting members, including the chairperson. The commissioner or a designated individual from widely knowledgeable authorities selects the members and chairperson. These authorities may come from any of the following fields:

- Immunology: the branch of medicine and biology concerned with immunity
- Molecular biology: the study of the chemical and physical structure of biological macromolecules
- rDNA: the study of **ribosomal DNA**, which codes for the rRNAs used in the production of ribosomes, the sites of cellular protein synthesis
- Virology: the study of viruses and virus-like agents, including their **taxonomy**, disease-producing properties, cultivation, and genetics
- Bacteriology: the study of bacteria
- Epidemiology: the study of the incidence, distribution, and possible control of diseases and other factors relating to health
- Biostatistics (**biometry**): the development and application of statistical methods to many biological topics
- Vaccine policy: vaccination requirements and laws
- Vaccine safety science: research and safety studies concerning the safe use of vaccines in the public forum
- Federal immunization activities: governmental practices concerning vaccinations
- Vaccine development (including translational and clinical evaluation programs): a combination of public and private involvement; drug development along with proteomics, genomics, genetics, metabolomics, and animal models are all examples of translational research; clinical evaluation studies in humans demonstrate safety and efficacy of vaccines before they are released for widespread use
- Allergy: the study of allergic disease and its related symptoms and reactions
- Preventive medicine: the practice of promoting preventive healthcare to improve patient well-being
- Infectious diseases: the study of complex relationships between hosts and contagious agents
- Pediatrics: the branch of medicine that involves the medical care of infants, children, adolescents, and, in some cases, young adults (including age 18)

- Microbiology: the branch of science that deals with microorganisms
- Biochemistry: the branch of science concerned with the chemical and physiochemical processes and substances occurring in living organisms

CENTER FOR BIOLOGICS EVALUATION AND RESEARCH

Under applicable federal laws, this part of the FDA regulates biological products for human use. These include the Public Health Service Act and the Federal Food, Drug, and Cosmetic Act. The CBER protects and advances public health by ensuring that biological products are safe, effective, and available to people needing them. It also provides the public with information to promote the safe and appropriate use of natural products.

The Public Health Service Act gave the US Public Health Service responsibility for preventing the introduction, transmission, and spreading of infectious diseases from foreign countries into the United States. The Federal Food, Drug, and Cosmetic Act brought cosmetics and medical devices under control and required drugs to be labeled with adequate directions for safe use.

You Should Remember

The mission of the CBER is to ensure the safety, purity, potency, and effectiveness of biological products. The CBER facilitates the availability of safe, effective natural products through regulatory work and applied scientific research. It also plays a vital role in maintaining US preparedness against threats caused by terrorism, pandemics, and other emerging infectious diseases. The CBER also strives to improve public health through international collaborations concerning research and information sharing.

TEST YOUR KNOWLEDGE

1. What does the VRBPAC do?
2. Which disciplines may be represented by VRBPAC members?
3. What are the functions of the CBER?

PRECLINICAL RESEARCH AND TESTING FOR VACCINES

Before a vaccine can be used to protect humans from a specific disease, there is a long, careful process involving extensive research and testing to determine whether the vaccine works and is safe for people. The exploratory phase of vaccine research involves laboratory research and can last several years. Once scientists have identified a target disease and obtained the necessary funding, they attempt to identify natural or synthetic antigens that could prevent or treat that disease.

In preclinical research, scientists test their ideas for new biomedical prevention strategies in laboratory experiments or animals. Clinical research refers to studies in humans. Preclinical research encompasses everything before a vaccine candidate is considered for human testing. Preclinical research answers a range of questions. First, scientists will see if their idea for a new strategy shows any promise. For example, they might take an experimental microbicide and combine it with HIV in a laboratory experiment to see if the microbicide stops HIV activity. If there is evidence that the testing strategy works during in ***vitro* experiments** animal experiments are conducted to gather additional information. This can include information on a practical candidate's safety, dosing strategy, toxicity, and whether the candidate might have an HIV risk reduction benefit. Mice, rabbits, guinea pigs, and monkeys are some animals used to evaluate potential candidates in preclinical *in vivo* experiments.

The exact questions asked during preclinical research depend on the tested strategy. Vaccine studies can look for immune responses in the animals' blood. Microbicide studies can look for any irritation in the rectal or vaginal linings of the animals. Studies in nonhuman primates are conducted to get a preliminary idea of whether the candidate might reduce the risk of HIV infection. These animals are then exposed to or "challenged" with strains of Simian immunodeficiency virus or Simian-human immunodeficiency virus (two families of HIV-like viruses that can cause disease in monkeys). Suppose animals that receive the experimental strategy have different responses to the challenge than animals that did not receive the experimental design. In that case, this is preliminary evidence of some risk reduction benefit. However, these animal studies cannot predict whether a product will protect people—nonhuman primates and humans differ in their immune systems and responses to HIV or HIV-like viruses. This is one reason why research in humans is so important and the research process is so uncertain.

CLINICAL DEVELOPMENT OF VACCINES

The clinical vaccine development process has been refined for over a century to meet society's need for safe and productive vaccines. Like chemical drugs, a vaccine's clinical evaluation typically comprises three phases. The process takes 10–15 years and requires a budget of about 1 billion US dollars. A vaccine-specific developmental plan should be established to ensure efficient and successful development before clinical evaluation. This includes identification of the target population (mostly healthy people with particular demographic characteristics) and their sociocultural factors, risk assessment of the target disease and the vaccine itself, understanding of the incidence of the target disease and environmental factors, identification of the dose and route of administration, plans to induce herd immunity, and regulatory strategies. Human studies of a vaccine candidate's acceptable safety and **reactogenicity** are achieved in phase I clinical trials.

In this phase, safety and tolerability are evaluated at the local and systemic levels as the primary endpoint. Dose-ranging and repeated-dose studies are often performed. Preliminary information on immunogenicity and efficacy may be collected. These trials are often designed as randomized, double-masked, placebo-controlled, single-center studies. A crossover or parallel design may be chosen according to the product's characteristics. The statistical analysis is generally descriptive and exploratory because the trials involve only small numbers of participants (20–80). Therefore more information is needed for confirmatory tests. In the "first-in-human" setting, more attention should be given to live attenuated vaccines because the risks tend to be higher than those of inactivated vaccines.

In phase II, the proof of concept of the vaccine product should be ensured. Clinical trials of this phase demonstrate the **immunogenicity** of the relevant active components and the safety profile of a candidate vaccine within the target population. Practices should also define the optimal dose, initial vaccination schedule, and safety profile of a candidate vaccine. Separating clinical trials into phase IIA and IIB often accomplishes these purposes. In designing these clinical trials, multiple variables associated with the host immune response are considered. Determinants of clinically applicable vaccine regimens are also included, such as the dose and number of doses, interval between doses, and route of administration. Vaccine efficacy may be evaluated using well-defined surrogate parameters. Most clinical trials include parallel group comparisons with **placebo** or active control groups. Prospective and confirmatory statistical analyses are performed, and the percentage of responders should be defined and described based on predefined criteria of an immune response.

The final step in the clinical evaluation before the product license is the phase III trial. This stage is intended to provide a vital conclusion needed for marketing approval, and the efficacy and safety of formulations of the immunologically active components must be assessed in the large-scale target population. The clinical outcome is strongly recommended for comparing efficacy against a placebo. Therefore serological data are usually collected from at least a subset of the immunized population at predefined intervals. The designs of phase II and phase III clinical trials are similar, but the size of a phase III trial is much larger. Considering the modern vaccination strategy—administration of multiple vaccines at the same time—interaction or interference with other vaccines is evaluated routinely. Conducting a confirmatory study to determine the protective efficacy of products containing the same antigens is sometimes impossible.

You Should Remember

One of the most critical aspects of vaccinology in the 21st century is the extension of the target population by developing new vaccines against emerging infections, tumors, and chronic diseases. Ultimately, the goal of modern vaccination may be expressed as to prevent or cure as many diseases as possible.

TEST YOUR KNOWLEDGE

1. What are the differences between preclinical and clinical vaccine research?
2. What should be ensured during phase II of vaccine development?
3. What is a phase III trial intended to provide?

SPECIAL CONSIDERATIONS AND EMERGENCY VACCINE DEVELOPMENT

The FDA is globally respected for its scientific vaccine safety, effectiveness, and quality standards. The agency provides scientific and regulatory advice to vaccine developers. It undertakes a rigorous evaluation of scientific information through all phases of clinical trials. This continues after a vaccine has been approved by the FDA or authorized for emergency use. The FDA recognizes the gravity of current public health emergencies and the importance of facilitating the fast availability of new vaccines that the public will trust and have confidence in receiving.

An **emergency use authorization** (EUA) is a mechanism to facilitate the availability and use of medical countermeasures, including vaccines, during public health emergencies, such as the COVID-19 pandemic. Under an EUA, the FDA may allow the use of unapproved medical products or unapproved uses of approved medical products in an emergency to diagnose, treat, or prevent serious or life-threatening diseases or conditions when specific statutory criteria have been met, including that there are no adequate, approved, and available alternatives. Considering input from the FDA, manufacturers decide whether and when to submit an EUA request to the FDA. Once presented, the FDA will evaluate an EUA request and determine whether the relevant statutory criteria are met, considering the totality of the scientific evidence about the vaccine available to the FDA.

From a safety perspective, the FDA expects an EUA submission will include all safety data accumulated from phase I and II studies conducted with the vaccine, with an expectation that phase III data will consist of a median follow-up of at least 2 months (meaning that at least half of vaccine recipients in phase 3 clinical trials have at least 2 months of follow-up) after completion of the entire vaccination regimen. In addition, the FDA expects that an EUA request will include a phase III safety database of well over 3000 vaccine recipients, representing a high proportion of participants enrolled in the phase 3 study who have been followed for severe adverse events and adverse events of particular interest for at least 1 month after completion of the entire vaccination regimen.

Part of the FDA's evaluation of an EUA request for a COVID-19 vaccine includes an assessment of the vaccine's chemistry, manufacturing, and control information. Sufficient data should be submitted to ensure the quality and consistency of the vaccine product. The FDA will use all available tools and information, including records reviews, site visits, and previous compliance history, to assess compliance with current good manufacturing practices.

You Should Remember

The FDA must ensure that recipients of the vaccine under an EUA are informed, to the extent possible given the applicable circumstances, (1) that the FDA has authorized the emergency use of the vaccine, (2) of the known and potential benefits and risks, the time to which such benefits and risks are unknown, and (3) that they have the option to accept or refuse the vaccine and of any available alternatives to the product. Typically, this information is communicated in a patient "fact sheet." The FDA posts these fact sheets on its website.

TEST YOUR KNOWLEDGE

1. What is an EUA?
2. From a safety perspective, what does the FDA expect an EUA application to include?

MANUFACTURING, SAFETY, AND QUALITY CONTROL OF VACCINES

Once a vaccine has reached the preapproval stage following clinical trials, it is assessed by the relevant regulatory body for compliance with quality, safety, and efficacy criteria. Following regulatory approval, manufacturers can submit a vaccine to the WHO for prequalification. This assessment process ensures quality, safety, and efficacy and helps the United Nations (UN) and other international procurement organizations determine the programmatic suitability of a vaccine.

During global health emergencies, the WHO Emergency Use Listing Procedure (EUL) may be used to allow emergency use of the vaccine. The EUL exists because, in a pandemic, products that could benefit people's lives worldwide may be prevented from coming to market with sufficient speed. The EUL is a fast-tracked but rigorous process designed to bring impactful products to all those in need as quickly as possible on a time-limited basis and based on a risk-versus-benefit evaluation. The WHO recommendation may be used by UN agencies such as UNICEF and the Pan American Health Organization Revolving Fund for procurement decisions in low- and middle-income countries.

Once the vaccine has been made in bulk, it is bottled in glass vials and carefully packaged for safe cold storage and transport. Vaccine packaging must be able to withstand extreme temperatures as well as the risks involved in being transported globally. Therefore vaccine vials are most commonly made from glass, as it is durable and able to maintain its integrity in extreme temperatures. A vaccine becomes less effective or inactive when it is too hot or cold. Vaccines can be ruined or unsafe if stored at the incorrect temperature. Most vaccines require refrigerated storage at between 2°C and 8°C. Some vaccines require temperatures as cold as −20°C. Some of the newer vaccines need to be kept ultracold at −70°C.

Some frozen vaccines can be safely stored for a limited time between 2°C and 8°C. Regular refrigerators cannot maintain an even temperature consistently, so specialized medical refrigerators are required for these precious products.

To maintain this cold chain, vaccines are shipped using specialized equipment that does not compromise the integrity of the product. Once shipments land in the destination country, refrigerated lorries transport the vaccines from the airport to the warehouse cold room. From there, portable iceboxes transport vaccines from the cold room to regional centers, storing them in refrigerators. If vaccination occurs outside the regional facility, the final step often requires portable iceboxes to transport the goods to local areas for vaccination campaigns. New technologies have invented mobile devices that can keep vaccines at their cold temperature for several days without electricity.

Once vaccines are administered, national authorities and WHO constantly monitor for and establish the severity of any possible adverse side effects and responses from people who have received the vaccine. The vaccine's safety is paramount, with regular assessments and postapproval clinical studies to report on its safety and effectiveness. Studies are often conducted to determine how long a given vaccine remains protective.

FDA REVIEW OF VACCINE LABELING REQUIREMENTS

All labels must be designed and applied to devices and containers so that the labels remain in place and legible during the customary distribution, storage, and use conditions. Likewise, other labeling, such as user instructions, should remain legible during average storage and use.

The FDA routinely assesses the warnings, use instructions, and precautionary information provided for licensed vaccines based on its surveillance of adverse event reporting and other data sources to manufacturers. This guidance document provides the FDA's current thinking about its vaccine labeling and surveillance review. The review of vaccine labeling completed by the FDA offers a helpful description of some methods of the warnings, use instructions, and precautionary information found in vaccine package inserts.

TEST YOUR KNOWLEDGE

1. What is the World Health Organization's EUL?
2. How are vaccines usually stored during transport?
3. What are the requirements for vaccine labeling?

KEY TERMS

Biometry
Biotechnology
Emergency Use Authorization
Immunogenicity
In vitro experiments
Placebo
Reactogenicity
Ribosomal DNA
Taxonomy
Viral vector

FURTHER READING

1. Barrett, J.S., 2022. Fundamentals of Drug Development. Wiley.
2. Blass, B.E., 2021. Basic Principles of Drug Discovery and Development, 2nd Edition. Academic Press.
3. Borrell, B., 2021. The First Shots: The Epic Rivalries and Heroic Science Behind the Race to the Coronavirus Vaccine. Mariner Books.
4. Chow, S.C., 2022. Innovative Methods for Rare Disease Drug Development (Biostatistics Series). CRC Press.
5. Consoli, D., Mina, A., Nelson, R.R., Ramlogan, R., 2015. Medical Innovation: Science, Technology, and Practice (International Studies in Health Economics). Routledge.
6. Ellis, R.W., 2000. Combination Vaccines: Development, Clinical Research, and Approval. Humana Press.
7. Faqi, A.S., 2016. A Comprehensive Guide to Toxicology in Nonclinical Drug Development, 2nd Edition. Academic Press.
8. Feng, X., Xie, H.G., Malhotra, A., Yang, C.F., 2022. Biologics and Biosimilars: Drug Discovery and Clinical Applications. CRC Press.
9. Hill, R.G., Richards, D.B., 2021. Drug Discovery and Development: Technology in Transition, 3rd Edition. Elsevier.
10. Hussain, K., 2020. The Drug Discovery and Development Cycle: A Concise Overview of the Key Steps from Concept to Launch. Hussain.
11. Ng, R., 2015. Drugs: From Discovery to Approval, 3rd Edition. Wiley Blackwell.
12. O'Donnell, J.J., Somberg, J., Idemyor, V., O'Donnell, J.T., 2021. Drug Discovery and Development, 3rd Edition. CRC Press.
13. Offit, P.A., Hoban, J.N., 2021. You Bet Your Life: From Blood Transfusions to Mass Vaccination – The Long and Risky History of Medical Innovation. Basic Books.
14. Rosenberg, Z., 2021. The COVID-19 Vaccine: An Expert's Medical Guide for All. Rosenberg.
15. Sheets, R., 2017. Fundamentals of Biologicals Regulation: Vaccines and Biotechnology Medicines. Academic Press.

Chapter 6

Prevention and Eradication of Infectious Diseases

Chapter Outline

Learning Objectives

After study of this chapter, readers should be able to:

1. Describe the transmission of microorganisms to humans.
2. Explain the importance of food safety techniques.
3. Identify the way to prevent sexually transmitted infections.
4. Describe community immunity or herd immunity.
5. Discuss the prevention of insect bites.
6. Explain Lyme disease and how it can be transmitted to humans.
7. Describe the concept of boosting immunity.
8. Explain the meaning of immunosenescence.
9. Discuss the mosquito-borne parasites that transmit the infectious disease.
10. Explain global infectious disease eradication.

Vaccinology and Immunizations. http://doi.org/10.1016/B978-0-443-23915-1.00006-8

OVERVIEW

Prevention and eradication of human infectious diseases have been the subject of conferences, symposia, workshops, planning sessions, and public health initiatives for over 100 years. While malaria, yellow fever, and other eradication programs of earlier years were unsuccessful, they contributed significantly to a better understanding of the many complexities of achieving the ultimate goal of disease control. Smallpox has been eradicated, and programs are underway to eradicate poliomyelitis and guinea worm disease. In 1993, the International Task Force for Disease Eradication evaluated more than 80 potential infectious diseases and concluded that six were eradicable. In 1997, the World Health Assembly passed a resolution to eliminate lymphatic filariasis as a public health problem. Preventing and eradicating infectious diseases is a significant goal for the world. Prevention focuses on restricting the circulation of contagious agents beyond levels resulting from spontaneous and individual behaviors. Eradication describes the total absence of human cases of a disease, the lack of a reservoir for causative organisms, and the full containment of any infectious source.

PROTECTING AGAINST INFECTIONS

Infections are caused by microscopic organisms known as pathogens—bacteria, viruses, fungi, or parasites—that enter the body, multiply, and interfere with normal functions. Infectious diseases are one of the leading causes of illness and death in the United States and worldwide. For certain people, particularly those with underlying conditions such as heart disease or cancer, serious injuries, or taking medications that weaken the immune system, it is more difficult to avoid getting sick with an infection. Living in a wealthy country like the United States, the threat of deadly viruses, bacteria, and parasites can seem remote, but these infectious microbes are ever present among us.

Transmission of Microorganisms

Not long ago, no one understood that infectious diseases were caused by tiny organisms that are transmitted from person to person. Even now, although some microorganisms may cause contagious diseases, we know that most microbes enter through openings in the body—the nose, mouth, ears, anus, and genital passages. They can also be transmitted through the skin through insect or animal bites. The best way to prevent infections is to block pathogens from entering the body.

Personal Hygiene

Good hygiene is the primary way to prevent infections. The first line of defense is to have good personal hygiene habits. Diseases can be stopped before they begin. These easy measures help prevent the spread of diseases to others:

- Wash your hands well, especially after using the bathroom, preparing food, gardening, or performing other potentially dirty tasks. People should also wash up after blowing their nose, coughing, or sneezing; feeding or stroking their pet; or visiting or caring for a sick person. Lather with soap or cleanser and rub it into the palms and backs of the hands and wrists. Clean the fingertips, under the nails, and between the fingers. Handwashing is the most essential way to prevent infectious diseases.
- Cover the mouth and nose with a tissue when sneezing or coughing. If no tissue is handy, cough or sneeze into your elbow rather than into the hands.
- Wash and bandage all cuts or wounds.
- Do not pick at healing wounds or squeeze pimples.
- Keep dishes, glasses, or eating utensils separate from other people's.
- Avoid direct contact with napkins, tissues, handkerchiefs, or similar items others use.

Food Safety Techniques

Although most cases of foodborne infection are not dangerous, some can lead to severe medical conditions, including **kidney failure** and meningitis. Individuals can prevent infections by foodborne pathogens in their households by preparing and storing foods safely. The following precautions will help kill microbes that are present in the food you buy:

- Rinse all fruits and vegetables under water before cooking or serving them.
- Wash hands with soap and water before and after handling raw meat.
- Separate raw foods and cooked foods. Use different utensils or cutting boards for raw and cooked meat.
- Cook foods thoroughly, using a meat thermometer to ensure that whole poultry is cooked to 180 °F, roasts and steaks to 145 °F, and ground meats to 160 °F. Cook fish until it is opaque.
- Defrost foods only in the refrigerator or in the microwave.

You Should Remember

Escherichia coli poisoning in foods can result in blood clots that block the kidneys' filtering system. This condition, called hemolytic uremic syndrome, results in the sudden failure of the kidneys to filter waste from the blood. Less often, other bacteria or viruses may cause this condition. Kidney failure can also result from food poisoning caused by the *Shigella* bacteria or from eating toxic mushrooms.

Immunizations

Vaccines are essential for protecting humans against infections. They help the immune system work better—and faster. Vaccines protect against potentially serious infectious diseases. They "alert" the immune system so that the body fights off pathogens and remembers them for the future. Because vaccines are made from tiny amounts of weakened or killed microorganisms, they do not cause the diseases they protect against. Vaccines often provide long-lasting immunity to serious diseases without the risk of serious illness.

When we receive recommended vaccines, they also protect unvaccinated people around us. This is known as **community immunity**, or herd immunity. It is essential to stay up to date on all recommended vaccines. Vaccines are constantly monitored for adverse effects after being introduced. Mild side effects, such as a temporary sore arm or low fever, may occur for a few days.

Traveling Precautions

If people are planning a trip, they may need immunizations (see Chapter 12). They must discuss the travel plans with their physician at least 3 months before they leave.

- If people travel to an area where insect-borne disease is present, take and use an insect repellent containing DEET. In many tropical regions, mosquitoes can carry malaria, dengue, yellow fever, Japanese encephalitis, or other serious infections.
- Get your shots before you leave the United States. Avoid getting any unnecessary, immunizations, or tattoos abroad. Needles and syringes (even disposable ones) are reused in some parts of the world.
- Do not consume ice while traveling. Freezing does not kill all waterborne infectious microbes.
- Drink only bottled drinks with secure caps, such as soft or bottled water. Be aware that some fruit juices may be made with impure local water.
- Boil all tap water before drinking or drink only bottled water; use bottled or boiled water to brush your teeth.
- Refrain from eating uncooked vegetables, including lettuce; only eat fruit you have peeled yourself.
- Do not consume dairy products (milk may not be pasteurized).

Preventing Sexually Transmitted Infections

The only sure way to prevent sexually transmitted infections is to avoid sexual intercourse or other sexual contact. That is not an option for most people, so the next best choice is to follow these safe sex guidelines:

- Engage in sexual contact only with one partner who is sexually exclusive with you.

- Both you and your partner should be tested for HIV and other sexually transmitted diseases.

If you do have sex with a new partner, make sure the partner is tested, and take the following precautions:

- For vaginal sex, use a latex or **polyurethane condom** or a female condom.
- For oral sex, use a latex or polyurethane male condom or a female condom.
- For anal sex, use a latex or polyurethane male condom.

Preventing Insect Bites

Both mosquitoes and ticks are carriers of viruses and bacteria. Both have been associated with severe epidemics in the last decade. While it is true that most mosquitoes in northern climates do not transmit disease, some do. Within one decade, West Nile virus spread throughout the United States and parts of Canada. Mosquitoes in North America also carry several other forms of mosquito-borne **encephalitis**. Tropical diseases pose a threat if the mosquitoes that carry them hitch a ride in boats or expand their range northward from Central America. In the United States, mosquito-borne disease is geographically widespread and occurs in several forms: West Nile disease, **La Crosse encephalitis**, eastern equine encephalitis, **Jamestown Canyon virus**, and others.

Ticks are widespread and can transmit **Lyme disease** (Figure 6.1). They live in grassy and brushy areas and are most prevalent during wet seasons. A common hiding place is in wet leaves. They often infest animals, including field mice and deer. They may be transported into people's homes by their pets. The following can help prevent infections from an insect bite:

- Use insect repellents approved by the Environmental Protection Agency, including those containing DEET, picaridin, or oil of lemon eucalyptus. If mosquitoes are biting you, reapply the repellent.
- Limit outdoor activity during peak mosquito hours of early morning and evening.

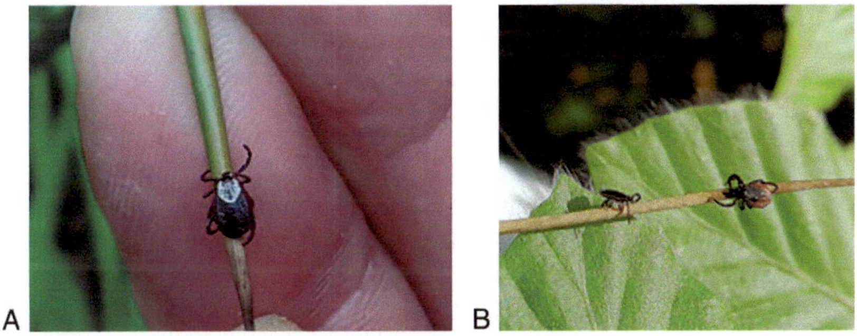

FIGURE 6.1 A tick that commonly transmits Lyme disease.

- Drain any standing water near your home to prevent mosquitoes from breeding.
- Check your neighborhood and pick up trash, discarded cans, bottles, and other containers containing enough water to allow mosquitoes to breed.
- If you plan to spend time in an area where ticks are common (even your backyard), wear light-colored clothing so ticks can be spotted and removed before they attach. When hiking on trails, stay in the center of the course to avoid picking up ticks from bushes and brush. When you return, check your clothing and body for ticks. Check your pet before allowing it indoors.
- If a tick has attached itself to you or your pet, grasp it firmly with tweezers close to the tick's mouth and pull steadily. Cleanse the area of the tick bite thoroughly with an antiseptic. Watch the site closely for signs of rash or swelling for a few weeks.

You Should Remember

Vaccines do not cause autism, allergies, overload, or immune system weakening. Almost all childhood vaccines do not contain mercury. However, some flu vaccines with more than one dose in the vial contain thimerosal, a mercury-based preservative. The small amount of thimerosal used to preserve vaccines is safe.

You Should Remember

The WHO has listed vaccine hesitancy as one of the most significant threats to global health. Vaccine hesitancy is when people with access to vaccines delay or refuse to be vaccinated.

TEST YOUR KNOWLEDGE

1. What types of infections are carried by mosquitoes?
2. What is the description of Lyme disease, which is carried by ticks?
3. What ingredients do approved insect repellents contain?

BOOSTING IMMUNITY

Vaccines work by imitating an infection to engage the body's natural defenses. This boosts immunity. The active ingredient in every vaccine is an antigen. This antigen can be either weakened or killed bacteria or viruses, small pieces of their exterior surface or genetic material, or a bacterial toxin treated to make it nontoxic. A single vaccine dose provides only partial protection.

In some cases, the number of doses required to achieve immunity depends on if the antigen is alive or dead. Live attenuated vaccines provide long-lasting protection with only two doses because they contain living bacteria or viruses. Nonlive vaccines usually require at least three doses to achieve security, but this fades over time and must be restored with *booster doses*. For example, the DTaP vaccine (against diphtheria, tetanus, and pertussis) is given to infants in four doses (at 2, 4, 6, and 18 months). Children receive one booster dose around the time of entering school and another during the start of middle school. Another example concerns the tetanus vaccine. Adults should get a tetanus booster once every 10 years or during each pregnancy. Additional criteria include the seasonal influenza vaccine. It is reformulated annually to target the four strains expected to be most common and dangerous. This is why annual boosters are needed.

New research shows that vaccines may not only protect against the disease for which they are manufactured. They may prime the immune system to prepare it better to fight other disease-causing bacteria or viruses. This is known as *immune fitness*. Being vaccinated at all stages of life helps to build immune fitness. For example, health system employees vaccinated against tuberculosis were significantly less likely to test positive for COVID-19 or to have reported COVID-19 symptoms than those without the tuberculosis vaccine (Bacille Calmette-Guérin, or BCG). Vaccines may prompt natural responses that improve immunity by reprogramming immune cells (*trained immunity*) or causing a "memory" by boosting preexisting memory cells generated by previous vaccinations. Much study is ongoing on boosting immunity against various diseases using the currently recommended vaccines.

TEST YOUR KNOWLEDGE

1. Why are vaccines necessary?
2. What is herd immunity?
3. What are the antigens used in vaccines?

PHYSICAL ACTIVITY AND NUTRITIONAL INFLUENCE ON IMMUNE FUNCTION

Physical activity (PA) and nutrition are the essential components of a healthy lifestyle. They can influence energy balance, promote the functional ability of various systems, and improve immunity. Infections and associated symptoms are common and frequent challenges to human health, causing severe economic and social consequences worldwide.

During aging, the human immune system undergoes dramatic changes and dysfunctions known as **immunosenescence**. Clinically, immunosenescence refers to the gradual deterioration of the immune system, increasing exposure to infections and reducing vaccine efficacy. Such a phenomenon is linked to impaired immune responses that lead to dysfunction of multiple organs. At the same time, lack of PA, progressive loss of muscle mass, and a concomitant decline in muscle strength facilitate immunosenescence and inflammation. Nutrition and PA can synergistically boost the immune system.

Evidence suggests that long-term PA is beneficial in improving the immune system and preventing infections. Regarding interactions with food intake, PA does not tend to increase energy intake over the short term. However, overcoming nutritional deficiencies is an efficient recommendation. A balanced, nutritious diet can fulfill optimal nutrition requirements and significantly impact the immune system. Supplementation of a single nutrient as food is generally not advisable. Instead, incorporating various fruits and vegetables, whole grains, proteins, and probiotics may ensure adequate nutrient intake. Therefore multinutrient supplements may benefit people with a deficiency despite a sufficient diet. Along with PA, supplementation of **probiotics**, plant-derived products, **bovine colostrum**, and functional foods may improve the immune system.

The invading pathogens lead to loss of appetite, malabsorption, increased nutrient demand, and loss of critical endogenous nutrients. The risk and severity of infection differ according to immune competence, development, maturation, and the immune system's decline. Therefore nutrition is one of the significant factors impacting the body's immune system or defense mechanism. Thus nutrition, primarily adequate and appropriate nutrition, is an essential determinant of optimal immune functions such as the trigger of immune cells, interaction, differentiation, or functional expression of these cells. **Malnutrition** deteriorates the immune system and increases the vulnerability to infectious pathogens. Nutrition can play a role in effective responses against pathogens and modulate immune functions to combat stress, disease, and injury.

Nutrition can come from either an exogenous or endogenous source. **Exogenous** sources are diets that provide vitamins or **micronutrients**. Some micronutrients and dietary components, such as activating immune functions, play specific immune roles. **Endogenous** sources, such as the stored form of energy in body cells or tissues, become instantaneous sources that can be derived through various mechanisms, such as when required, in the absence or insufficiency of exogenous nutrients.

TEST YOUR KNOWLEDGE

1. What is immunosenescence?
2. Aside from PA, what supplements may improve the immune system?
3. What are exogenous and endogenous sources of nutrition?

EMERGENCY PREPAREDNESS FOR OUTBREAKS

During an outbreak of infections, the Immunization Safety Office (ISO) of the CDC prepares for emergencies by ensuring that solid systems are in place that can quickly monitor vaccine safety. In an emergency that involves mass vaccination, it is essential to monitor vaccine safety for the following reasons:

- The vaccines used may be new: initial safety data can be limited. It is essential to monitor safety to detect concerning or unexpected patterns closely.
- Large numbers of vaccines may be given over a short period: this means that more adverse events or side effects may need to be reported to the Vaccine Adverse Event Reporting System (VAERS).
- Public awareness of vaccination programs may increase reporting: during an emergency, reporting adverse events or side effects to VAERS may result in a higher reporting volume than during nonemergency situations.

VAERS accepts vaccine adverse event reports from patients, parents, healthcare professionals, vaccine manufacturers, and other entities. CDC and FDA scientists review reports using statistical techniques to detect unusual or unexpected patterns because these could indicate a safety problem with a vaccine.

The Clinical Immunization Safety Assessment (CISA) project is a national network of vaccine safety experts. It focuses on vaccine safety issues, conducts clinical research, and assesses complex adverse events after vaccinations. The **Vaccine Safety Datalink (VSD)** project collects information on vaccines administered to members of specific healthcare organizations in the United States. A "rapid cycle analysis" system allows the CDC to address vaccine-related health problems quickly. Vaccine safety coordinators in 62 different health departments carry out vaccine safety and emergency preparedness activities, coordinating with the CDC.

THE EFFECT OF IMMUNIZATION

In the 20th century, the development, licensing, and implementation of vaccines as part of large, systematic immunization programs started to address global health inequities. However, access to vaccines that prevent life-threatening infectious diseases remains unequal to all infants, children, adults, and older adults worldwide. This is a problem that many individuals and agencies are working hard to address globally. After learning of the emergence of the SARS-CoV-2 virus in December 2019 and its potential for global dissemination to cause COVID-19, there was an urgent need to develop vaccines at an unprecedented rate and scale. As we appreciate and quantify the health, economic, and social benefits of vaccines and immunization programs to individuals and society, we should endeavor to communicate this to the public and policymakers for the use of endemic, epidemic, and pandemic diseases.

The development of safe and efficacious vaccination against diseases that cause substantial morbidity and mortality has been one of the foremost scientific advances of the 21st century. Vaccinations, sanitation, and clean drinking water are public health interventions undeniably responsible for improved health outcomes globally. It is estimated that vaccines have prevented 6 million deaths from vaccine-preventable diseases annually, partly due to effective vaccines that prevent disease and prolong life expectancy across all continents. However, much must be done to ensure vaccine financing, provision, distribution, and administration to all populations, particularly those difficult to reach, including those skeptical about their protective value and those living in civil disruption. Agencies including the WHO, The United Nations International Children's Emergency Fund (UNICEF), the Vaccine Alliance, The Bill & Melinda Gates Foundation, and the Coalition for Epidemic Preparedness Initiative (CEPI), with their multiple funding streams, have been instrumental in expanding vaccine benefits to all. The importance of these organizations in global cooperation and participation was essential in the setting of the 2019 global pandemic of SARS-CoV-2 in light of the health and economic impact of COVID-19 on societies in high-, middle-, and low-income countries.

Immunization is a worldwide health and development story of success, with millions of lives saved annually. Some vaccines prevent over 20 life-threatening diseases. Immunization prevents 3.5 to 5 million deaths yearly from diphtheria, tetanus, pertussis, influenza, and measles. Immunization is a crucial component of primary healthcare. Vaccines are critical to the prevention and control of infectious disease outbreaks.

Immunizations also help prevent disease, disability, and death from vaccine-preventable diseases. These include cervical cancer, measles, poliomyelitis, parotitis, rubella, diphtheria, pertussis, tetanus, bacterial pneumonia, hepatitis A and B, bacterial meningitis, and rotavirus diarrheal diseases. Key facts about new vaccines are summarized in Table 6.1.

However, there are also some adverse facts. For example, 2.7 million American children must complete their essential vaccinations. Also, in the countries of America, 12 out of 42 reporting countries reported less than 80% coverage with the first dose of the measles, mumps, and rubella vaccine. Regional coverage for the third dose of the vaccine that contains antigens against diphtheria, tetanus, and pertussis fell from 89% in 2018 to 85% in 2021.

TABLE 6.1 Key facts about new vaccines.

Vaccine	Facts
Human papillomavirus	45 countries and territories have now introduced the HPV vaccine.
Pneumococcal	37 countries and territories have now introduced this vaccine.
Rotavirus	22 countries and territories have now introduced this vaccine.
Tetanus	Haiti (a priority country) has certified the elimination of neonatal tetanus.

Vaccines are highly beneficial on a population level and are cost effective compared to other public health interventions. Government departments must perform systematic economic analyses of vaccines and vaccine programs to justify their purchase, given the global pressure on public and private finances; the 2008 financial crash exacerbated this. A vaccination program has precise direct costs, including vaccine purchase, **infrastructure** to run the program and maintain the cold chain, and healthcare/administration personnel. Often supported by charities and nongovernmental organizations, governments invest in these to improve health. The reduction in morbidity and mortality associated with successful vaccine programs, through a combination of direct and indirect protection, has reduced disease incidence. This potentially leads to economic growth, with less money spent owing to the costs averted through fewer medical tests, procedures, treatments, and less time off work by patients or parents. Additionally, the use of combination vaccines, for example, DTaP/IPV/Hib/HepB, protects an increased number of diseases, with no additional infrastructure costs, that is, the same number of injections per child within existing immunization programs.

You Should Remember

Vaccines effectively prevent disease, but they do not always work. According to the CDC, most recommended childhood immunizations are 90% to 100% effective. However, for reasons that are not entirely understood, sometimes a child will not become fully immunized against a disease after receiving a vaccine. This is all the more reason to get children vaccinated. Children in whom the vaccine is 100% effective protect those few who have not been completely immunized. This lessens everyone's chance of exposure to the disease.

You Should Remember

The most common side effects after vaccination are mild. They include pain, swelling, or redness where the shot was given. Sometimes, a mild fever, chills, headache, tiredness, and muscle and joint aches occur. Serious side effects from vaccines are infrequent. For example, if 1 million vaccine doses are given, one to two people may have a severe allergic reaction.

TEST YOUR KNOWLEDGE

1. What is immunosenescence?
2. Why is it vital to monitor vaccine safety when mass vaccinations are required?
3. How many diseases and deaths are prevented by vaccines?

CHILD DEVELOPMENT AND SCREENING

Vaccines have the potential to not only prevent specific diseases during childhood but can strengthen a child's overall future health. There is a proven link between vaccination and improved cognitive functions, education, and productivity during adulthood. Vaccination may help enhance a child's ability to learn, think, and develop due to educational success, cognitive reasoning, and thinking skills. Vaccinated children miss fewer school days. For example, children vaccinated against the flu miss 1.5 fewer days of school per 100 school days compared to those who do not receive the flu vaccine.

Before the pneumococcal conjugate vaccine era in the United States, pneumococcus was the most common cause of severe and recurring ear infections in children. Multiple ear infections in early childhood increase the risks of hearing loss. Plus, speech and language develop during the same period. These factors may explain why children with recurrent ear infections during early childhood have lower cognitive, speech, language development, and overall intelligence than children with fewer ear infections. Another example concerns severe brain and brain-related infections such as meningitis or encephalitis. These life-threatening infections are highly associated with impaired thinking and learning after illness, which may be lifelong. About half of those who develop and survive encephalitis have permanent cognitive, psychological, or neurological disabilities.

Some vaccines are linked to gains in cognitive and learning tests in later childhood. For example, children vaccinated against measles scored better on **cognitive tests** of language development, math, and reading than those not vaccinated. Healthy, vaccinated children are more likely to attend school, perform better while there, and attend for longer than children who are often sick or suffering permanent illness-related disabilities.

Screening for children concerning vaccinations takes into account a variety of factors, which include the following:

- Is the child currently sick?
- Does the child have allergies (medications, foods, vaccine components, or latex)?
- Has the child had a severe reaction to a vaccine previously?
- Does the child have a long-term condition (lung disease, heart disease, kidney disease, **metabolic diseases** such as diabetes mellitus, asthma, a blood disorder, lack of a spleen, complement component deficiency, a cochlear implant, or a spinal fluid leak), and is the child on long-term aspirin therapy?
- If the child is 2–4 years of age, has a healthcare provider told the parent or caregiver that the child had wheezing or asthma in the past 12 months?
- If the child is an infant, has the parent or caregiver been told the infant has had intussusception?
- Has the child, a sibling, or a parent had seizures? Has the child had brain or other nervous system problems?

- Does the child have cancer, leukemia, HIV/AIDS, or other immune system problems?
- Does the child have a parent, brother, or sister with an immune system problem?
- Over the past 3 months, has the child taken medications that affect the immune system (prednisone or other steroids, or anticancer drugs), drugs to treat rheumatoid arthritis, Crohn disease, or psoriasis, or had radiation treatments?
- Over the past year, has the child received a transfusion of blood or blood products or received immune globulin or an antiviral drug?
- Is the teen pregnant, or is there a chance of pregnancy during the next month?
- Has the child received any vaccinations over the past 4 weeks?

TEST YOUR KNOWLEDGE

1. How can childhood vaccines continue to have effects into adulthood?
2. How can recurrent ear infections in children affect later life?
3. How are childhood vaccines linked to better cognitive and learning tests?

ELIMINATION AND CONTROL OF INFECTIOUS DISEASES

Elimination of an infectious disease refers to the deliberate effort that leads to the reduction to zero of the incidence of infection caused by a specific pathogen in a defined geographic area. A disease can be eliminated from a particular region without being eradicated globally. Malaria is an excellent example of a condition that can be controlled locally. People cannot eliminate it because the **mosquito-borne parasites** that transmit the disease can develop drug resistance. But you can handle it through healthcare and prevention strategies such as aggressive mosquito control, bed nets, and antimalaria medications. Often the first step toward disease elimination is disease control.

Significant progress has also been made to eliminate polio, which is now endemic in only Afghanistan and Pakistan. With highly contagious diseases such as polio, as long as the infection exists anywhere, its ability to spread means it remains a global threat. The poliovirus can easily be imported into a polio-free country and spread rapidly among unimmunized populations, making the polio vaccine crucial, especially for children.

Another example of a disease on the path to elimination and potentially eradication is pediatric HIV. During the past year, several countries, including Thailand, Cuba, and a few others, have received official validation from the WHO that they have eliminated mother-to-child transmission of HIV—a pivotal step to ending the entire AIDS epidemic.

ERADICATION OF INFECTIOUS DISEASES

Global infectious disease eradication can be achieved for pathogens restricted to human reservoirs. To eradicate infectious diseases, high levels of population immunity are required globally to ensure no ongoing transmission in our well-connected world. Furthermore, **surveillance systems** must be in place to monitor the decline in disease, with accurate and reliable diagnostic testing to monitor ongoing cases. The only infectious disease eradicated in humans by vaccination is smallpox, which was announced by the World Health Assembly in 1980, a historic public health achievement. The second example of eradication was the rinderpest virus in livestock. This infection indirectly led to human loss of life through loss of agriculture and humanitarian crises through famine and poverty. Rinderpest virus infects cattle, buffalo, and numerous other domestic species, with widespread disease affecting parts of Africa and Europe in the 19th century. The Plowright tissue culture rinderpest vaccine, developed during the 1950s, was used for mass vaccination campaigns alongside other public health measures, leading to eradication in 2011.

The subsequent infection targeted for eradication is wild poliovirus. This devastating paralytic disease routinely afflicted children and adults in both industrialized and developing settings before the development of vaccines. Both vaccines have been used globally, with oral poliovirus vaccines being much cheaper and easier to administer. In 1998, the Global Polio Eradication Initiative, the most significant public-private partnership led by national governments in collaboration with the WHO, Rotary International, US CDC, and UNICEF, was launched with the aim of global polio eradication by 2000. Although this target still needs to be met due to a lack of funding, political will, and competing health initiatives, there was a 99% reduction in polio incidence by 2000.

By 2003, there were only six endemic countries with new cases: Egypt, Niger, India, Nigeria, Afghanistan, and Pakistan, of which only the latter four had new issues by 2005. Eradication in India was problematic due to the high birth rates and poor sanitation among densely populated regions with marginalized communities and increased population mobility. India was declared polio free in 2014. Wild poliovirus type 2 was eradicated in 2015, the last case of wild type 3 was in 2012, and eradication was announced in 2019, with uncontrolled type 1 virus remaining in two countries, Pakistan and Afghanistan. In 2019, Nigeria was declared 3 years free of wild polio, the last African country to see any cases. In the first 6 months of 2020, 51 and 17 wild type 1 polio cases were reported in Pakistan and Afghanistan, respectively. Ongoing programs to roll out universal vaccination in both countries still need to be improved because of armed conflict, political instability, remote communities, and underdeveloped infrastructure.

You Should Remember

It is important to remember that some infectious diseases, especially those that infect animals, such as swine influenza or rabies, may never be entirely eradicated. With the proper education and interventions in place, healthcare professionals can help to ensure that people, especially those living in areas with limited resources, will soon see the end of some of the most severe public health threats the world has ever known.

TEST YOUR KNOWLEDGE

1. How is malaria controlled?
2. What is required for the eradication of infectious disease?
3. Why was the eradication of polio in India problematic?

KEY TERMS

Bovine colostrum
Cognitive tests
Community immunity
Encephalitis
Endogenous
Exogenous
Immunosenescence
Infrastructure
Jamestown Canyon virus
Kidney failure
La Crosse encephalitis
Lyme disease
Malnutrition
Metabolic diseases
Micronutrients
Mosquito-borne parasites
Polyurethane condom
Probiotics
Surveillance systems
Vaccine Safety Datalink

FURTHER READING

1. Adelman, Z.N., 2015. Genetic Control of Malaria and Dengue. Academic Press.
2. Bricker, D., Macy, M., Squires, J., Marks, K., 2013. Developmental Screening in Your Community: An Integrated Approach for Connecting Children with Services. Brookes Publishing.
3. Cochi, S.L., Dowdle, W.R., 2011. Disease Eradication in the 21st Century: Implications for Global Health, Volume 7. The MIT Press.
4. Cowan, T., Fallon Morell, S., 2018. Vaccines, Autoimmunity, and the Changing Nature of Childhood Illness. Chelsea Green Publishing.
5. Gabrielsen, E., 2013. Emergency Preparedness: A Practical Guide for Preparing Your Family, 2nd Edition. Cedar Fort, Inc.
6. Katz, R., Banaski, J., 2018. Essentials of Public Health Preparedness and Emergency Management (Essential Public Health), 2nd Edition. Jones & Bartlett Learning.
7. Leys Stepan, N., 2012. Eradication: Ridding the World of Diseases Forever?. Reaktion Books.
8. Life Extension, 2013. Disease Prevention & Treatment, 5th Edition. Life Extension.
9. Lin, B., Ratna, B., 2021. Virus Hybrids as Nanomaterials: Methods and Protocols. Humana Press.
10. Loomis, J., 2020. Epidemics: The Impact of Germs and Their Power over Humanity. Turner.
11. Miller, N.Z., 2016. Miller's Review of Critical Vaccine Studies: 400 Important Scientific Papers Summarized for Parents and Researchers. New Atlantean Press.
12. Munyua, A., 2023. Immunizations and Vaccines. Munyua.
13. Sears, R.W., 2011. The Vaccine Book: Making the Right Decision for Your Child (Parenting Library). Little Brown Spark.
14. Shank Coviello, J., 2019. Health Promotion and Disease Prevention in Clinical Practice, 3rd Edition. Wolters Kluwer.
15. Wallace, J., Hunt Wallace, C.L., 2016. Physianthropy. Palala Press.

Chapter 7

Vaccine Safety and Errors

Chapter Outline

Learning Objectives

After study of this chapter, readers should be able to:

1. Describe the concept of vaccination errors.
2. Explain the reasons that patient identification errors occur.
3. Discuss the medication administration record.
4. Describe the items included in the vaccine documentation.
5. Explain the information about vaccines given to you in the Pink Book.
6. Identify the refrigerated and frozen vaccines.
7. Describe the three main categories of adverse reactions.
8. Explain the six items that must be documented for each vaccination in a patient's medical chart.
9. Describe vaccine expiration and its negative effects.
10. Discuss a vaccination screening questionnaire.

Vaccinology and Immunizations. http://doi.org/10.1016/B978-0-443-23915-1.00007-X

OVERVIEW

Vaccination is an excellent way to prevent disease and is estimated to save 2 to 3 million lives annually globally. The most commonly used vaccines have been used for decades, and millions have received them safely every year. New vaccines are under development that will help prevent more life-threatening diseases or improve the effectiveness of existing vaccines. However, safety issues must still be considered so that vaccines are continually monitored concerning their safe use. Vaccine safety monitoring utilizes many local, regional, national, and international resources. Organizations such as the Centers for Disease Control and Prevention, Food and Drug Administration, and World Health Organization are concerned with vaccine safety and preventing errors. Vaccine errors still occur and are linked to causes such as insufficient staff training, distractions, changes in recommendations, lack of standardized protocols, patient misidentification, use of nonstandard or error-prone abbreviations, and easily misidentified products. However, with constant monitoring of errors and the establishment of better protocols to prevent them, the safety of vaccine delivery is continually improving.

VACCINATION ERRORS

A vaccine administration error is any preventable event that may cause or lead to inappropriate vaccine use or patient harm. Like other medical practices, errors related to vaccine administration also can occur. Vaccination practices and the programmatic factors that influence them are essential for public health. Several barriers impact vaccination efforts, including vaccination errors, which pose the risk of reduced population-wide vaccination efficacy and individual adverse drug events. Pooled vaccination error prevalence was calculated to be 1.15 per 10,000 vaccine doses. The most commonly reported vaccination errors were "wrong vaccine administered" and "off-schedule administration." Unfortunately, vaccine administration errors occur too frequently in medical practices. Most of the time, these errors go unreported or, even worse, may not be recognized. Inadequate training in vaccine administration is a core problem for many medical practices.

Patient safety is always the most crucial consideration. Vaccination errors usually do not cause direct harm to patients, but subtherapeutic doses, incorrect vaccines, or expired vaccines can make patients more susceptible to disease. Learning and understanding vaccination errors that have previously been reported is essential. The **Institute for Safe Medication Practices (ISMP)** published a 2017 analysis of vaccine errors and identified the most commonly reported errors as wrong vaccine, wrong dose, wrong age, and administration of expired, contaminated, or deteriorated vaccines.

Immunization is one of the most outstanding public health achievements, but its continued success relies on the quality of the process, including how vaccines are stored, prescribed, dispensed, and administered. Many of the underlying causes of vaccine-related errors are ongoing issues. For example, healthcare providers who plan to stock and administer COVID-19 vaccines should anticipate the types of mistakes that can and do happen and take the necessary steps to prepare and mitigate the risk of COVID-19 vaccine errors.

A recent analysis of more than 160 COVID-19-related event reports submitted to the ISMP and National Vaccine Errors Reporting Program (VERP) from December 2020 through April 2021 emphasizes that more needs to be done to reduce the risk of vaccination errors because they can lead to inadequate immunity, increased cost, and reduced confidence in the healthcare delivery system. These brief descriptions of commonly reported COVID-19 vaccine errors are meant to help healthcare providers anticipate risk during the most considerable vaccination effort in US history.

Healthcare professionals must, every time that they give an immunization, write down the **lot number** of the vaccine and the **expiration date** of the vaccine. An expired vaccine cannot cause harm but will not work. Live viruses, such as measles or chickenpox, cease to work and do not become dangerous.

You Should Remember

Given the reliance on spontaneous reporting, it is impossible to determine the frequency of vaccination errors from current error reporting programs. However, estimates from systematic reviews of vaccination records indicate that errors occur in 27% to 35% of all vaccinations.

TEST YOUR KNOWLEDGE

1. What are the most commonly reported vaccination errors?
2. Which vaccination errors can make patients more susceptible to disease?
3. What must be written down by healthcare professionals when immunization is given?

Wrong Patient Identification Error

Patient identification errors happen for many reasons, including physical proximity within a healthcare facility. These errors can cause significant harm or distress to patients or families. Imagine getting a call that a loved one who has been hospitalized has died or finding out shortly after that a mistake was made due to a similar name and that the loved one is still alive.

"Wrong patient" errors can occur at any point in patient encounters or during any phase of the medication use process. During prescribing, wrong patient errors can result in order entry mix-ups or reliance upon incorrect patient data. During transcription, telephone orders can be mistranscribed, and patient labels can be mixed up. During dispensing, there can be data entry errors or coupled drug delivery in which one patient receives another patient's drug because both medications may be transported within the same chemotherapy bag. During administration, there must always be reliance on the correct name and date of birth to prevent errors.

The Joint Commission National Patient Safety Goal requires healthcare practitioners to use patient identifiers three times to reliably identify the individual as the person for whom the service or treatment is intended and to match the service or treatment to that patient. Patient verification using two identifiers must be accomplished whenever any of the following occurs:

- Physicians prescribe medications.
- Pharmacists or technicians enter or verify orders and dispense medications.
- Unit secretaries, nurses, or other authorized staff members transcribe medication orders.
- Nurses or other qualified providers administer medications.
- Healthcare workers set up, obtain, receive, give, document, or file diagnostic test results (which are often required for medication prescribing).
- Healthcare practitioners participate in any other critical processes.

The **medication administration record (MAR)** or electronic MAR (eMAR) should be at the patient's bedside to verify two unique identifiers. Anyone ordering medications via a pharmacy computer must select the patient profile using the patient's medical record number and never a hospital room number or by scanning the barcode on the patient's label on an order set and then confirming the name and number on the screen with the orders. Unit secretaries and nurses must compare patient information on the order form and MAR when transcribing. Computerized prescriber order entry systems can be designed so logged-on physicians can select the name from a list of assigned patients.

You Should Remember

MAR reports detail the drugs administered to a patient by a healthcare professional at a treatment facility. They are also known as drug charts. The electronic versions are sometimes referred to as eMARs. They aim to accurately record medication usage to reduce dosing errors and potentially harmful interactions. The MAR is filled out every time a patient receives a dose of medication and is a component of the medical chart.

Wrong Time

Vaccinations must be given within the correct time frame, yet parents have many reasons for delaying them. These include children who cry every time they get a shot or parents feeling that a child is too young to get "so many" vaccines. However, a child's immune system is more vulnerable without vaccinations being given at the correct time. They can become seriously ill or die from measles, mumps, or whooping cough. Parents should be advised that while a child being upset at having to receive a vaccination is a temporary situation, the potential long-term consequences of contracting a disease without vaccination are much more severe.

Recommended immunization schedules are safe and effective for protecting patients based on how the immune system responds at various ages and how likely exposure is. Following the recommended programs during childhood ensures that young patients are protected from 14 potentially severe diseases at precisely the right time. No data support that spacing out vaccines offers safe or adequate protection from these diseases. Delaying vaccines could leave a child vulnerable to infection when they are most likely to have serious complications. Vaccinating before a child is exposed to dangerous conditions is always best. If a parent waits until a child is exposed, such as when starting daycare or during a disease outbreak, there may be insufficient time for a vaccine to work. The experts who create immunization schedules pay meticulous attention to the correct time to receive each vaccine.

Some parents wonder if the number of vaccines and doses their children receive can be too much for their young bodies to handle. The answer is *no*. Extensive research has been done to ensure the safety of vaccines for children. Children are exposed to microorganisms every day. The amount they are exposed to by getting a vaccine (150 for the entire schedule) is a tiny fraction of the antigens they encounter daily (2000–6000).

TEST YOUR KNOWLEDGE

1. When can wrong patient identification errors occur?
2. What is a MAR?
3. What do the recommended immunization schedules ensure for children?

Wrong Vaccine

Confusion often occurs due to a misunderstanding of vaccine names, abbreviations, and components of combination products. For example, Tdap is mistaken for DTaP, and MMRV is mistaken for MMR. Pneumococcal vaccine errors have occurred from administering the incorrect PPSV23 product when PCV13 was intended. Protein conjugates have also been confused. They are used to produce vaccines to improve immune system responses to antigens. Conjugates are used along with polysaccharide antigens, including those of *Haemophilus* b, meningococcal, and pneumococcal vaccines. For example, the *Haemophilus* b vaccine label reads "Haemophilus b Conjugate Vaccine (Tetanus Toxoid Conjugate)." The vaccine protects against *Haemophilus influenzae* type b (Hib), and the formulation uses the tetanus toxoid conjugate to assist the immune system in providing a solid response to the antigen. Vaccination with this product does not protect against tetanus. Another Hib vaccine label reads "Haemophilus b Conjugate Vaccine (Meningococcal Protein Conjugate)." It only protects against Hib, using a meningococcal protein to assist the immune system in responding better to the Hib antigen. It does not protect against meningococcal disease. Both vaccines have been administered in error to protect against Hib and tetanus, or Hib and meningococcal disease.

Vaccine administration errors can have many consequences, including inadequate immunological protection, possible injury to the patient, cost, inconvenience, and reduced confidence in the healthcare delivery system.

You Should Remember

Vaccine safety starts with how the products are stored and labeled. Different vaccines must be kept in other storage areas if they look similar. Overall, vaccine mix-ups are rare. Should a patient receive the wrong vaccine, clear communication between the patient and provider must be made about what happened. This must occur immediately, and steps must be taken to seek needed care and receive the correct vaccine appropriately.

Wrong Dose and Age

Several vaccine types have different formulations available with various indications of age. For example, there are about four different manufacturers that make influenza vaccines. Certain products are indicated only for patients 65 and older and are designed with higher doses for that age group. Other influenza vaccine products are only meant for children 5 years or older. Furthermore, certain influenza products are indicated for persons 6 months of age and older. Errors in which a provider administers the incorrect product for the age group have been reported. Hepatitis B, meningococcal, tetanus-diphtheria-pertussis, and many combination vaccines indicate specific age groups. Close attention should be given to the stated age group for all vaccines.

Wrong Route, Needle Length, and Technique

Using the wrong route for a vaccine can result in various outcomes. To avoid this error, reference materials should be posted in the vaccine preparation area that shows the site and route for each vaccine for each age group. The route information should be highlighted or marked on the vaccine package. Care must be taken for deltoid muscle injections to avoid injections too high on the upper arm and to avoid injury to the shoulder. The gluteus muscle should not be used for hepatitis B, rabies, or HPV vaccines. Suppose a vaccine is given by the wrong route, such as subcutaneously instead of intramuscularly (IM) (or vice versa).

In that case, the vaccine does not need to be repeated except for these four exceptions: hepatitis B, rabies, HPV, and the inactivated influenza vaccine.

For the COVID-19 vaccines, the preferred site is the deltoid muscle, while the alternate location is the vastus lateralis muscle. If another site is used, the dose should not be repeated. The recipient must be informed of the potential for local and systemic adverse events. This is also true if the vaccine is given subcutaneously.

Vaccines must reach the desired tissue to provide the best immune response and reduce the likelihood of injection site reactions. Needle selection is based on the route, age, injection site, and, for adults, gender and weight. Table 7.1 summarizes recommended needle gauges and lengths. Clinical judgment should be used when selecting needles to administer injectable vaccines.

The wrong vaccination technique could be a reason behind clotting following inoculation by certain vaccines, such as the adenovirus-based COVID-19 vaccines. The incorrect approach could lead to the injection accidentally being given into a blood vessel instead of a muscle. It could be a potential mechanism for postvaccination thrombocytopenic syndrome, also known as vaccine-induced immune thrombotic **thrombocytopenia**.

The vaccine can reach into the bloodstream if the needle tip does not get the muscle or hits a blood vessel. This can occur if an inadequately trained provider pinches the skin up. If the skin is pinched, an IM injection needle's tip only reaches the subcutaneous tissue. The vaccine is then not absorbed correctly. In rare cases, it can hit one of the blood vessels in the layer between the skin and muscle, which contains a network of blood vessels. The correct method for IM injection is not to pinch the skin up. Instead, gently stretch the skin before

TABLE 7.1 Recommended vaccine needle gauges and lengths.

Route	Age	Gauge and length	Injection site
Subcutaneous injection	All ages	23 to 25 gauge 5/8 inch (16 mm)	Vastus lateralis muscle (for infants younger than 12 months of age, may be administered into the upper outer triceps area if necessary); upper outer triceps area (for those 12 months of age and older)

(Continued)

TABLE 7.1 Recommended vaccine needle gauges and lengths—cont'd

Route	Age	Gauge and length	Injection site
Intramuscular injection	Neonates, 28 days, and infants	22 to 25 gauge 5/8 inch (16 mm; if the skin is stretched tightly and subcutaneous tissues are not bunched)	Vastus lateralis muscle
	Infants, 1 to 12 months	22 to 25 gauge 1 inch (25 mm)	Vastus lateralis muscle
	Toddlers, 1 to 2 years	22 to 25 gauge 1.25 inches (25 to 32 mm)	Vastus lateralis muscle (preferred site)
		22 to 25 gauge 5/8 (if the skin is stretched tightly and subcutaneous tissues are not bunched) to 1 inch (16 to 25 mm)	Deltoid muscle of arm
	Children, 3 to 10 years	22 to 25 gauge 5/8 (if the skin is stretched tightly and subcutaneous tissues are not bunched) to 1 inch (16 to 25 mm)	Deltoid muscle of arm (preferred site)
		22 to 25 gauge 1 to 1.25 inches (25 to 32 mm)	Vastus lateralis muscle
	Children, 11 to 18 years	22 to 25 gauge 5/8 (if the skin is stretched tightly and subcutaneous tissues are not bunched) to 1 inch (16 to 25 mm)	Deltoid muscle of arm (preferred site), but the vastus lateralis muscle can also be used.
	Adults 19 years and older – 130 lbs (60 kg) or less – 130 to 152 lbs (60 to 70 kg) – Males 152 to 260 lbs (70 to 118 kg) – Females 152 to 200 lbs (70 to 90 kg) – Males 260 lbs (118 kg) or more – Females 200 lbs (90 kg) or more	22 to 25 gauge 1 inch (25 mm, though some experts recommend a 5/8-inch need for those weighing less than 60 kg; if used, skin must be stretched tightly, and subcutaneous tissues must not be bunched) 1 inch (25 mm) 1 to 1.5 inches (25 to 38 mm) 1 to 1.5 inches (25 to 38 mm) 1.5 inches (38 mm) 1.5 inches (38 mm)	Deltoid muscle of arm

plunging the needle at 90 degrees. The syringe must be aspirated gently to check for blood before injecting the vaccine. This ensures that a blood vessel has not been hit.

TEST YOUR KNOWLEDGE

1. Which vaccines are commonly confused with each other?
2. For deltoid muscle injections, what care must be taken?
3. What wrong vaccination technique causes adverse effects with the adenovirus COVID-19 vaccine?

Wrong Documentation

It is always best to follow federal law and thoroughly document each immunization. The items to be included are the vaccine manufacturer; lot number; date of administration; name, office, address, and title of the provider administering the vaccine; the date printed on the vaccine immunization schedule; and the date the vaccine immunization schedule was given to the patient, parent, or guardian. An immunization record should also be provided to them. Never forget to submit vaccine information to the appropriate state or local immunization information system.

When reporting **adverse events** after immunization, information about which vaccine was given, how it was administered, and if it was issued within the expiration date is often incomplete. To improve immunization practice, a standardized uniform procedure is required.

THE PINK BOOK IN PHARMACY

The **Pink Book** is an excellent source of information about vaccine administration, individual vaccines, and the diseases they prevent. It provides physicians, nurse practitioners, physician assistants, pharmacists, nurses, and other healthcare professionals comprehensive information on routinely used vaccines and the diseases they prevent. The 14th edition of the Pink Book includes:

- General immunization recommendations
- Vaccine safety, storage and handling, and administration information
- Detailed information about vaccine-preventable diseases, including disease **pathogenesis**, clinical features, epidemiology, and secular trends in the United States
- Detailed information about vaccines, including vaccine characteristics, schedule and use, efficacy, safety, and contraindications and precautions

Four appendices provide reference materials, including vaccine minimum age and intervals, vaccine excipients, catch-up schedules, and more.

PREVENTING VACCINATION ERRORS

Education about **immunization protocols**, vaccine preparation, and administration is essential to prevent vaccination errors. Following standard protocols helps identify issues concerning patient evaluation before a mistake can be made. Because there are so many formulations and names of vaccines, it is essential to use the standard abbreviation of the vaccine and brand name on eMARs, dispensing system screens, and pharmacy labels. Labeling on vaccine storage bins should also indicate standard abbreviations and brand names. Conjugate vaccine labeling should emphasize the active vaccine and not the conjugate component.

TEST YOUR KNOWLEDGE

1. What items should be included when documenting a vaccination?
2. What is the Pink Book?
3. What types of abbreviations must be used concerning vaccines?

REPORTING VACCINATION ERRORS

The frequency of errors reported to the Vaccine Errors Reporting Program is reflected in the following percentages:

- Wrong age: 24%
- Wrong vaccine: 24%
- Extra dose: 10%
- Too large a quantity: 10%
- Expired vaccine: 8%
- Wrong interval: 7%
- Component omission: 5%

VACCINE STORAGE

Many vaccines have particular storage requirements that, if not met, can reduce their **potency** significantly, rendering them completely ineffective. Vaccines must be stored correctly from the moment they are manufactured until they are ultimately administered, and this is the shared responsibility of the manufacturer, distributor, and healthcare provider. Most vaccines should be stored between 2°C and 8°C in a refrigerator, with a preferred average of 5°C, though some should remain frozen between −15°C and −50°C. Storage and transportation of freeze-sensitive vaccines (such as DTP, tetanus toxoid, hepatitis B, and Hib vaccines) require careful temperature control, where the risk of reaching a freezing temperature is higher than exposure to excessive heat.

Additionally, many vaccines should be protected from light and packaged appropriately, as UV light can damage them. Human papillomavirus, Hib, inactivated polio, Japanese encephalitis, meningococcal, MMR, MMRV, rabies, rotavirus, varicella, and herpes zoster are sensitive to light, causing loss of potency.

Many live virus vaccines can tolerate freezing temperatures and rapidly deteriorate once defrosted, while activated vaccines more commonly require temperatures of 2°C to 8°C and are damaged at temperature extremes. The typically administered MMR vaccine can be stored frozen or refrigerated, while the MMRV vaccine, which also contains the live varicella virus, must be frozen. Other vaccines that must be frozen include chickenpox and shingles. All Pfizer-BioNTech COVID-19 vaccine products can be stored at ultracold frozen temperatures until expiration. Use storage labels to help staff quickly identify the correct product based on the recipient's age and refrigerate it for up to 10 weeks.

In some cases, manufacturers may recommend storing the concentrated form as provided at one temperature and the prepared diluted form, if any such steps are necessary, at another, though generally, the latter should be prepared at most 30 minutes in advance. In cases where a frozen vaccine must be prepared, most manufacturers recommend slowly defrosting in a refrigerator. For example, all vaccines that contain varicella, the live virus chickenpox vaccine, should be stored frozen but can be defrosted in a refrigerator for 72 hours before use.

Several studies have highlighted key issues in vaccine storage, with the most common errors including the storage of vaccines past their expiration date, deep freezers being too warm (−14°C or higher), and refrigerators being too warm (over 8°C). Major risk factors have been identified, such as lacking a thermometer in freezers, and less commonly in refrigerators, or using a combination refrigerator/freezer, as the freezer compartment inside such devices keeps poor temperature **homeostasis**. Additionally, the chambers frequently affect one another's temperature, particularly in smaller appliances, where setting the freezer compartment to the desired −14°C lowers the fridge to below 2°C, damaging the refrigerated vaccines.

All refrigerators and freezers should be free-standing and dedicated to the purpose. Most consumer appliances do not offer the stability in temperature required to store vaccines, both in terms of hourly fluctuations and across seasons. The cooling coil accessible on the interior of many refrigerators also poses a potential hazard, and units with exposed rings are banned from storing vaccines in many countries. Similarly, refrigerator walls, cooling vents, doors, floors, and ceilings are more prone to temperature fluctuations than the unit's center, where vaccines should be stored in complete packaging.

Each unit should also possess an independent thermometer calibrated regularly, preferably with an external temperature display that can be viewed without opening the door. As a best practice, most storage locations will likely utilize an automatic temperature logger to review historical temperatures. However, this may be done manually where a digital option is unavailable.

Surge protectors and other electronic safety equipment should be utilized to lower the risk of power interruption or loss of power to the storage unit, and all inventory should be carefully logged, taking special note of the expiration date. As a practical point, the CDC additionally recommends not storing "sound-alike" or "look-alike" vaccines in the exact location to avoid the incorrect vaccine being selected. If a refrigerator must also keep other biologics, the vaccines should be placed on the highest shelf to avoid contamination, and food or drink should never be stored in the same unit.

You Should Remember

Proper vaccine storage and handling play a vital role in protecting the public from vaccine-preventable diseases. Vaccine quality is the responsibility of everyone involved, from the time the vaccine is manufactured until it is administered to a patient.

TEST YOUR KNOWLEDGE

1. What are the top three most commonly reported vaccination errors?
2. At what temperatures should most vaccines be stored?
3. Which refrigerator parts are more prone to temperature fluctuations than the unit's center?

PREPARATION FOR VACCINATION

Patients must be assessed for vaccine contraindications and precautions before administering a vaccine. A screening questionnaire is used and should be filled out by each patient or guardian before the vaccine is given. These questionnaires ask about past and current illnesses or health conditions that could be a reason not to provide the vaccine. There are also questions about allergies, the use of medications or blood products that could interfere with the effects of the vaccine, and past reactions to vaccines. The answers to all questions must be evaluated before the vaccine is administered.

PREPARING FOR ADVERSE REACTIONS

Adverse reactions can occur after administration of a vaccine. These reactions have three main categories: local, systemic, and allergic. Local reactions, including pain, swelling, and redness at the injection site, are widespread. They are often mild and occur within hours of the injection. Systemic reactions include fever, headache, a general feeling of discomfort or unease, and muscle pains. These symptoms are usually mild and can occur 3 to 21 days after vaccination. Allergic reactions can occur because of the vaccine or one of its **ingredients**. Although rare, allergic reactions can be severe. Anaphylaxis is a life-threatening allergic reaction that sometimes happens.

Psychological reactions rarely occur. Patients receiving a vaccine may fear the injection and respond with paleness, sweating, nausea, dizziness, lightheadedness, weakness, visual disturbances, and fainting. Therefore, following the facility's protocol, the patient must be seated or lying down during vaccination and monitored after immunization.

Each facility should have an immunization protocol that describes the management of vaccine reactions. For anaphylactic reactions, autoinjectors or vials of epinephrine should be available. Other medications that are used include diphenhydramine and hydroxyzine.

DOCUMENTATION AND REPORTING

According to the National Childhood Vaccine Injury Act (NCVIA), six items must be documented for each vaccination in a patient's medical chart. These include the date of administration, name and title of the vaccinator, lot number, manufacturer, address of the facility where the permanent record resides, and the vaccine immunization schedule. Both the date of the program and the date it was given to the patient or guardian must be documented. Additional documentation, sometimes but not always required, includes the vaccine type, route, dose volume, site, and whether any vaccine was refused.

Once a vaccine is given, it must be reported to the patient's primary care provider and the state immunization information systems (IIS) if applicable. Any adverse events following the vaccine should be documented and reported to the primary care provider. Documentation of vaccination should also be provided to the patient or guardian. The IIS is an immunization registry, a database containing vaccination information for each individual in a state or other region. Vaccination information from multiple providers can be entered into this central database, allowing providers to check immunization status or the date of the last vaccination in a series. Pharmacies that immunize people can participate in the IIS, following state instructions.

All adverse events after a vaccine should be reported using the Vaccine Adverse Event Reporting System (VAERS). New or more frequent adverse events may be noticed as vaccines are used more often or when a new vaccine is released to the general population. The CDC and FDA monitor VAERS and work to identify new side effects or side effect patterns related to vaccines. Cause and effect studies are then performed to determine if the vaccine caused the adverse events. If so, changes may be implemented, including updating the manufacturer's package insert and the vaccine information sheet. Also, new recommendations may be made concerning the risk of side effects and the vaccine's benefit in preventing disease. Adverse events can be reported by anyone using the VAERS website. Reporting helps identify possible problems with vaccines and is essential for public safety. Reporting adverse events through institutional adverse event programs and to the patient's primary care physician is also important.

TEST YOUR KNOWLEDGE

1. What does a vaccination screening questionnaire ask about?
2. What are the three main categories of adverse reactions after a vaccine?
3. Once a vaccine is given, to whom must it be reported?

Expired or Impure Products

Suppose an expired vaccine is inadvertently administered. In that case, it is considered a vaccine administration error. It requires remediation, including a VAERS report and contacting the recipient to inform them of the error. It may or may not require revaccination based on the manufacturer's guidance. Please promptly report any expired vaccine that has been administered. This helps the CDC and DPH accurately monitor the amount of vaccine in the field. Remember that reporting waste has no negative consequences and will not negatively impact future vaccine shipments. The CDC recognizes that unused, expired vaccine is a normal part of any vaccination program.

It is essential to pay attention to expiration dates on vaccines. Certain ingredients can stop working after expiry, which could render a vaccine less effective. Using an expired vaccine could cause harmful reactions, but not many documented cases exist. There are no existing data that taking a inactivated COVID-19 vaccine is dangerous.

Most vaccines have an expiration date of about 2 to 3 years. Vaccines can also expire if they are not kept at the correct temperature. Several COVID-19 vaccines have specific storage requirements that include refrigerators and freezers.

Suppose a dose of an expired vaccine is given to a patient. The amount of a nonexpired identical vaccine should be repeated. If the expired quantity was a live virus vaccine, you should wait at least 4 weeks after the expired dose was given before repeating it with an unexpired live virus vaccine.

Vaccines should be inspected for expiration before they are administered or transported to other facilities. Facility vaccine coordinators need to be aware of the standard expiration date of June 30 for IIV and make plans for the safe disposal or return of any remaining doses of IIV after that date. Sometimes unused vaccines may be returned for credit, even if the amounts must be discarded. State immunization programs or vaccine manufacturers should be contacted to determine whether such provisions apply. Any person who receives an expired influenza vaccine should be revaccinated with the current season's influenza vaccine.

You Should Remember

If an expired vaccine is accidentally administered, it is considered a vaccine administration error. There must be remediation that includes a VAERS report, contacting the patient to inform them about the error, and, in some cases, revaccination based on the manufacturer's guidance.

Vaccine Administration

It is essential to document and record vaccine administration correctly. It should be noted if any of the following occur during vaccine administration:

- A vaccine is administered after it has expired.
- Vaccines were not given within the prescribed periods following reconstitution.
- Vaccines were drawn into syringes a long time before administration (they should be drawn into the syringe immediately before administration).
- Vaccines were mixed in the same syringe and were not the types of vaccines approved by the FDA for this technique.

Adverse Effects

An undesired drug or vaccine effect can range from mild to severe and can be life-threatening. Most **side effects** from vaccination are mild, such as pain, swelling, or redness at the injection site. The other adverse effects include chills, mild fever, headache, muscle pain, and tiredness. Serious side effects are rare but may cause seizures or life-threatening allergic reactions. A possible side effect of vaccination is known as an adverse event.

TEST YOUR KNOWLEDGE

1. How long does it take most vaccines to expire?
2. What improper occurrences must be documented if they happened during vaccine administration?
3. How serious are most side effects from vaccinations?

KEY TERMS

Adverse events
Adverse reactions
Expiration date
Homeostasis
Ingredients
Immunization protocols
Institute for Safe Medication Practices
Lot number
Medication administration record
Pathogenesis
Potency
Side effects
Thrombocytopenia

CASE STUDIES

Case Study 1

A 3-year-old girl was brought by her mother to receive her first chickenpox vaccination. Before the procedure, the nurse removes the vial from the refrigerator and draws up the vaccine in an area that the little girl cannot see so as not to frighten her. The vaccine is given without any problem. Later in the day, as the physician writes up his notes, he finds that he mistakenly gave the girl an MMR vaccine instead of varicella. Both vials were kept close together in the refrigerator, were made by the same manufacturer, and had similar packaging. The nurse calls the girl's mother to apologize and reassure her that there should be no harm or adverse effects due to the mix-up. A study is carried out to determine what went wrong and future measures to ensure it never happens again. In a few weeks, the girl receives her chickenpox vaccine.

Critical Thinking Questions

1. How prevalent are vaccine errors, and which errors are most common?
2. Are these errors regularly reported?
3. Do vaccination errors usually cause direct harm to patients?

Case Study 2

An 11-year-old boy who lived in India needed his hepatitis B vaccination, which had somehow been missed. The boy's father gave consent for his son to receive the vaccine. It was soon discovered that due to a labeling error, the boy had been given the hepatitis A vaccine instead of hepatitis B. The supervising physician quickly explained the mistake to the boy's father and that the incorrectly given vaccine would not cause any harm and could even protect the boy against hepatitis A in the future. The father became furious, reported the incident to the clinic administrator, and refused to let his son receive the hepatitis B vaccine.

Critical Thinking Questions

1. What are the most commonly reported vaccine errors?
2. What must healthcare professionals do every time they give an immunization?
3. What are the possible consequences of vaccine administration errors?

FURTHER READING

1. Agency for Healthcare Research and Quality, U.S. Department of Health and Human Services, 2015. Safety of Vaccines Used for Routine Immunization in the United States. CreateSpace Independent Publishing Platform.
2. Caulfield, T., 2017. The Vaccination Picture. Viking.
3. Committee on the Review of the National Immunization Program's Research Procedures and Data Sharing Program, 2013. Vaccine Safety Research, Data Access, and Public Trust. National Academy of Sciences.
4. Congressional Research Service, Sekar, K., Dabrowska, A., 2020. Vaccine Safety in the United States: Overview and Considerations for COVID-19 Vaccines. Congressional Research Service.
5. Cowan, T., Fallon Morell, S., 2018. Vaccines, Autoimmunity, and the Changing Nature of Childhood Illness. Chelsea Green Publishing.

6. Dudley, M.Z., Salmon, D.A., Halsey, N.A., Orenstein, W.A., Limaye, R.J., O'Leary, S.T., Omer, S.B., 2018. The Clinician's Vaccine Safety Resource Guide – Optimizing Prevention of Vaccine-Preventable Diseases Across the Lifespan. Springer.
7. Edwards, K.M., Orenstein, W.A., Stephens, D.S., 2021. The COVID-19 Vaccine Guide: The Quest for Implementation of Safe and Effective Vaccinations. Skyhorse.
8. Franklin, M., 2019. Everything You Need To Know About Vaccines. Franklin.
9. Institute of Medicine, Board on Population Health and Public Health Practice, and Committee on the Assessment of Studies of Health Outcomes Related to the Recommended Childhood Immunization Schedule, 2018. The Childhood Immunization Schedule and Safety – Stakeholder Concerns, Scientific Evidence, and Future Studies. National Academies Press.
10. Kuca, M., 2020. mRNA COVID-19 Vaccine – The Human GM Frontier: Safety/Efficiency/ Future Applications. Kuca.
11. Miller, N.Z., 2016. Miller's Review of Critical Vaccine Studies: 400 Important Scientific Papers Summarized for Parents and Researchers. New Atlantean Press.
12. Miller, N.Z., Blaylock, R., 2011. Vaccine Safety Manual for Concerned Families and Health Practitioners (Guide to Immunization Risks and Protection), 2nd Edition. New Atlantean Press.
13. Morrow, W.J.W., Sheikh, N.A., Schmidt, C.S., Davies, D.H., 2012. Vaccinology: Principles and Practice. Wiley-Blackwell.
14. Rappuoli, R., Vozza, L., 2022. Vaccines in the Global Era: How to Deal Safely and Effectively with the Pandemics of Our Time. WSPC.
15. Thomas, P., Margulis, J., 2016. The Vaccine-Friendly Plan: Dr. Paul's Safe and Effective Approach to Immunity and Health – from Pregnancy Through Your Child's Teen Years. Ballantine Books.
16. Wailoo, K., Livingston, J., Epstein, S., Aronowitz, R., 2010. Three Shots at Prevention: The HPV Vaccine and the Politics of Medicine's Simple Solutions. Johns Hopkins Press.
17. WHO Regional Office for the Western Pacific, 2016. Vaccine Safety Communication for Immunization Programme Managers and National Regulatory Authorities (An WPRO Publication). World Health Organization.

Chapter 8

Preventable Childhood Infections

Chapter Outline

Vaccinology and Immunizations. http://doi.org/10.1016/B978-0-443-23915-1.00008-1

Learning Objectives

After study of this chapter, readers should be able to:

1. Describe the four different types of influenza.
2. Explain the etiology and risk factors for diphtheria.
3. Discuss the three stages of pertussis.
4. Describe the diagnosis of rotavirus infection.
5. Identify the most common pathogenic species of *Haemophilus*.
6. Explain the specific clinical manifestations of measles.
7. Identify the risk factors for pneumococcal infections.
8. Describe the etiology and risk factors for meningococcal meningitis.
9. Explain the diagnosis of acute viral hepatitis.
10. Discuss dengue disease and its clinical manifestations.

OVERVIEW

Infectious diseases are illnesses caused by microbes. It is essential to realize that not all microorganisms (bacteria, viruses, fungi, and parasites) cause disease. Many microorganisms are pathogenic, causing acute or chronic infections and even death. The record of human suffering and death caused by smallpox, cholera, typhus, influenza, dysentery, malaria, and others establishes the importance of infectious diseases. Despite the outstanding successes in control afforded by improved sanitation, immunization, and antimicrobial therapy, infectious diseases remain a common and significant problem. The most prevalent disease of humanity, the common cold, is contagious, as is the modern disease called AIDS (caused by HIV). Some chronic neurological diseases that were previously thought to be degenerative diseases have proven to be infectious. There is little doubt that the future will continue to have contagious diseases as major medical problems.

INFLUENZA

Influenza is a contagious viral infection that can cause mild to severe symptoms and life-threatening complications, including death, even in healthy children and adults. It is commonly known as the "flu." There are four types of influenza viruses: A, B, C, and D. Aquatic birds are the primary source of influenza A virus (IAV), which is also widespread in various mammals, including humans and pigs. Influenza B virus (IBV) and influenza C virus mainly infect humans, and influenza D virus is found in cattle and pigs. IAV and IBV circulate in humans and cause seasonal epidemics, and influenza C virus causes a mild infection, primarily in children. Influenza D virus can infect humans but is not known to cause illness. In humans, influenza viruses are usually transmitted through respiratory droplets produced from coughing and sneezing. Transmission also occurs through aerosols, intermediate objects, and surfaces contaminated by the virus.

Epidemiology

In a typical year, 5% to 15% of the population contracts influenza. There are 3 to 5 million severe cases annually, with up to 650,000 respiratory-related deaths globally. Deaths most commonly occur in high-risk groups, including young children, older adults, and people with chronic health conditions. In temperate regions, the number of influenza cases peaks during winter, whereas in the tropics, influenza can occur year-round. Since the late 1800s, large outbreaks of novel influenza strains that spread globally, called pandemics, have occurred every 10 to 50 years. These are known as *seasonal epidemics* caused by IAV and IBV. Pandemics are rarer, and there have been six major influenza pandemics, occurring in Russia (1889), Hong Kong (1900 and 1968), Spain and other countries (1918), Asia (1957), and in multiple countries in what was known as **swine influenza** (2009). In 2009 and 2010, the H1N1 flu pandemic spread to over 70 countries and all 50 US states, with most deaths occurring in Mexico.

Etiology and Risk Factors

Since 1968, most seasonal influenza epidemics have been caused by H3N2, an IAV. The IBVs may cause milder cases but often cause epidemics with moderate to severe disease, either as the primary circulating virus or along with influenza A. A predominant serotype causes the majority of influenza epidemics. Yet different viruses can appear in sequence, in one location, or simultaneously, with one virus predominating in one area and another prevailing in other regions. Certain patients are at high risk of influenza complications. These include the following:

- Children under 5 years of age, with those under 2 years of age being at the highest risk
- Adults over 65 years of age
- People with chronic cardiopulmonary disease, diabetes mellitus, renal or hepatic insufficiency, hemoglobinopathies, or immunodeficiencies
- Females in the second or third trimester of pregnancy
- Patients with disorders that impair how respiratory secretions are handled, such as cognitive dysfunction, neuromuscular disorders, seizure disorders, and stroke
- Patients less than 18 years taking aspirin because **Reye syndrome** is a risk factor

Morbidity and mortality may increase because of a worsening underlying illness, acute respiratory distress syndrome, primary influenza pneumonia, or secondary bacterial pneumonia.

Clinical Manifestations

The incubation period for influenza is 1 to 4 days. When mild, symptoms are similar to the common cold, with rhinorrhea, sore throat, and, sometimes, mild conjunctivitis. Children may develop significant nausea, vomiting, or abdominal pain, and infants may develop **septicemia**. After 2 to 3 days, acute symptoms quickly subside, though the fever can last up to 5 days. Some patients have weeks of persistent coughing, fatigue, sweating, and weakness. A worsening cough, **hemoptysis**, dyspnea, and rales indicate pneumonia. Secondary bacterial **pneumonia** is characterized by persistent or recurrent fever and coughing after the main illness resolves. Less commonly, encephalitis, myocarditis, and **myoglobinuria** can develop. Reye syndrome often occurs during influenza B epidemics, especially in children who have been given aspirin. Encephalopathy, elevated liver enzymes, fatty liver, elevated ammonia, hypoglycemia, and lipidemia characterize Reye syndrome.

Diagnosis

The diagnosis of influenza is usually made clinically based on signs and symptoms when it is known to be present in the community. Sensitivities of rapid diagnostic molecular (antigen detection) tests vary widely. Diagnostic tests should be performed when results will directly affect clinical decisions. Reverse transcriptase polymerase chain reaction (RT-PCR) studies are accurate and can differentiate between influenza types and subtypes. If these tests are readily available, results can be used to choose antiviral therapy. These tests should also be done when influenza is suspected in a hospitalized patient because antiviral treatment is usually required. The tests can prevent the unnecessary use of antibacterial agents. Identification of the actual influenza virus is essential for infection control. The tests help determine if outbreaks of respiratory disease are caused by influenza. If a patient has lower respiratory tract signs and symptoms (dyspnea or rales), pulse oximetry and a chest X-ray should be done so that hypoxemia and pneumonia can be assessed. Primary influenza pneumonia develops as focal or diffuse interstitial infiltrates or acute respiratory distress syndrome. Secondary bacterial pneumonia is often lobar or segmental.

Treatment

The treatment for most influenza patients is based on symptoms and includes hydration, rest, and antipyretics as needed. Aspirin is avoided in children. Appropriate antibiotics are required for any complicating bacterial infections that develop. Antivirals are given 1 to 2 days after symptoms start to decrease the duration of fever, symptom severity, and time needed to return to normal activities. Antivirals are recommended for high-risk patients who develop influenza symptoms, and early treatment can prevent complications. Drugs used to treat influenza include the following:

- Oseltamivir (a neuraminidase inhibitor): given orally twice daily, 75 mg per dose, to children older than 12. Lower doses can be used in children as young as 1 year. The drug can cause nausea and vomiting and may decrease the incidence of otitis media. No data clearly shows that its use will prevent complications of influenza.

- Zanamivir (a neuraminidase inhibitor): given by an inhaler, with two puffs of 10mg each twice daily. It can be used in children aged 7 or older. It sometimes causes bronchospasm and should not be given to patients with reactive airway disease. Some people cannot use the inhalation device.
- Peramivir (a neuraminidase inhibitor): given IV as a single dose for patients older than 2 years of age who cannot tolerate oral or inhaled drugs. However, studies of its use for influenza B are limited.
- Baloxavir (an endonuclease inhibitor) is given orally as one 40-mg dose to patients 12 years of age or older who weigh 40 to 80kg or as a single 80-mg dose for patients who weigh more than 80kg. It can be used in patients aged 12 or older with uncomplicated influenza who have been symptomatic for 48hours or less and are otherwise healthy or at a high risk of developing complications.

Prevention

Annual vaccination is the primary and most effective way to prevent influenza and its complications, especially for high-risk groups. Vaccines against the flu are trivalent or quadrivalent, providing protection against an H1N1 strain, an H3N2 strain, and one or two IBV strains. Two types of vaccines are in use: vaccines that contain "killed" (inactivated) viruses and live attenuated influenza vaccines that contain weakened viruses. There are three types of inactivated vaccines: whole virus, split virus (in which a detergent disrupts the virus), and subunit, which only contains the viral antigens hemagglutinin (HA) and neuraminidase (NA). Most flu vaccines are inactivated and administered via intramuscular (IM) injection. Live attenuated influenza vaccines are sprayed into the nasal cavity.

Vaccination recommendations vary by country. Some recommend vaccinations for people above a certain age, such as 6 months and older. Other countries' offers are limited for high-risk groups, such as pregnant females, young children (excluding newborns), older adults, people with chronic medical conditions, healthcare workers, people who come into contact with high-risk people, and people who transmit the virus quickly. Young infants cannot receive flu vaccines for safety reasons, but they can inherit passive immunity from their mother if inactivated vaccines are administered to the mother during pregnancy. Influenza vaccination also helps to reduce the probability of reassortment. Virus reassortment is a process of genetic recombination exclusive to segmented RNA viruses in which the coinfection of a host cell with multiple viruses may cause the shuffling of gene segments. This generates "offspring" viruses with novel genome combinations. Reassortment is primarily described for influenza viruses as a primary mechanism for transmission between species and the emergence of pandemic virus strains.

You Should Remember

High-risk patients include institutionalized, very young or old, those with cardiopulmonary abnormalities, or females in the late stages of pregnancy. Young and healthy patients can die from influenza during pandemics.

TEST YOUR KNOWLEDGE

1. Which age group of children is at the highest risk of having influenza complications?
2. In humans, how are influenza viruses transmitted?
3. What are the clinical manifestations of influenza in children?

DIPHTHERIA

Diphtheria is a severe bacterial infection that produces a toxin. It can result in dyspnea, arrhythmias, and death. The disease is spread between people from coughing or sneezing. The condition can also be spread by touching infected open sores or ulcers. Those at increased risk for contracting diphtheria include people in the same household or individuals working in healthcare with close contact with a patient.

Epidemiology

Diphtheria is rare today. From 1996 through 2018, there were only 14 cases reported in the United States, an average of less than one per year. However, it is endemic in many countries in Asia, the South Pacific, the Middle East, Eastern Europe, Haiti, and the Dominican Republic. In 2017, a total of 8819 cases were reported worldwide, which was the most since 2004. On average, there were 4300 to 5700 reported cases per year (from 2006 to 2013).

Etiology and Risk Factors

Diphtheria is a severe infection caused by strains of *Corynebacterium diphtheriae* that produce the toxin that causes the disease. Diphtheria risk factors include crowded environments, poor hygiene, and lack of immunization.

Clinical Manifestations

Signs and symptoms are based on the affected body part. The incubation period is between 2 to 5 days after exposure. The clinical presentation of diphtheria includes weakness, sore throat, mild fever, and enlargement of lymph nodes in the neck. The bacterial toxin kills healthy tissues in the respiratory system. Within 2 to 3 days, the dead tissue forms a thick gray coating that can build up in the throat or nose. It is a *pseudomembrane* and can cover tissues in the nose, tonsils, larynx, and throat, making it difficult to breathe and swallow. The toxin can cause heart, nerve, and kidney damage if it enters the bloodstream.

Diagnosis

The diagnosis of diphtheria is confirmed by isolating *C. diphtheriae* and testing the isolate for toxin production using the **Elek test**, an *in vitro* immunoprecipitation (immunodiffusion) assay. Specimens for culture should be obtained from the nares of the nose and the oropharynx or any mucosal or cutaneous lesion. The material should be obtained from beneath the membrane (if present) or a portion. Specimens are more likely to be culture positive if brought before the patient receives antibiotic treatment. Infection with other pathogens could result in a similar clinical presentation as diphtheria, so testing for other pathogens should be considered. Pathogens include group A beta-hemolytic *Streptococcus*, *Staphylococcus aureus*, ***Candida albicans***, **Epstein-Barr virus**, cytomegalovirus, adenovirus, and herpes.

Treatment

Diphtheria treatment involves using diphtheria antitoxin to stop the bacterial toxin from damaging the body. This treatment is essential for respiratory diphtheria infections but is rarely used for skin infections. Also, antibiotics such as erythromycin or penicillin are used to kill the bacteria. This is important for respiratory diphtheria infections and skin, eye, or blood disease. Finishing the entire course of antibiotics is essential to remove the bacteria from the body. After this, tests will be conducted to ensure the bacteria are gone.

Even though the disease is usually not contagious 48 hours after antibiotic treatment begins, droplet precautions are maintained until the patient has completed the antibiotic course and is culture negative. Once antibiotic therapy is completed, elimination of the organism is documented by obtaining two consecutive negative cultures 24 hours apart. Having diphtheria may not confer immunity. Persons recovering from diphtheria should begin or complete vaccination with diphtheria toxoid during convalescence if not up to date with vaccination.

Prevention

In the United States, there have been four vaccines used to prevent diphtheria, which include the following:

- DTaP (diphtheria, tetanus, pertussis): only for children younger than 7 years of age
- Tdap (tetanus, diphtheria, pertussis): for children 7 years and older, adolescents, and adults
- DT (diphtheria, tetanus): discontinued by the manufacturer in 2023, but it is being evaluated for future use in infants and children who should not receive acellular pertussis–containing vaccines.

- Td (tetanus, diphtheria): usually given as a booster dose every 10 years, or after 5 years in the case of a severe or dirty wound or burn—for children 7 years and older, adolescents, and adults

All vaccines for diphtheria are given intramuscularly (IM). The preferred injection site in infants and young children is the vastus lateralis muscle of the thigh. The selected injection site in older children and adults is the deltoid muscle of the upper arm.

For prophylaxis purposes, anyone having close contact with patients must receive antibiotics to prevent disease.

You Should Remember

Management of close contacts should include monitoring for possible respiratory or cutaneous diphtheria for 7 to 10 days from the last exposure to the diphtheria patient and obtaining nasal and throat cultures for *C. diphtheriae*. Close contacts should also receive erythromycin or penicillin as prophylaxis. For compliance reasons, if the health department cannot monitor close contacts, the close contacts should receive a dose of IM benzathine penicillin. The health department should also direct close connections to obtain a diphtheria toxoid booster appropriate for their ages if they are not up to date with diphtheria vaccination.

You Should Remember

Most complications of respiratory diphtheria, including death, are attributable to the effects of the toxin. The most frequent complications of respiratory diphtheria are myocarditis and neuritis. Other complications include otitis media and respiratory insufficiency due to airway obstruction, especially in infants.

TEST YOUR KNOWLEDGE

1. What is the "pseudomembrane" of diphtheria?
2. What is the treatment used for diphtheria?
3. Which diphtheria vaccine is used in children younger than 7 years of age?

TETANUS

Tetanus is an infection caused by a bacterium called *Clostridium tetani*. When the bacteria enter the body, they produce a toxin that causes painful muscle contractions. Spasms of the masseter muscles result (lockjaw), a hallmark of the disease. The tetanus bacilli form durable spores in soil and animal feces, remaining viable for years.

Epidemiology

Globally, tetanus is estimated to cause more than 200,000 deaths yearly, primarily in neonates and young children. However, the disease is so rarely reported that only rough estimates can be made. From 2009 to 2017, 264 cases of tetanus and 19 deaths were reported in the United States. Age distribution was 64% (in people aged 20 to 64), 23% (in those aged 65 or older), and 13% (in people less than 20 years of age, which included three cases of **tetanus neonatorum**). All tetanus-related deaths were in people older than 55 years. Disease incidence is related to immunizations in a given population, proving the effectiveness of preventive efforts. In the United States, immunity levels are usually lower in older age groups. Tetanus has an approximately 50% fatality rate worldwide. It has a 15%–60% fatality rate in untreated adults, but in neonates, 80% to 90% will die even with treatment. Mortality is highest for the young, very old, and drug abusers.

Etiology and Risk Factors

The cause of tetanus is infection with *C. tetani*. The spores usually enter through contaminated wounds. The toxin enters the peripheral nerve endings and irreversibly binds there. Next, it travels retrograde along axons and synapses, eventually joining the central nervous system (CNS). The release of inhibitory transmitters from nerve terminals is blocked. This causes unopposed muscle stimulation by **acetylcholine** and generalized tonic spasticity, usually accompanied by intermittent tonic seizures; disinhibited autonomic neurons and loss of control of **adrenal catecholamine** release cause autonomic instability and a hypersympathetic state. The toxin cannot be neutralized after being bound.

Risk factors for tetanus include burn or crush injuries, surgical wounds, deep punctures, or a history of abusing injected drugs. Tetanus can also follow minor or inapparent wounds. It can develop postpartum in the uterus (maternal tetanus) or within an infant's umbilicus (tetanus neonatorum) from unsanitary delivery methods or poor umbilical cord care. Other risk factors include diabetes mellitus and a history of immunosuppression. Nearly all cases of tetanus within the United States reported today are among those who have never been vaccinated against tetanus or did not stay up to date on their tetanus booster doses.

Clinical Manifestations

Manifestations of tetanus are caused by *tetanospasmin*, an exotoxin produced when bacteria lyse. Tetanus is usually generalized and affects skeletal muscles throughout the body but can be localized to muscles close to an entry wound. The incubation period is usually 10 days but can range from 3 to 21 days. Signs and symptoms begin gradually and then progressively worsen over 2 weeks. They typically start at the jaw and progress downward on the body. Signs and symptoms include **dysphagia**, restlessness, irritability, stiffness (neck, arms, or legs), arching of the back, headache, sore throat, and tonic spasms. Over time, the affected patient has problems opening the jaw.

Facial muscle spasms cause the smile to appear "fixed" and the eyebrows to be elevated, known as **risus sardonicus**. Sphincter spasms may cause urinary retention or constipation. Dysphagia may interfere with getting adequate nutrition. Painful and generalized tonic spasms with extreme sweating can be caused by minor factors such as drafts, noises, or movements. The mental status is usually normal, but repeated spasms may result in a coma. As generalized cramps occur, the patient cannot speak or cry out due to the rigidity of the chest wall or spasm of the **glottis**. In rare cases, sustained spasms cause bone fractures. The spasms also interfere with respiration and can result in **cyanosis** or fatal **asphyxia**. The temperature is slightly elevated unless a complicating infection is present. There are hyperpnea, tachycardia, and hyperreflexia. Chronic tetanus may cause overactivity of the sympathetic nervous system with myocardial irritability.

Respiratory failure is the most common cause of death. Laryngeal spasms, rigidity, and spasms of the abdominal wall, chest wall, and diaphragm muscles can cause asphyxiation. Hypoxemia can result in cardiac arrest. Pharyngeal spasms lead to aspiration of oral secretions, leading to pneumonia and a hypoxemic death. Pulmonary embolism sometimes occurs. Often, a patient's cause of death is not apparent.

Localized tetanus causes spasticity of muscles near the entry wound without **trismus**. The spasticity can continue over weeks. **Cephalic tetanus** affects the cranial nerves and is more common in children, occurring with chronic otitis media or after a head wound. This form is most common in Africa and India. The seventh cranial nerve is mainly involved, but all can be affected, and tetanus may become generalized. Tetanus in neonates is usually generalized and often fatal, beginning in a poorly cleaned umbilical stump after the infant was born to an insufficiently immunized mother. Onset over the first 2 weeks features rigidity, spasms, and poor feeding. Surviving children may become deaf in both ears.

Diagnosis

Tetanus is considered when there is sudden, unexplained muscle stiffness or spasms, especially after a recent wound or other tetanus risk factors. The disease can be confused with meningoencephalitis. However, this combination is suggestive of tetanus:

- Intact sensorium
- Normal cerebrospinal fluid (CSF)
- Muscle spasms

Trismus must be differentiated from a peritonsillar, retropharyngeal abscess, or another localized cause. Phenothiazines, antipsychotic medications, can cause tetanus-like rigidity, with dystonic reactions and **neuroleptic malignant syndrome**. The causative bacterium can sometimes be cultured from the wound but lacks sensitivity. Only 30% of tetanus patients have positive cultures. False-positive cultures can occur in patients who do not have the disease.

Treatment

The treatment of tetanus requires adequate ventilation, early and thorough use of human tetanus immune globulin (TIG), prevention of additional toxin production, sedation, control of symptoms (muscle spasms, hypertonicity, fluid imbalance, and recurrent infections), and continuous nursing care. If TIG is unavailable, IV immune globulin can be used because it contains tetanus antitoxin. Wounds must be debrided to prevent further toxin release, followed by administration of antibiotics. The unbound toxin outside the CNS is neutralized with TIG. **Tetanus toxoid** is used for immunization, injected into a different body site than the antitoxin. Steps are taken to minimize the effect of the toxin already in the CNS. Muscle spasms are managed with benzodiazepines (diazepam, midazolam, lorazepam), paralytic drugs (vecuronium, pancuronium, rocuronium), intrathecal baclofen, and dantrolene. Autonomic dysfunction is managed with morphine, esmolol, atropine, clonidine, magnesium sulfate, pyridoxine, sodium valproate, angiotensin-converting enzyme inhibitors, dexmedetomidine, and adenosine. Typical antibiotics include penicillin G, doxycycline, and metronidazole. Supportive care includes intubation for mechanical ventilation, IV hyperalimentation, stool softeners, rectal intubation, bladder catheterization, chest physiotherapy, frequent turning, forced coughing, and opioids.

Prevention

A primary series of tetanus vaccinations, then regular booster doses, is required. Children younger than 7 years require five primary vaccinations. Unimmunized patients under 7 require three prior vaccinations. The vaccine may be tetanus toxoid alone, though toxoid is usually combined with diphtheria and pertussis. Children's vaccines have higher doses of the diphtheria and pertussis components than the adult vaccines. Children are given DTaP at ages 2 months, 4 months, 6 months, 15 to 18 months, and 4 to 6 years. They should receive a Tdap booster at 11 to 12 years and Td every 10 years after that. Pregnant females should be given Tdap during each pregnancy (27 to 36 weeks, gestation), regardless of their last vaccination. The fetus can develop passive immunity from this.

You Should Remember

Tetanus (lockjaw) causes tightening of the jaw muscles, muscle spasms, stiffness, and seizures. Muscle spasms make it difficult to swallow or breathe, potentially leading to respiratory failure and death.

TEST YOUR KNOWLEDGE

1. How fatal is tetanus in children on a global scale?
2. In which group of children is cephalic tetanus most common?
3. What quantities of tetanus vaccine are used in various age groups of children?

PERTUSSIS

Pertussis is a respiratory infection capable of causing violent and rapid coughing fits that sometimes result in vomiting. The disease is named because of the "whooping" noise made as the affected person tries to breathe in after coughing. It is highly contagious and can affect anyone, but it is most serious in unvaccinated infants. Transmission is mostly via droplets of secretions that contain *Bordetella pertussis*, a gram-negative bacterium. More than 80% of people in close contact with an infected person will become infected.

Epidemiology

Pertussis only occurs in humans and is endemic throughout the world. The rates are highest among young children in countries with lower vaccination coverage. In 2018, the WHO reported 151,074 pertussis cases globally. Based on 2008 data, the WHO estimated that there were 89,000 deaths. However, a publication modeling pertussis cases ends with data from 2014 estimates that there were 24.1 million pertussis cases and 160,700 deaths in children younger than 5 years worldwide. Despite high vaccination coverage, pertussis remains one of the leading causes of vaccine-preventable deaths worldwide. WHO has reported that most pertussis cases occur in developed countries. In 2019, China had the highest number of pertussis cases globally, with 30,027 patients; Japan, Russia, Australia, and India followed with 16,845, 14,407, 12,021, and 11,875 patients, respectively.

In the United States, its incidence cycles every 3 to 5 years. During the 1980s, pertussis was at an all-time low, affecting 1 in every 100,000 people. By 2014, this had increased to 10 in every 100,000. By 2019, it had lowered again, affecting 5.7 of every 100,000. In 2019, there were 18,617 cases and 7 deaths. The incidence per 100,000 was higher in infants younger than 6 months (76.5). Also, four of the seven deaths occurred in infants younger than 1 year. The increase since the 1980s was due to immunity becoming reduced in previously vaccinated individuals and parents refusing to vaccinate their children (vaccine hesitancy). Epidemiology may also be affected because the virulence of outbreak strains may be increasing.

Etiology and Risk Factors

The causative bacterium is *B. pertussis*, which spreads between individuals. The bacteria is described as a small, aerobic gram-negative rod that requires special media for isolation. Pertussis is primarily a toxin-mediated disease in which the bacteria produce toxins that lead to respiratory tract inflammation and interfere with clearing pulmonary secretions. Secondary bacterial pneumonia is the most common complication and the cause of most related deaths. Risk factors for pertussis include not being vaccinated, contact with infected individuals, epidemic exposures, and pregnancy.

Clinical Manifestations

Pertussis is characterized initially by rhinorrhea, mild fever, and a mild, occasional cough. There may be apnea and cyanosis. As the cough worsens, symptoms include intensified coughing with the whooping sound, vomiting during or after coughing, and exhaustion. Anorexia, weight loss, and a cough that worsens at night may also occur. The incubation period is 7–14 days and a maximum of 3 weeks. As the respiratory mucosa is invaded, mucus secretion increases (at first, it is thin, but later becomes viscid and tenacious). The uncomplicated disease lasts 6–10 weeks, in three stages, as follows:

- *Catarrhal stage*: starts insidiously, with sneezing, tearing, and other signs of **coryza**; **anorexia**; listlessness; and a hacking nocturnal cough that slowly becomes diurnal; hoarseness may occur, but fever is rare.
- *Paroxysmal stage*: after 10–14 days, this starts with increased cough severity and frequency; there are repeated consecutive forceful coughs during expiration, followed by a fast and deep inspiration known as the *whoop*; copious viscid mucus can be expelled or bubble from the nostrils during or after the paroxysms; vomiting is common; infants may choke, with or without cyanosis, more often than whooping.
- *Convalescent stage*: symptoms start to resolve in this stage, usually within 4 weeks of onset; average illness duration is 7 weeks (in a range of 3 weeks to 3 months or longer); the paroxysmal coughing can recur for months; it is usually induced by irritation from an upper respiratory infection.

Respiratory complications, including asphyxia and otitis media, may occur. Bronchopneumonia can be fatal at any age. Seizures are common in infants but rare in older children. Severe paroxysmal and anoxia can lead to bleeding in the brain, eyes, skin, and mucous membranes, leading to cerebral hemorrhage, edema, intellectual disability, or other neurologic problems. Sometimes, **umbilical hernia** and rectal prolapse occur.

Diagnosis

The catarrhal stage may be difficult to differentiate from influenza, bronchitis, adenovirus infections, or tuberculosis. In more than 80% of cases in the catarrhal and early paroxysmal stages, cultures of nasopharyngeal specimens will be positive for *B. pertussis*. Samples should be collected during the first 2 weeks of illness following cough onset. This is when viable bacteria are still present in the nasopharynx. Sensitivity decreases after the first 2 weeks, and the risk of false negatives increases. The culture of *B. pertussis* is considered the gold standard for diagnosis because it is the only 100% specific method for identifying the disease. Thorough fluorescent antibody testing of the smears provides an accurate diagnosis but is less sensitive than culture. Convalescent serologic testing can also be helpful. PCR testing of nasopharyngeal samples is the preferred test given that it is the most rapid. However, PCR tests vary in specificity, and results should be interpreted along with clinical symptoms. Leukocytosis typically indicates the presence of infection or inflammation. Parapertussis may be differentiated by culture or with the fluorescent antibody method.

Treatment

Early treatment of pertussis most effectively reduces symptom severity during the disease course. For seriously ill infants, hospitalization with respiratory isolation should be undertaken and continued until antibiotics have been administered for 5 days. Suction to remove excess throat mucus can be lifesaving. Some infants require oxygen, **tracheostomy**, or **nasotracheal intubation**. To avoid disturbances, the seriously ill infant is kept in a dark, quiet room with minimal disruptions. Patients treated at home must be isolated, especially from susceptible infants, for 4 weeks or more until symptoms have subsided. In the catarrhal stage, antibiotics may lessen symptoms, but once paroxysms are established, they are only used to limit disease spread. Preferred antibiotics include azithromycin, erythromycin, clarithromycin, and trimethoprim-sulfamethoxazole. Antibiotics are also used for bacterial complications such as bronchopneumonia or otitis media.

Prevention

Active immunization against pertussis is part of standard childhood vaccinations. Five doses of acellular pertussis vaccine are given, usually combined with diphtheria and tetanus, at 2 months, 4 months, 6 months, 15 to 18 months, and 4 to 6 years. After a natural pertussis infection, immunity lasts about 20 years. Close contacts younger than 7 with less than four vaccine doses must complete the recommended childhood vaccination schedule.

Postexposure antibiotics are given to household contacts within 21 days of coughing onset in the primary patient, regardless of vaccination status. These antibiotics are also provided to people at high risk irrespective of vaccination status, which may include:

- Infants younger than 12 months
- Females in the third trimester of pregnancy
- People with conditions worsened by pertussis (chronic lung disease, immunodeficiency, moderate to severe asthma)
- Those in close contact with infants under 12 months of age, pregnant females, or those with conditions that may result in severe illness or complications
- All high-risk people in childcare centers, maternity wards, or neonatal intensive care units

A 7- to 14-day course of oral erythromycin is given four times daily. Other antibiotics include clarithromycin and azithromycin. For infants younger than 1 month, azithromycin is preferred for postexposure prophylaxis.

You Should Remember

Parapertussis is similar to pertussis but is less severe and less common. It occurs most frequently among children less than 10 years of age. All infants under 6 months of age should receive antibiotics as a preventive measure if they have been in contact with someone with parapertussis.

You Should Remember

Whooping cough is usually spread by coughing, sneezing, or breathing very close to an infected person. Still, it sometimes is transmitted by an uninfected person touching an infected surface and then touching their mucous membranes. Whooping cough is contagious for about 2 weeks after coughing begins, but antibiotics can shorten the time of being contagious.

TEST YOUR KNOWLEDGE

1. Where are the rates of childhood pertussis highest?
2. What are the three stages of pertussis?
3. What is the treatment for seriously ill people with pertussis?

POLIOMYELITIS

Poliomyelitis (polio) is a disabling and life-threatening disease. It is caused by the *poliovirus*, which spreads between individuals and is highly contagious. It can invade the spinal cord, causing **paralysis**. There are three types of wild poliovirus (WPV). People must protect themselves against all three virus types to prevent polio disease. Polio vaccination provides the best protection. Types 2 and 3 WPVs were declared eradicated in September 2015 and October 2019, respectively, and only type 1 WPV remains.

Epidemiology

WPV cases have decreased by over 99% since 1988, from 350,000 patients in more than 125 endemic countries to six reported cases in 2021. Extensive vaccination has nearly eradicated poliomyelitis globally. Even so, cases still occur in areas with incomplete immunization, such as sub-Saharan Africa and southern Asia. In 2020, there were 140 reported wild-type poliovirus type 1 (84 cases in Pakistan and 56 in Afghanistan). Nearly 1000 cases of circulating vaccine-derived poliovirus also occurred, mainly in Pakistan, Afghanistan, Chad, and the Democratic Republic of the Congo.

Etiology and Risk Factors

The causative poliovirus has three serotypes. Type 1 is the most paralytogenic and was formerly the most common cause of epidemics. Humans are the only natural hosts of polio. Immunity to one serotype does not produce significant immunity to the other serotypes. Infection is highly transmissible via direct contact. The virus enters through the fecal-oral or respiratory route, multiplying in the oropharyngeal and lower GI tract mucosa. The virus is secreted into saliva and feces, which can be transmitted to other people. The virus next enters the cervical and mesenteric lymph nodes. A primary but minor **viremia** occurs as the virus spreads to the **reticuloendothelial system**. The infection may be contained, or the virus can multiply further, causing several days of secondary viremia, after which symptoms and antibodies develop.

In paralytic infections, the virus enters the CNS. Significant damage occurs in the spinal cord and brain, mainly in the nerves that control motor and autonomic function. Inflammation worsens the damage. The risk factors of severe neurologic damage include the following:

- Increased age
- Recent IM injection or tonsillectomy
- Pregnancy
- Impaired B-lymphocyte function
- Physical exertion that is concurrent with the onset of the CNS phase

Clinical Manifestations

Most infections (70%–75%) cause no symptoms. The symptomatic disease may be either abortive poliomyelitis or paralytic or nonparalytic poliomyelitis. Most symptomatic infections, especially in young children, are minor. There are 1–3 days of mild fever, malaise, headache, sore throat, and vomiting, which develop 3–5 days following exposure. Physical examination is unremarkable except for the malaise. Approximately 4% of cases develop nonparalytic CNS involvement with aseptic meningitis. There is usually a stiff neck, back, or both, plus a headache appearing after several days of **prodrome**, similar to abortive poliomyelitis. Symptoms continue for 2–10 days.

Paralytic poliomyelitis occurs in under 1% of all poliovirus infections. It may appear as a biphasic illness in infants and young children. There is a paralytic phase, several days after abortive poliomyelitis symptoms resolve. Incubation is usually 7–21 days. Common manifestations of paralytic poliomyelitis include deep muscle pain, paresthesias, and hyperesthesias. During active myelitis, there are urinary retention and muscle spasms. Asymmetric **flaccid paralysis** can appear, progressing over 2–3 days. Sometimes, the encephalitis signs predominate.

The earliest signs of bulbar involvement usually include dysphagia, nasal regurgitation, and a nasal-sounding voice. Some patients have pharyngeal paralysis and are unable to control their oral secretions. Bulbar involvement and skeletal muscle paralysis may worsen over 2–3 days. Sometimes the respiratory and circulatory centers of the brainstem are affected, leading to respiratory compromise. Rarely, respiratory failure develops from the diaphragm or intercostal muscles being affected. Postpoliomyelitis syndrome develops in some patients years or decades after paralytic poliomyelitis. It is characterized by muscle fatigue, decreased endurance, weakness, fasciculations, and atrophy.

Diagnosis

Immunization history, patient age, recent travel, and the year's season help suggest the cause. Poliovirus can be detected in specimens from the throat, stool, and occasionally CSF by isolating the virus in cell culture or by detecting the virus by PCR.

Treatment

Standard treatment is supportive, including rest, analgesics, and antipyretics as needed. There is no specific antiviral therapy available. During active myelitis, precautions may be required to avoid deep venous thrombosis, atelectasis, urinary tract infections, and contractures. Mechanical ventilation is needed in patients with respiratory failure. In nonparalytic poliomyelitis, recovery is complete. In paralytic poliomyelitis, about 66% of patients will have a residual permanent weakness. **Bulbar paralysis** is more likely to resolve than peripheral paralysis.

Prevention

There is no cure for polio, but safe and effective vaccines can prevent it. Polio vaccination has become part of routine immunizations in the United States and many other countries. Since 2000, the inactivated polio vaccine has been the only type given via an injection into the arm or leg, based on the patient's age. The oral polio vaccine is used in other countries. Most infected individuals have no symptoms, and about 24% have minor flulike signs that are only temporary. A sore throat, fever, nausea, tiredness, headache, or stomach pain may occur. Only a few cases will develop into meningitis or paralysis of the arms or legs.

You Should Remember

Between 2 and 10 out of every 100 people with paralysis caused by the poliovirus infection will die because it affects the respiratory muscles. Children who appear to recover fully can develop new muscle pain, weakness, or paralysis as adults, even 15 to 40 years later.

TEST YOUR KNOWLEDGE

1. What are the common manifestations of paralytic poliomyelitis?
2. What are the risk factors of neurologic damage in polio?
3. Which polio vaccines are used in various countries?

ROTAVIRUS INFECTION

Rotavirus infection is a very contagious virus that causes severe diarrhea. Before the development of a vaccine, most children had been infected with the virus at least once by age 5. Good hygiene, such as washing your hands regularly, is essential. However, vaccination is the best way to prevent rotavirus infection.

Epidemiology

Since the introduction of routine rotavirus immunization, rotavirus incidence has decreased by about 80% in the United States. Rotavirus gastroenteritis is common in infants and young children. Those under 5 (especially 6 months to 2 years of age) are most vulnerable. Rotavirus occurs globally. Before the rotavirus vaccine, about 35% to 40% of children under age 5 in developed and developing countries contracted rotavirus. Most infections occur in the winter. Every year in the United States, a wave of rotavirus illness starts in the Southwest in November and ends in the Northeast in March.

Etiology and Risk Factors

Rotavirus is often spread through the fecal-oral route because children do not wash their hands properly or often enough. It can also be caused by eating or drinking contaminated food or water. The virus may live on surfaces such as doorknobs, toys, and other complex objects for an extended period. Risk factors include a long time spent in childcare settings, babysitting, and winter and spring seasons. It is possible to be infected with rotavirus more than once, even if a patient has been vaccinated. However, repeat infections are typically less severe.

Clinical Manifestations

Rotavirus infection usually starts within 2 days of exposure to the virus. It lasts 5–7 days in infants and young children. Early signs and symptoms include fever, abdominal pain, vomiting, and 3–7 days of watery diarrhea. Children are more likely than older patients to have severe dehydration and death. In healthy adults, a rotavirus infection may cause only mild signs and symptoms or none at all. The incubation period is approximately 2 days. Severe diarrhea can lead to dehydration, particularly in young children. Left untreated, dehydration can become a life-threatening condition regardless of its cause.

Diagnosis

The diagnosis of rotavirus involves stool tests to identify the virus. This test is only routinely done to diagnose outbreaks. Two commonly used tests are the enzyme-linked immunosorbent assay and latex agglutination. Nucleic acid testing (PCR) is often done in a multiplex PCR panel that includes a variety of causes of gastroenteritis.

Treatment

Treatment for rotavirus gastroenteritis is primarily supportive, with fluid rehydration and electrolytes. Oral glucose-electrolyte solutions, broth, or bouillon may prevent or treat mild dehydration. Children can quickly dehydrate, so an appropriate rehydration solution must be given. If vomiting makes this problematic, an antiemetic such as ondansetron may be offered. Ringer lactate or standard saline solution (isotonic IV fluids) is given when there is severe dehydration, shock, altered mental status, failure of oral rehydration therapy, or ileus. IV rehydration is continued for severe dehydration until pulse, perfusion, and mental status are normal. Antidiarrheal agents are avoided in children with acute diarrhea.

Prevention

To reduce the spread of rotavirus, washing your hands thoroughly and often, especially after using the toilet, changing an infant's diaper, or helping a child use the bathroom, is essential. However, even strict handwashing does not offer guarantees, and commonly used alcohol-based hand sanitizers have little effect on rotavirus. The WHO recommends that all infants should be given a rotavirus vaccine. There are two vaccines available: RotaTeq and Rotarix. The RotaTeq vaccine is given orally in three doses, usually at 2, 4, and 6 months. The vaccine is not approved for use in older children or adults. The Rotarix vaccine is a liquid given twice to infants at 2 and 4 months. They are safe and effective against most strains that cause rotavirus gastroenteritis. Rotavirus immunization is part of the recommended infant vaccination schedule. Children with intussusception are more likely to have it again after receiving the rotavirus vaccine. The US Food and Drug Administration recommends that the vaccine not be given to children with a history of intussusception.

You Should Remember

Rotavirus infection usually starts within 2 days of exposure to the virus. Fever and vomiting appear first, followed by 3–7 days of watery diarrhea. Abdominal pain is present as well. Most children recover by resting and drinking fluids, but when severe, treatment of a rotavirus infection may require intravenous fluid administration.

TEST YOUR KNOWLEDGE

1. In which age groups of children is rotavirus gastroenteritis common?
2. In children, how is rotavirus often spread?
3. Which vaccines are used to prevent rotavirus infection?

HAEMOPHILUS INFLUENZAE B

Haemophilus influenzae type B (Hib) is a gram-negative bacteria of the *Haemophilus* species that causes many mild to severe infections. These species are often normal flora in the upper respiratory tract, rarely causing disease. Pathogenic strains enter the upper respiratory tract via droplet inhalation or direct contact. In nonimmune populations, it spreads rapidly.

Epidemiology

Hib occurs globally. In 2018, cases were at 0.08 per 100,000 population in children younger than 5 years, with 38 cases of invasive disease due to Hib reported in the United States. The number of cases and deaths of invasive infections increased from 3400 in 1997 to 6840 in 2018, with 11.8% of patients being fatal. The case fatality rate of Hib meningitis is about 5%. In survivors, severe neurologic sequelae occur in 10%–15% and deafness in 15%–20%.

Etiology and Risk Factors

The most common pathogenic species of Hib is *H. influenzae* bacteria. It has six distinct encapsulated serotypes (A through F) and many nonencapsulated, nontypeable strains. Before using the Hib conjugate vaccine, most cases of the severe and invasive disease were caused by type B. Risk factors include being under age 5 years old or over 65 years old, male gender, and the African American or Native American ethnic or racial groups. Other risk factors include overcrowded living conditions, attendance in daycare centers, immunodeficiency, **asplenia**, and **sickle cell disease**.

Clinical Manifestations

The most common diseases that result from Hib infection include meningitis, bacteremia, epiglottitis, pneumonia, arthritis, and cellulitis. The clinical manifestations of Hib include fever, chills, fatigue, abdominal pain, nausea with or without vomiting, diarrhea, anxiety, shortness of breath, difficulty breathing, and confusion. There may be a severe headache, stiff neck, convulsions, seizures, extreme drowsiness, difficulty awakening, or loss of consciousness.

Diagnosis

Diagnosis of Hib infections is based on an examination and medical history. Specific tests depend on the location of the disease. Sometimes, a fluid culture is taken from the eyes, ears, throat, CSF, or blood. Chest X-rays and blood tests are helpful.

Treatment

Treatment is based on the type and location of the infection. Beta-lactam/beta-lactamase inhibitors, fluoroquinolones, and second- or third-generation cephalosporins are used for invasive diseases. The Hib conjugate vaccines have significantly reduced rates of bacteremia. Children with serious illnesses are hospitalized with contact and respiratory isolation for 24 hours after starting antibiotics. The choice of antibiotic is based on the site of infection and requires susceptibility testing. Many isolates in the United States produce beta-lactamase, and more than 50% are resistant to ampicillin. For invasive diseases (including meningitis), cefotaxime or ceftriaxone is recommended. Oral cephalosporins, azithromycin, other macrolides, amoxicillin-clavulanate, omadacycline, and lefamulin are usually effective if the infection is less severe. Cefotaxime and ceftriaxone eliminate the respiratory impact of the bacterium. Because other antibiotics used for systemic disease do not do this, children not treated with either of these two drugs should be given rifampin immediately after completing treatment and before resuming contact with other children.

Prevention

Hib conjugate vaccines are available for children 2 months or older and have reduced invasive infections by 99%. Infants 2 through 6 months of age should receive either a three-dose series of ActHIB, Hiberix, Pentacel, or Vaxelis or a two-dose series of PedvaxHIB. The initial dose of Hib vaccine can be administered as early as 6 weeks. Based on the chosen vaccine, a primary series is given at 2, 4, and 6 months or at ages 2 and 4. A booster is needed at 12–15 months. Unimmunized or incompletely immunized household contacts under 4 years of age should receive a dose of vaccine. All household members except pregnant females should receive prophylaxis with oral rifampin once a day for 4 days. Nursery or daycare contacts must receive prophylaxis if two or more cases of invasive disease occur over 60 days.

You Should Remember

Hib can result in potentially deadly encephalitis in young children. It may also cause meningitis, septicemia, **epiglottitis**, sinusitis, otitis media, pneumonia, cellulitis, and **septic arthritis**.

TEST YOUR KNOWLEDGE

1. What are the complications of Hib infection?
2. What are the common manifestations of Hib infection?
3. What are potential antibiotic treatment options for a severe Hib infection?

MEASLES

Measles is a highly contagious and severe disease caused by a virus. Before the introduction of the measles vaccine in 1963 and widespread vaccination, there were significant epidemics worldwide; it is considered one of the most contagious infectious diseases.

Epidemiology

Before the measles vaccine was introduced, significant epidemics occurred every 2–3 years, with 2.6 million related deaths occurring annually. One of the first documented accounts of measles was in Persia (Iran) in the 9th century. Measles remains a leading cause of mortality, especially among children less than 5 years of age. Worldwide incidence estimates are difficult to obtain because of heterogeneous surveillance systems and probable underreporting.

The availability of measles vaccination beginning in the 1960s immediately impacted disease incidence, reduced associated mortality rates, and altered global distribution. In 2000, the United States declared measles eliminated. Measles occurs predominantly in areas with low vaccination rates, particularly in resource-limited settings. However, even in resource-rich settings, measles outbreaks have occurred where vaccination uptake has declined, allowing for transmission of imported measles virus from unvaccinated and infected travelers. In 2019, 1274 reported measles cases drew concern, as this was the highest registered number of cases in the United States since 1992. Cases were primarily unvaccinated individuals. In 2022, cases decreased to only 121 reported cases in the United States.

Etiology and Risk Factors

A paramyxovirus causes measles, usually passed through airborne transmission or direct contact. The virus infects the respiratory tract and then spreads throughout the body.

Individuals at risk for measles include children too young to be vaccinated, those who have not been vaccinated for medical or other reasons, those who have not received a second dose of the measles vaccine, and those who failed to elicit a protective immune response from the vaccine (a tiny fraction of those immunized with two doses of vaccine).

Clinical Manifestations

The initial sign of measles is a high fever (as high as 105 °F), starting 10 to 12 days after exposure and lasting up to 7 days. Other signs and symptoms include rhinorrhea, sore throat, coughing, red and watery eyes, tiredness, and **Koplik spots**. After a few days, a rash erupts, usually on the face and upper neck, and then spreads over 3 days to reach the hands and feet. It lasts for up to 6 days and then fades. Most related deaths are due to complications, mostly under age 5 or over 30. Complications include blindness, encephalitis, severe diarrhea and dehydration, ear infections, and pneumonia. Severe measles is most common in poorly nourished young children or those with weakened immunity. Accelerated immunization activities have significantly reduced measles deaths.

Diagnosis

Measles is generally diagnosed based on clinical signs and symptoms, though a complete blood count can show **leukopenia** with a relative lymphocytosis. Laboratory confirmation is required for public health purposes and to control outbreaks. It is done by showing the presence of the measles IgM antibody in serum specimens or via viral culture or RT-PCR of blood, throat swabs, nasopharyngeal swabs, or urine samples. Increased IgG antibody levels between acute and convalescent sera are highly accurate, but the time required to obtain the information delays diagnosis. All suspected measles cases must be reported to the local health department before being confirmed in the laboratory. The signs and symptoms resemble **Kawasaki disease** in areas where measles is an infrequent and complicated diagnosis.

Treatment

The treatment for measles is supportive. Hospitalized patients are managed with standard and airborne precautions utilizing appropriate equipment. For 4 days after the development of the rash, contact with other people must be severely limited. Vitamin A supplementation reduces morbidity and mortality in children in areas that lack sufficient medical supplies. Because low serum levels of vitamin A are related to severe disease, vitamin A treatment is recommended for children with measles. The dose is given orally once daily for 2 days, based on the child's age. If there are clinical signs of vitamin A deficiency, another age-specific amount of vitamin A is given 2 to 4 weeks later.

Prevention

In most countries, children are routinely given a live-attenuated virus vaccine containing measles, mumps, and rubella (MMR). The first dose is best at 12–15 months but can be given as young as 6 months during outbreaks or before international travel. The second dose is given at ages 4–6 years. Infants immunized under 12 months of age require two additional doses after the first birthday. People without immunity to measles, including infants, may be vaccinated within 72 hours of exposure. If measles still develops, it usually has milder symptoms and lasts longer. Pregnant females, infants, and people with weakened immune systems who are exposed to the virus may receive an injection of immune serum globulin. When given within 6 days of exposure to the virus, these antibodies can prevent measles or worsen symptoms.

You Should Remember

The measles vaccine is contraindicated in patients with severe immunodeficiency (leukemia, lymphoma, solid tumors), use of immunosuppressants (corticosteroids, alkylating agents, irradiation, antimetabolites), or severe HIV infection, and those who are pregnant.

TEST YOUR KNOWLEDGE

1. What is the cause of measles, and how is it spread?
2. Is laboratory confirmation required for measles?
3. What type of vaccine is used to prevent measles, and how many doses are given?

MUMPS

Mumps is a viral infection that previously was most common in children and adolescents, leading to inflammation in salivary glands and organs that could result in chronic problems. It usually causes painful enlargement of the salivary glands (**parotitis**).

Epidemiology

Mumps occurs mainly in unimmunized populations, though outbreaks in largely immunized populations have occurred. In 2006, there was a resurgence of mumps in the United States, with 6584 cases, mostly in younger people who had previously been vaccinated. Sporadic outbreaks have also occurred in schools and other areas of close contact. More recent cases have ranged from only 229 in 2012 to 6366 in 2016. Peak incidence is in the late winter and early spring. The disease occurs at any age but is rare in children younger than 2 years. Globally, about 500,000 cases of mumps were reported to the WHO annually between 1999 and 2019. The actual incidence is difficult to estimate because mumps is not a notifiable disease in many countries.

Etiology and Risk Factors

The causative agent of mumps is a *paramyxovirus* spread by droplets or saliva, usually entering through the nose or mouth. It remains in the saliva up to 7 days before inflammation begins and is most transmissible just before parotitis begins. The virus is also found in the blood, urine, and CSF. Risk factors for mumps include living in or traveling where the disease is common, being exposed to anyone with the illness, being in crowded settings such as schools, not being immunized, and having a weakened immune system.

Clinical Manifestations

The manifestations of mumps occur about 2 to 3 weeks after being infected and last for up to 2 weeks. Mumps results in fever, cough, headache, and inflammation of the salivary glands and lymph node inflammation. The disease is usually spread by transmission of droplets via talking, coughing, or sneezing. Complications of mumps happen more often among adults than children and may include **orchitis**, **mastitis**, encephalitis, **oophoritis**, pancreatitis, or deafness.

Diagnosis

The diagnosis of mumps is based on salivary gland inflammation and typical systemic symptoms, especially if there is a known outbreak. Laboratory testing is not needed for diagnosis but should be done for public health. Mumps is also suspected if a patient has unexplained aseptic meningitis or encephalitis during a mumps outbreak. For patients with meningeal signs, a lumbar puncture is required. Laboratory diagnosis is necessary if the disease causes prominent involvement of tissues besides the salivary glands, occurs in a previously immunized patient, or is recurrent or unilateral. Testing is also recommended for patients with parotitis that lasts 2 days or longer with no identified cause via RT-PCR, serologic testing with complement fixation, or enzyme-linked immunosorbent assay, and viral culture of the throat, CSF, and, sometimes, the urine. IgM testing can be falsely negative in previously immunized people. Therefore RT-PCR should be done on saliva or throat-washing samples as early as possible.

Treatment

The treatment for mumps is supportive, with the patient being isolated until the swelling subsides. Sometimes, bed rest is necessary for the first few days. Pain caused by chewing is reduced with a soft diet. Citrus fruit juices should be avoided if they cause discomfort. Repeated vomiting related to pancreatitis may require IV hydration. If orchitis is present, bed rest and support of the scrotum in cotton with an adhesive tape bridge between the thighs helps reduce tension. Ice packs can be used to relieve pain.

Prevention

The prevention of mumps requires vaccination with a live mumps virus vaccine. The first dose, given as MMR, is recommended for children at 12–15 months of age, followed by the second dose at 4–6 years.

TEST YOUR KNOWLEDGE

1. What are the risk factors for mumps?
2. What are the clinical manifestations of mumps?
3. What is the diagnosis of mumps based on?

RUBELLA

Rubella is a mild contagious viral infection in children and nonimmune young adults. It was initially considered a variant of measles or **scarlet fever**, but this has been proven incorrect. Rubella is also called "German measles."

Epidemiology

Ten percent to 15% of unvaccinated young adults who did not have a childhood rubella infection are susceptible. Due to routine childhood vaccination, incidence in the United States is at a historic low point. All cases in the United States since 2004 have come from people who brought them back after traveling to another country. Rubella was previously a global infection. It has been eliminated in North, Central, and South America since 2009. However, an estimated 110,000 babies are born with rubella annually, mainly in Southeast Asia and Africa, followed by the Middle East.

Etiology and Risk Factors

Rubella is caused by the *rubella virus*, which is an RNA virus. Respiratory droplets spread through close contact with the air. The disease can be transmitted during asymptomatic infection or from 7 days before the rash appears until 15 days after the onset of the rash. It is most transmissible from a few days before the rash appears to 7 days after the start of the rash. Congenitally infected infants can transmit rubella for many months after birth. Although less contagious than measles, immunity to rubella appears to be lifelong after natural infection.

Clinical Manifestations

Many cases of rubella are mild. About 25%–50% of rubella infections are asymptomatic. After an incubation period of 14–21 days, there is a 1- to 5-day prodrome that usually consists of low fever, conjunctivitis, malaise, and lymphadenopathy. These symptoms are less evident in children than in adults. There can be tender swelling of the postauricular, posterior cervical, and suboccipital lymph nodes. The rash is less extensive than measles and more **evanescent**. It starts on the face and neck, quickly spreading to the trunk and extremities. An initial blanching, macular erythema may appear (usually on the front), which, on the second day, often becomes more pinpoint, with a reddish flush. **Petechiae**, known as *Forchheimer spots*, form on the soft palate and then coalesce into a red blush. The rash lasts for 3–5 days. Children may then develop mild malaise or arthralgias. Complete resolution usually occurs, though encephalitis can be fatal. In rare cases, thrombocytopenic purpura and otitis media arise.

Diagnosis

The diagnosis of rubella is based on the signs and symptoms. Laboratory diagnosis is required for neonates, patients with encephalitis, and pregnant females. It is also encouraged for all suspected rubella cases to be reported for public health purposes. Diagnosis is confirmed by a fourfold increase between acute and convalescent (4- to 8-week) antibody titers. Confirmation can also be done with serum rubella IgM antibody testing. Another method is the detection of viral RNA via RT-PCR testing.

Treatment

The treatment of rubella is mainly supportive. In pregnant females, management depends on the fetal gestational age at the onset of infection. Suppose the condition occurs before 18 weeks of gestation. In that case, the fetus is at high risk for disease and subsequent malformation, and management should consider pregnancy termination according to local ethical and legislative regulations. If the condition occurs after 18 weeks of gestation, the pregnancy could be continued with ultrasound monitoring and specific neonatal management. Treatment of children with congenital rubella syndrome should be symptomatic and organ specific. It usually involves a multidisciplinary approach and requires pediatric, ophthalmologic, cardiac, audiological, and neurodevelopmental evaluation. Long-term follow-up is needed to monitor for delayed manifestations.

Prevention

For rubella, a live virus vaccine is routinely given that produces immunity for 15 or more years in 95% of patients. Vaccination is given to children as two doses of the MMR vaccine (at 12–15 months and again at 4–6 years). The use of the vaccine is contraindicated during pregnancy. Vaccinated children rarely develop adverse effects, including low-grade fever, lymphadenopathy, rash, **polyneuropathy**, **arthralgia**, and arthritis.

You Should Remember

In nonpregnant individuals, rubella is generally a self-limited and benign infection. However, maternal rubella infection, especially during the first 10 weeks of gestation, can result in miscarriage, fetal death, or severe congenital disabilities, collectively known as congenital rubella syndrome.

TEST YOUR KNOWLEDGE

1. Where does rubella still occur?
2. How does the rash of rubella spread across the body?
3. What is the treatment of children with congenital rubella syndrome?

VARICELLA

Varicella (chickenpox) is a highly contagious disease caused by the varicella-zoster virus, also known as human herpesvirus type 3, or *primary varicella infection*. In most cases, chickenpox is contracted during childhood, spread by mucosal droplets or particles or direct contact with skin lesions. After primary infection, the virus stays in the body as a latent infection. Later reactivation of the latent phase is known as **shingles**.

Epidemiology

Over 95% of American adults have had chickenpox, and about 4 million people get chickenpox every year. Traditionally, varicella epidemics have occurred in the winter and early spring in 3- to 4-year cycles. It still appears globally. In areas of temperate climate, it mainly affects children under 10 years. In tropical climates, children acquire it at older ages, resulting in a higher proportion of young adults remaining susceptible. The annual global incidence is estimated at 80–90 million cases. Most developing countries have low immunization rates because of cost factors, so varicella is a risk for travelers who visit these countries.

Etiology and Risk Factors

Varicella spreads from person to person by direct contact or through the air. Family members who have never had chickenpox have a 90% chance of becoming infected when another family member is infected. Most individuals with chickenpox will be immune to the disease for the rest of their lives. However, there is a chance of developing shingles later in life. It is communicable from 48 hours before the first lesions appear on the skin until the final lesions have crusted. The incubation period is typically 14–16 days after exposure to the virus. Risk factors include being nonimmunized, having never had chickenpox, and having close contact with infected people.

Clinical Manifestations

Signs and symptoms are usually mild among children but may be life-threatening to adults and people with weak immune systems. While symptoms vary from child to child, the most common include fever, fatigue, muscle pain, cough, runny nose, and itching. A blister-like rash initially appears on the chest, back, and face before spreading over the entire body. Serious complications include secondary bacterial infections, encephalitis, and, in rare cases, death.

Diagnosis

The diagnosis of varicella is based on the unique rash seen during physical examination. Laboratory confirmation requires a PCR test for viral DNA, immunofluorescent detection of the viral antigen in lesions, serologic tests, viral culture, or a **Tzanck smear**. In serologic tests, detecting IgM antibodies to the virus, or seroconversion from negative to positive for antibodies to the virus, indicates an acute infection. Usually, samples are obtained by scraping the bases of the lesions and transporting them to the lab in viral media. A Tzanck smear from grinding a ruptured **vesicle**, stained with Wright-Giemsa or toluidine blue stain, will show multinucleated giant cells and epithelial cells with eosinophilic intranuclear inclusion bodies. Cultures have less sensitivity than PCR and take longer to complete (1–2 weeks).

Treatment

There is no specific treatment for chickenpox, but there are pharmacy remedies that can alleviate symptoms. These include acetaminophen to relieve fever, calamine lotion, and cooling gels to ease itching. In most children, the blisters crumble and fall off naturally within 1 to 2 weeks. Therapy with intravenous acyclovir every 8 hours for 7–10 days should be initiated at the first sign of infection for people requiring hospitalization with severe disease. A switch to oral antiviral therapy (acyclovir, valacyclovir, or famciclovir) can be considered when the patient is afebrile and new lesion formation has ceased.

Prevention

The best way to prevent the disease is to get the varicella vaccine, which became available in the United States in 1995. It is a live attenuated vaccine with three different formulations: standard dose, combination measles-mumps-rubella-varicella, and a higher-dose vaccine to prevent herpes zoster. Healthy children receive two doses of the vaccine. Vaccination is contraindicated in patients with moderate to severe acute concurrent illness, immunocompromised patients, patients taking high doses of systemic corticosteroids, and those taking aspirin. Postexposure prophylaxis using IM varicella-zoster immune globulin is used for neonates whose mothers developed chickenpox within 5 days before or 2 days after delivery and neonates born at less than 28 weeks who were exposed to a nonmaternal source even if their mothers have evidence of immunity. Exposed neonates born at 28 or more weeks should receive immune globulin if their mothers have no proof of immunity. Varicella-zoster immune globulin is given as soon as possible and within 10 days of exposure. Vaccination is delivered as quickly as possible to exposed, susceptible, healthy patients of 1 or more years with no contraindications. Infection with varicella confers lifelong protection. Potentially sensitive individuals require strict precautions to avoid others who could transmit the infection. The vaccine is very safe and effective at preventing the disease.

TEST YOUR KNOWLEDGE

1. What are the signs and symptoms of chickenpox?
2. What does laboratory confirmation of chickenpox require?
3. What is the best way to prevent chickenpox?

PNEUMOCOCCAL DISEASE

Pneumococcal disease is caused by *Streptococcus pneumoniae*, which can attack different parts of the body. Pneumococcus is a gram-positive bacteria. Pneumococcal infections range from ear or sinus infections to pneumonia and septicemia.

Epidemiology

Pneumococcal infections affect people of all ages, but children younger than 2 years of age and adults aged 65 years and older are at higher risk. The prevalence and distribution of invasive *S. pneumoniae* serotypes differ across populations and geographical areas. The incidence of pneumococcal diseases peaks in the winter months in temperate climates. Seasonality is attributed to lower humidity, indoor crowding, associated viral infections, cold weather, and air pollution. Pneumococcal disease occurs globally.

Etiology and Risk Factors

Pneumococcal disease is spread through contact with respiratory secretions such as saliva or mucus. Children often have the causative bacteria in their noses or throats without signs of infection and can transmit it to others. Risk factors for developing pneumococcal disease include cardiorespiratory disease, type 1 diabetes, liver disease, immunodeficiency or immunosuppression, asplenia, sickle cell disease, cochlear implant, CSF leak, smoking, and alcoholism. People from Aboriginal, Alaskan, or specific Native American populations are also at increased risk. Pneumococcal disease may result in long-term hospitalization.

Clinical Manifestations

Signs and symptoms of pneumococcal pneumonia include fever, chills, coughing, tachypnea, dyspnea, and chest pain. Complications include **empyema**, pericarditis, abscess, and atelectasis. Symptoms of pneumococcal meningitis include a stiff neck, fever, headache, **photophobia**, and confusion. In infants, it may cause poor eating and drinking, low alertness, and vomiting.

Diagnosis

Depending on the symptoms, pneumococcal disease is diagnosed using several tests, including physical examination, chest X-ray, sputum test, blood test, and CSF test. Microscopically, diagnosis of pneumococcal disease is based on the appearance during Gram staining of the lancet-shaped diplococci. Using the **Quellung test**, there is an application of antiserum followed by staining with India ink, which causes the bacterium's capsule to appear like a surrounding "halo." It is also visible in smears stained with methylene blue. Culture is confirmatory, and antimicrobial susceptibility testing is needed. A urine antigen detection test is more than 90% specific but only 50% to 80% sensitive. The positive predictive value is more than 95%. Still, the negative predictive value—the number of patients with a disease-free negative test—is low, so negative urine antigen tests do not rule out pneumococcal disease. Radiographic appearances considered classic for pneumococcal pneumonia include lobar consolidations, air bronchograms in adults, and round pneumonia in children. However, the bacterial capsule of pneumococcal pneumonia can have many different appearances. CT may reveal lymphadenopathy and complications.

Treatment

Noninvasive pneumococcal infections are usually mild and go away without needing treatment. Rest, fluids, and over-the-counter painkillers such as acetaminophen are typically advised. More invasive types of pneumococcal infections can be treated with antibiotics at home or in the hospital. However, initial therapy is chosen based on local resistance patterns. The preferred treatment is with a beta-lactam or macrolide antibiotic, though resistant strains have emerged that complicate treatment. Worldwide, strains highly resistant to penicillin or ampicillin are common. Resistance to macrolide antibiotics has also significantly increased. Intermediately resistant bacteria can be treated with usual or high doses of beta-lactams such as penicillin G. Extremely ill patients with nonmeningeal infections caused by penicillin-resistant organisms may be treated with ceftaroline, ceftriaxone, or cefotaxime. Extremely high doses of parenteral penicillin G can also be effective. The mortality rate for bacteremic pneumococcal pneumonia is lower when combination therapy is used, such as a macrolide with beta-lactam. Vancomycin is also an option and can be used with ceftriaxone, cefotaxime, and rifampin in patients with meningitis.

Prevention

Prevention involves vaccination and prophylactic antibiotics. Two pneumococcal vaccines are available (pneumococcal conjugated vaccine [PCV13] and pneumococcal polysaccharide vaccine [PPSV23]). All children 2 months through 6 years of age should receive PCV13 as part of the routine childhood vaccination schedule. Prophylactic penicillin V is given orally twice daily for asplenic children under 5. Sometimes prophylaxis is continued throughout childhood and into adulthood. For older children and adolescents, oral penicillin is recommended, dosed twice daily for at least 1 year after splenectomy.

You Should Remember

Pneumococcal diseases include pneumonia, bacteremia, endocarditis, meningitis, otitis media, septic arthritis, sinusitis, and, rarely, peritonitis. Pneumococcal pneumonia is fatal in about 5% of cases. Pneumococcal meningitis is fatal in 1 of every 12 children who contract it. Pneumococcal bacteremia is fatal in 1 of every 30 children.

TEST YOUR KNOWLEDGE

1. When does the incidence of pneumococcal diseases peak?
2. What are the risk factors for pneumococcal disease?
3. Which pneumococcal vaccines are available?

MENINGOCOCCAL DISEASE

Meningococcal disease is a rare but very serious and often deadly disease caused by a bacterium called Neisseria *meningitidis*, a gram-negative diplococcus that causes meningitis and **meningococcemia**.

Epidemiology

The global incidence of endemic meningococcal disease is 0.5–5 cases per 100,000 population, with higher incidence during the winter and spring in temperate climates. Local outbreaks are most common in sub-Saharan Africa as part of the *sub-Saharan (African) meningitis belt*, which includes 26 countries. In major African epidemics, cases ranged from 100–800 per 100,000 population, affecting as many as 200,000 people yearly. In the United States, the annual incidence varies from 0.12–1.1 per 100,000. Over the past 20 years, the incidence of meningococcal disease has declined annually. Most cases are sporadic, usually in children under 2 years of age. Outbreaks are rare, with only about 5% of cases. They mainly occur in enclosed communities such as schools or daycare centers, usually involving children aged 16 or 17.

Etiology and Risk Factors

About 1 in 10 people have *N. meningitidis* in the back of their nose and throat without being ill. These individuals are carriers of the disease. Sometimes, the bacteria invade the body and cause meningococcal disease. Risk factors for meningococcal disease include infants younger than 1 year old, adolescents and young adults aged 16 through 23, college students living in residence halls, and people with certain medical conditions that affect the immune system, such as HIV.

Clinical Manifestations

Common signs and symptoms of meningococcal meningitis include sudden fever, headache, and stiff neck. Other symptoms may include nausea, vomiting, photophobia, and confusion. Children and infants may show different signs and symptoms such as inactivity, irritability, vomiting, poor reflexes, photophobia, lethargy, a maculopapular or hemorrhagic petechial rash on the palms of the hands, soles of the feet, roof of the mouth, and abdomen. Fulminant meningococcemia syndromes include **Waterhouse-Friderichsen syndrome**, sepsis with multiple organ failure, shock, and disseminated intravascular coagulation.

Less common infections target the lungs, joints, respiratory passageways, genitourinary organs, rectum, eyes, endocardium, and pericardium. *N. meningitidis* can cause cervicitis and urethritis. The incidence of meningococcal urethritis and proctitis has been increasing in male homosexuals.

Diagnosis

The diagnosis of meningitis is based on a medical history, a physical exam, and specific tests. Standard tests to diagnose meningitis include blood cultures, CT scans, and head MRIs. A definitive diagnosis of meningitis requires a spinal tap to collect CSF. In patients with meningitis, the fluid often shows a low sugar level, increased white blood cell count, and increased protein. Analyzing the fluid also may help identify which bacterium caused the meningitis. If viral meningitis is suspected, a DNA-based test known as a PCR amplification may be performed on a CSF sample. Another test checks for antibodies against certain viruses to determine the specific cause and proper treatment.

You Should Remember

From January 2013 to May 2018, 10 university-based meningococcal disease outbreaks caused by serogroup B were reported in seven states. These outbreaks resulted in a total of 39 cases and two deaths.

Treatment

Acute bacterial meningitis must be treated immediately with IV antibiotics and sometimes corticosteroids. This helps to ensure recovery and reduce the risk of complications such as brain edema and seizures. The antibiotic or combination depends on the type of bacteria causing the infection. Antibiotics such as ceftriaxone or penicillin G must be given. While penicillin G is often the first choice for invasive disease, some countries prefer a third-generation cephalosporin initially (ceftriaxone or cefotaxime). Additional treatment with ceftriaxone, ciprofloxacin, or rifampin is required when penicillin is used to eliminate nasopharyngeal carriage. Corticosteroids such as dexamethasone are used carefully based on the causative organism and are given with or before the first dose of antibiotics.

Prevention

Antibiotic prophylaxis for close contact with patients with meningococcal disease includes rifampin, ciprofloxacin, or ceftriaxone. If these are contraindicated, a single dose of azithromycin can be an alternative. There are two types of meningococcal vaccines licensed in the United States: meningococcal conjugate vaccines and serogroup B meningococcal (MenB) vaccines. These vaccines help protect against all three serogroups (B, C, and Y) of *N. meningitidis* bacteria, most seen in the United States. Like with any vaccine, meningococcal vaccines are not 100% effective. This means there is still a chance someone can develop meningococcal disease after vaccination. People should know the signs and symptoms of meningococcal disease because early recognition and quick medical attention are extremely important. The CDC recommends that all 11- to 12-year-olds receive a meningococcal vaccine with a booster dose at 16 years. Healthy adolescents between 16 and 23 years may also receive a MenB vaccine. Specific at-risk populations, including adolescents and young adults with asplenia or complement component deficiency, or those on a complement inhibitor, should receive the MenB vaccine.

You Should Remember

Treatment for chronic meningitis is based on the underlying cause. While antifungal medications are used for fungal meningitis, a combination of specific antibiotics can treat tuberculous meningitis. However, these medicines can have serious side effects, so treatment may be deferred until a laboratory can confirm if the cause is fungal.

TEST YOUR KNOWLEDGE

1. What are the risk factors for meningococcal disease?
2. What does a definitive diagnosis of meningitis require?
3. What are the two types of meningococcal vaccines licensed in the United States?

VIRAL HEPATITIS

Viral hepatitis is an inflammation of the liver that results in abnormal function of the organ. A virus often causes it, and there are five types of viral hepatitis, which include hepatitis A (hep A), B (hep B), C (hep C), D, and E. The most common types are hep A, hep B, and hep C. However, we discuss only hep A and B in this chapter because vaccines are available only for these two types (Chapter 3).

Epidemiology

Annually, about 8500 people in the United States become infected with the hep A virus (HAV), many of whom are children. At the same time, an estimated 880,000 to 1.89 million people are chronically infected with hep B. However, new cases of hep B infection have generally been decreasing. Since 2012, reported cases of acute hep B are approximately 3000 per year.

Etiology and Risk Factors

HAV is the most common cause of acute viral hepatitis and is very common in children and young adults. HAV mainly spreads by the fecal-oral route, so it often occurs in areas of poor hygiene. Waterborne and foodborne epidemics occur in countries lacking adequate and effective water treatment and sanitation facilities. Eating contaminated raw shellfish is sometimes responsible. Sporadic cases usually occur from person-to-person contact. Risk factors for hep A include poor sanitation, lack of safe drinking water, close contact with an infected person, having a sexual partner with acute hep A infection, use of recreational drugs, sexual contact between men, and traveling to endemic areas without being immunized.

Common ways that the hep B virus (HBV) can spread include sexual contact, sharing needles, accidental needlesticks, blood transfusion, and from mother to child during birth. Risk factors for hep B include unprotected sex with multiple sex partners or with an infected person, sharing needles, sexual contact between men, living with someone who has a chronic HBV infection, infants born to infected mothers, and working in a job that may involve exposure to human blood. However, the most common risk factor is the self-injection of drugs, which is related to the opioid crisis and heroin use.

Clinical Manifestations

In children under age 6, approximately 70% of hep A infections are asymptomatic. When a child does have symptoms, jaundice is rare. Most older children have the usual manifestations of viral hepatitis (anorexia, fever, malaise, nausea, vomiting), and jaundice appears in over 70%. Symptoms usually resolve after 2 months but sometimes continue or recur for up to 6 months. Some patients have cholestatic hepatitis caused by hep A, with signs including severe jaundice with pruritus, continued fever, weight loss, diarrhea, and malaise. Recovery is usually complete, and fulminant hepatitis is rare.

Symptoms of acute hep B range from mild to severe and usually appear about 1–4 months after infection. Symptoms may rarely appear as early as 2 weeks after the disease. Young children are often asymptomatic. Signs and symptoms include abdominal pain, dark urine, fever, joint pain, loss of appetite, nausea, vomiting, weakness, fatigue, and jaundice.

Diagnosis

When acute viral hepatitis of any subtype is suspected, screening for hep A and B requires testing for the IgM antibody to HAV (IgM anti-HAV), hep B surface antigen, and the IgM antibody to the hep B core. Acute hep A is diagnosed when the IgM anti-HAV test is positive. The IgG antibody to HAV (IgG anti-HAV) test is done to help distinguish acute from prior infection. A positive IgG anti-HAV test suggests previous HAV infection or acquired immunity. HAV is present in serum only during acute infection and cannot be detected by clinically available tests. The IgM antibody usually develops early in the disease, peaking about 1–2 weeks after jaundice develops. It reduces in several weeks and creates a protective IgG antibody (IgG anti-HAV), which usually continues throughout life. Liver tests (if not previously done) are required. They include serum alanine aminotransferase, aspartate aminotransferase, and alkaline phosphatase. Other liver function tests include serum albumin, bilirubin, and prothrombin time/international normalized ratio.

The diagnosis of hep B begins with patient history, physical examination, and assessment of jaundice or abdominal pain. Tests include blood tests, liver ultrasound (transient elastography), and a liver biopsy. Screening for hep B may be performed for pregnant females. A patient's history may help with the diagnosis to determine risk factors for infection, including people with many sexual partners, homosexual males, and anyone with an account of a sexually transmitted disease, HIV, or hepatitis B.

Treatment

There are no treatments except supportive care for acute viral hep A. Alcohol increases liver damage, so it should be avoided. Viral hep A must be reported to local or state health departments. For hep B, an immunoglobulin injection is given within 24 hours of exposure to the virus, followed by the hep B vaccine if it was never given previously. For acute hep B, treatment may only be supportive: rest, proper nutrition, plenty of fluids, and close monitoring. If the case is severe, antiviral drugs or hospitalization may be required. For chronic hep B, treatment is usually given throughout the individual's lifespan. Treatments include antiviral medications, interferon injections, and liver transplantation. New drugs to treat hepatitis B are being developed.

Prevention

Prevention of hep A includes good personal hygiene, barrier protection, and cleaning spills and contaminated surfaces with diluted household bleach. The hep A vaccine is recommended for all children beginning at 1 year of age, with a second dose 6 to 18 months later. Postexposure prophylaxis is given to family members and close contacts of infected patients. For healthy, unvaccinated contacts, one dose of the vaccine is given. The vaccine is strongly recommended for newborns, children, and adolescents to prevent hep B. It is also recommended for adults 19 to 59 years of age if there are no contraindications.

You Should Remember

Hep B is a potentially life-threatening liver infection caused by HBV. It is a major global health problem. Hep B may result in chronic disease and puts people at high risk of death from cirrhosis and liver cancer. The virus can survive outside the body for at least 7 days. During this time, the virus can still cause infection if it enters the body of a person not protected by the vaccine.

TEST YOUR KNOWLEDGE

1. What are the risk factors for hep A and B?
2. What are the signs and symptoms of acute hep B?
3. When should the hep A and B vaccines be given?

HUMAN PAPILLOMAVIRUS

Human papillomavirus (HPV) is the most common sexually transmitted infection in the United States. The HPV vaccine can prevent some of the adverse health outcomes caused by HPV. There are many different types of HPV. Some cause diseases such as genital warts and cancers, though the available vaccines can prevent these. Genital warts usually appear as a small bump or group of nodes in the genital area. They can be any size, flat or raised, or they resemble the shape of a cauliflower. HPV can cause cervical, vulvar, vaginal, penile, anal, or oropharyngeal cancer. Cancer usually takes years to decades to develop after being infected with HPV. Genital warts and cancers result from different types of HPV. Cervical cancers are caused mainly by HPV-16 and HPV-18. People with weak immune systems may be less able to fight off the effects of HPV and may be more likely to develop HPV-related health problems.

Epidemiology

There are more than 43 million HPV infections annually in the United States, often among people in their late teens or early 20s. Within 10 years after the HPV vaccine was introduced, the prevalence of HPV types 6, 11, 16, and 18 has decreased by 86% among females aged 14–19 and 71% among females aged 20–24.

Etiology and Risk Factors

HPV can be spread via vaginal, anal, or oral sex with an infected person. However, it is most commonly spread during vaginal or anal sex. It also spreads via close touching during intercourse. An infected person can pass HPV to others without signs or symptoms. Symptoms develop for some people years after having intercourse with an infected person. In 9 out of 10 people, HPV resolves within 2 years without health problems. The primary risk factor for HPV is becoming sexually active at an early age. Risks for a severe HPV infection that is persistent and will lead to cervical cancer are higher in people who became sexually active before age 18 and in those with multiple sex partners.

Clinical Manifestations

In most cases, HPV does not cause any symptoms, and patients may be unaware they have it. Sometimes, the virus causes painless genital warts. If the immune system cannot rid the body of HPV, which is oncogenic, it can eventually turn normal cells into abnormal cells and lead to cancer. About 10% of females with HPV infection of the cervix develop long-term HPV infections that increase the risks for cervical cancer.

Diagnosis

The essential methods to diagnose an HPV infection include the following:

- *Colposcopy and acetic acid test*: **colposcopy** is performed by specially trained clinicians on an outpatient basis, using a *colposcope*, a low-powered microscope to examine the cervix, vagina, and sometimes the vulva after *acetic acid solution* is applied. The acid solution causes genital warts, dysplastic, and neoplastic tissues to turn white. During colposcopy, all lesions suspected of representing **neoplasia** can be biopsied. False-positive results are expected. They can result from anything causing **parakeratosis**, such as candidiasis, **lichen planus**, **psoriasis**, a healing epithelium, or **sebaceous glands**.
- *Biopsy*: removing samples of abnormal areas is critical because treatment is based on the severity of the abnormality. If the biopsy shows dysplasia or cancer, treatment is started.
- *Pap smear*: a procedure in which a small brush is used to gently remove cells from the surface of the cervix and the area around it. Then, it can be examined under a microscope for cervical cancer.

Treatment

While there is no treatment for HPV, there are treatments for the conditions it may cause. Genital warts can be treated with topical medications such as imiquimod (which boosts the immune system), podophyllin and podofilox (a resin that destroys genital wart tissue), trichloroacetic acid (which "burns" off genital warts), and a cream called *sinecatechins*. For more prominent genital warts or those that do not respond to medications, surgery may be needed. Surgical options include **cryotherapy**, **electrocautery**, surgical excision, or laser surgery.

Prevention

The only preventive methods against HPV are to receive the vaccine, use condoms as much as possible during intercourse, avoid direct contact with anyone known to be infected, and get tested for HPV if any of the risk factors are present.

You Should Remember

HPV is a nonenveloped, double-stranded, circular DNA virus that is responsible for causing multiple epithelial lesions and cancers. Depending on the subtype, it can manifest as cutaneous and anogenital warts, which may progress to carcinoma.

TEST YOUR KNOWLEDGE

1. What types of cancer can be caused by HPV?
2. How is HPV spread?
3. How is a colposcopy performed?

DENGUE

Dengue is a mosquito-borne disease that is also known as **breakbone fever**. A flavivirus causes it and can lead to a fatal hemorrhagic fever. The virus is spread primarily through the bite of an infected *Aedes aegypti* or *Aedes albopictus* mosquito.

Epidemiology

About 50% of the world's population (4 billion people) live in areas with a dengue risk. Dengue outbreaks occur in many different countries. There are an estimated 100 to 400 million new infections of dengue annually. Dengue ranked as the second-most vector-borne severe disease worldwide, following malaria. The economic burden of dengue has reached 2 billion US dollars in five countries, including Brazil, El Salvador, Guatemala, Panama, and Venezuela, and three hyperendemic Southeast Asian countries, including Cambodia, Malaysia, and Thailand.

Etiology and Risk Factors

Dengue is caused by the dengue virus spread by mosquitoes, mostly in tropical and subtropical climates. Risk factors include lack of protection against mosquito bites, poor mosquito control, urbanization, excessive time spent outside, poor water storage practices, and lack of education about dengue.

Clinical Manifestations

Dengue may be asymptomatic. About 25% of cases reveal symptoms with nonspecific acute febrile illness. Infection with any of the four different dengue viruses will result in long-term immunity to the specific virus. However, because there are four viruses, people can be infected with dengue multiple times. About 1 in 20 patients with dengue progresses to severe disease, which is life-threatening. A second infection with dengue is a risk factor for developing severe dengue. Recognizing early signs of shock and then quickly starting intensive supportive therapy can reduce the risk of death from severe dengue. Severe dengue can cause extreme plasma leakage, bleeding, and organ impairment.

Diagnosis

Diagnostic testing includes nucleic acid amplification tests, serologic tests, and cross-reactive flavivirus tests. Nucleic acid amplification tests are performed on serum specimens collected up to 7 days after the onset of symptoms. Serologic tests include IgM antibody and plaque reduction neutralization tests. The IgM antibody is used for qualitatively detecting dengue virus IgM antibodies and tests the blood serum or CSF. The plaque reduction neutralization tests can detect specific neutralizing antibodies against dengue virus and other flaviviruses.

Treatment

No specific antiviral agents exist for dengue. Patients must stay well hydrated. They must avoid aspirin and other nonsteroidal antiinflammatory drugs because of their anticoagulant properties. Fever must be controlled with acetaminophen and slightly warm sponge baths. Mosquito protection is essential to reduce the risks of further dengue transmission.

Prevention

Avoiding mosquito bites must be emphasized. A dengue vaccine is approved for use in children aged 9–16 years when there is a confirmed previous dengue virus infection and the location is within an area where dengue is endemic. There are not enough data to show how well the vaccine works in a population that is visiting, but not living in, a place where dengue is common.

You Should Remember

The clinical diagnosis of dengue can be challenging, as many other illnesses can present similarly early in the disease course. Other considerations should include malaria, influenza, Zika, chikungunya, measles, and yellow fever. Obtain a detailed history of immunizations, travel, and potential exposures.

TEST YOUR KNOWLEDGE

1. What are the risk factors for dengue?
2. How common is severe dengue, and what symptoms does it cause?
3. If dengue develops, what drugs must be avoided and why?

KEY TERMS

Acetylcholine
Adrenal catecholamine
Anorexia
Arthralgia
Asphyxia
Asplenia
Breakbone fever
Bulbar paralysis
Candida albicans
Cephalic tetanus
Colposcopy
Coryza
Cyanosis
Dysphagia
Elek test
Epstein-Barr virus
Evanescent
Flaccid paralysis
Glottis
Hemoptysis
Kawasaki disease
Koplik spots
Leukopenia
Lichen planus
Mastitis
Meningococcal disease
Meningococcemia

Myoglobinuria
Nasotracheal intubation
Neoplasia
Oophoritis
Orchitis
Parakeratosis
Parotitis
Petechiae
Polyneuropathy
Prodrome
Psoriasis
Reticuloendothelial system
Reye syndrome
Risus sardonicus
Scarlet fever
Sebaceous glands
Septicemia
Sickle cell disease
Swine influenza
Tetanus neonatorum
Tetanus toxoid
Tracheostomy
Trismus
Tzanck smear
Umbilical hernia
Vesicle
Viremia
Waterhouse-Friderichsen syndrome

CASE STUDIES

Case Study 1

A 10-year-old boy was brought to the local hospital with anorexia, weight loss, and a persistent cough that was worse at night. The boy also had wheezing and chest tightness. A tuberculosis test was done, but it came back negative. Additional tests confirmed the presence of pertussis infection, and the boy was started on clarithromycin. After 2 weeks, all symptoms were resolved. Soon, two of his family members came down with the same symptoms and were treated successfully.

Critical Thinking Questions

1. What is the causative pathogen for pertussis?
2. What is the paroxysmal stage of pertussis?
3. What are the treatment options for pertussis?

Case Study 2

A 3-year-old girl started vomiting and quickly developed a fever. Her parents took her to the emergency department. The girl was not entirely responsive and did not recognize her parents. The girl was admitted and found to have tachypnea and tachycardia. Her pupillary responses were sluggish, and her capillary blood gas levels were lower than usual. Meningoencephalitis was considered, but additional testing revealed the correct diagnosis of acute bacterial meningitis.

Critical Thinking Questions

1. What are the risk factors for meningococcal disease?
2. How is acute bacterial meningitis treated?
3. What preventive measures are available for meningococcal disease?

Case Study 3

A 17-year-old girl underwent a routine gynecological examination and reported being sexually active for the past year. Condoms were occasionally used. The girl complained of chronic pelvic pain and sometimes experienced bleeding after sex.

Routine tests were performed, and the girl was unaware of HPV. She also had a tumor on her cervix that appeared to be cancerous.

Critical Thinking Questions

1. How common is the HPV infection?
2. What type of HPV results in cervical cancer?
3. Why is the biopsy of abnormal areas critical in cases of HPV?

FURTHER READING

1. American Academy of Pediatrics, Tan, T.Q., 2022. Red Book Atlas of Pediatric Infectious Diseases, 5th Edition. American Academy of Pediatrics.
2. Berkowitz, F.E., 2007. Case Studies in Pediatric Infectious Diseases. Cambridge University Press.
3. Boyce, T.G., 2018. Moffet's Board Review for Pediatric Infectious Disease. Wolters Kluwer.
4. Centers for Disease Control and Prevention, 2015. Epidemiology and Prevention of Vaccine-Preventable Diseases, 13th Edition. CDC.
5. Cherry, J., Demmler-Harrison, G.J., Kaplan, S.L., Steinbach, W.J., Hotez, P.J., 2017. Feigin and Cherry's Textbook of Pediatric Infectious Diseases, 8th Edition. Elsevier.
6. Cowan, T., Fallon Morell, S., 2018. Vaccines, Autoimmunity, and the Changing Nature of Childhood Illness. Chelsea Green Publishing.
7. Dudley, M.Z., Salmon, D.A., Halsey, N.A., Orenstein, W.A., Limaye, R.J., O'Leary, S.T., Omer, S.B., 2018. The Clinician's Vaccine Safety Resource Guide: Optimizing Prevention of Vaccine-preventable Diseases Across the Lifespan. Springer.
8. Feder, L., Hoang, L., 2017. The Parents' Concise Guide to Childhood Vaccinations, 2nd Edition: From Newborns to Teens, Practical Medical and Natural Ways to Protect Your Child. Hatherleigh Press.
9. Herron, S.P., 2016. Childhood Diseases. CreateSpace Independent Publishing Platform.
10. Kimberlin, D.W., 2021. Red Book Pediatric Infectious Diseases Clinical Decision Support Chart, 2nd Edition. American Academy of Pediatrics.
11. Kimberlin, D.W., Fischer, M., Long, S.S., Prober, C.G., 2022. Principles and Practice of Pediatric Infectious Diseases, 6th Edition. Elsevier.
12. Mukwela, J., Lupwenge, J., 2021. Monitoring Morbidity and Mortality of Preventable Childhood Diseases. Our Knowledge Publishing.
13. Roush, S.W., McIntyre, L., Baldy, L.M., the CDC, 2013. Manual for the Surveillance of Vaccine-preventable Diseases, 6th Edition. CreateSpace Independent Publishing Platform.
14. Shope, T.R., Hashikawa, A.N., 2023. Managing Infectious Diseases in Child Care and Schools: A Quick Reference Guide, 6th Edition. American Academy of Pediatrics.
15. Stiehm, E.R., McGhee, S.A., Yazdani, S., 2011. Chronic Complex Diseases of Childhood: A Practical Guide for Clinicians. BrownWalker Press.
16. Thompson, J., Camp, E., Boice, J., 2017. The Unvaccinated Child: A Treatment Guide for Parents and Caregivers. Vital Health Publishing, LLC.
17. Wilkins, C.G., Brovsky, C., 2017. Two Drops That Changed the World: A Polio Survivor's Journey with Rotary International to Eradicate Polio and Promote Childhood Immunization. Wilkins.

Chapter 9

Pediatric Immunizations

Chapter Outline

Learning Objectives

After study of this chapter, readers should be able to:

1. Describe vaccination preparation.
2. Identify vaccines that are given orally in the United States.
3. Discuss the types of vaccines that must be administered subcutaneously.
4. Describe the intramuscular vaccines available for infants.
5. Identify the most common sites for intradermal vaccine administration.
6. Explain how multiple vaccines are administered.
7. Identify the documentation listed in the patient's medical chart for each vaccination.
8. Describe the pediatric vaccinations for children 6 weeks through 6 years of age.
9. Explain the CDC vaccination schedules for children 7 years through 18.
10. Discuss contraindications and precautions for immunizations.

OVERVIEW

Vaccines have significantly contributed to global reductions in morbidity and mortality by reducing the incidence of serious infectious diseases. Today,

Vaccinology and Immunizations. http://doi.org/10.1016/B978-0-443-23915-1.00009-3

people worldwide experience the benefits of immunizations, beginning in infancy. Vaccines are considered one of the most significant advances in modern medicine. They have greatly improved the quality of life by reducing or eliminating many serious infectious diseases. The effect of vaccines on public health is highly remarkable. Vaccines have contributed to worldwide reductions in morbidity and mortality by reducing the incidence of serious infectious diseases. Childhood immunizations are an essential part of preventive healthcare. The Centers for Disease Control and Prevention (CDC) and the American Academy of Pediatrics (AAP) promote public awareness and education about childhood immunizations, encouraging complete vaccination. Failure to immunize may cause severe disease from vaccine-preventable illnesses. Increased levels of immunization are required for the immunity of the community. Children may receive up to 24 injections by 2 years of age and up to 5 injections in a single visit.

PREVENTING INFECTIOUS DISEASES

Vaccine development is one of the significant achievements in medicine. The concepts of modern immunization date back to the 1790s, with Edward Jenner's work concerning preventing smallpox through vaccination with the cowpox virus. In the late 1800s, Louis Pasteur created the first live attenuated (weakened) bacterial vaccine. He later developed the first rabies vaccine. Since then, vaccines for more than 26 diseases have been developed. Vaccines have saved many lives while preventing pain, suffering, and complications from previously untreatable diseases. The World Health Organization (WHO) estimates immunization prevents approximately 2 to 3 million deaths annually. With expanded global immunization, another 1.5 million deaths could be prevented.

PREPARING FOR VACCINATION

Patients should be assessed for vaccine contraindications and precautions before vaccine administration. A screening questionnaire is used, which should be filled out by each patient or guardian before the vaccine is given. Screening questionnaires ask about past and current illnesses or health conditions that could be a reason not to give a vaccine. The questionnaires also have questions about allergies, the use of medications or blood products that could interfere with the vaccine's effect, and past reactions to vaccines. The answers to these questions must be evaluated before any vaccine administration.

VACCINATION ROUTES

In most countries, including the United States, vaccines are available in five routes: oral, intranasal, subcutaneous (SQ), intramuscular (IM), and intradermal. Oral vaccines are administered as drops into the mouth. Intranasal vaccines are administered into each nostril using a nasal sprayer. SQ injections are administered into the fatty tissue below the dermis (the outer layer of skin) but above muscle tissue. Intramuscular injections are administered into the muscle through the skin and SQ tissue. Intradermal injections are administered into the dermis.

TEST YOUR KNOWLEDGE

1. What were the earliest vaccines ever developed?
2. What determines if a vaccine can be given to a patient?
3. What are the five available routes for vaccines?

Oral

Oral vaccines are safe, easy to administer, and convenient for all ages. They have been successfully developed to protect against many infectious diseases acquired through oral transmission. Oral delivery of vaccines represents the most attractive mode of administration over other delivery routes because oral vaccination is noninvasive, safe, and straightforward to execute, showing good patient compliance and clinical practicality. The guidelines of the oral vaccine manufacturer must always be followed. If multiple types of vaccines are required, oral vaccines should be administered first. They are given slowly to the inside of the mouth on one side or, if the patient is an infant, between the cheek and the gum. If the infant spits the dose out, it is not recommended to readminister. Rotavirus, adenovirus, cholera vaccine, and oral typhoid vaccines are the only vaccines administered orally in the United States. Oral typhoid capsules should be administered as directed by the manufacturer. The oral polio vaccine is administered in other countries. The rotavirus vaccine is contraindicated in infants with a history of **intussusception** or uncorrected congenital malformation of the gastrointestinal tract that would predispose them to intussusception.

Intranasal

The **live attenuated influenza vaccine** (**LAIV**) is the only vaccine administered intranasally in the United States, following manufacturer guidance. The vaccine syringe has a clip that separates the dose into two 0.1-mL sprays. Each spray is given in the left and right nostrils while the patient sits and breathes normally. The dose should be avoided if the patient sneezes or expels the quantity. Studies show that IM and nasal vaccine administration have similar efficacy.

Subcutaneous

Subcutaneous (SQ) injection is given in the fatty tissue, just under the skin. This contains fewer blood vessels than muscle, which releases the vaccine more slowly and consistently. Certain vaccines must be given via SQ injection. These vaccines include measles, mumps, and rubella (MMR), inactivated polio, and varicella (chickenpox). For an infant under 12 months of age, the preferred SQ site is the fatty tissue on the thigh (Figure 9.1). The upper outer triceps (posterior edge of the upper arm) may also be used if necessary. All possible SQ injection sites are shown in Figure 9.2. The upper outer triceps muscle is used for children 1 year and older. A 5/8-inch, 25-gauge needle should be used. The needle is inserted at a 45-degree angle into the SQ tissue.

TEST YOUR KNOWLEDGE

1. If multiple vaccines are required simultaneously, which type should be administered first?
2. What vaccines should be administered SQ?

Intramuscular

Most vaccines are injected into thick muscle tissue—usually a muscle in the upper arms or thighs. These muscles contain lots of blood vessels, which means the vaccine is dispersed into the general circulation relatively quickly, as well as immune cells called antigen-presenting cells that mediate lasting protective responses to vaccines. **Intramuscular injections** also tend to have few severe side effects besides mild pain and redness at the injection site. Even so, they are usually only given by trained healthcare professionals to avoid damage to nerves or blood vessels. Intramuscular vaccines include diphtheria-tetanus-pertussis, inactivated influenza, and human papillomavirus.

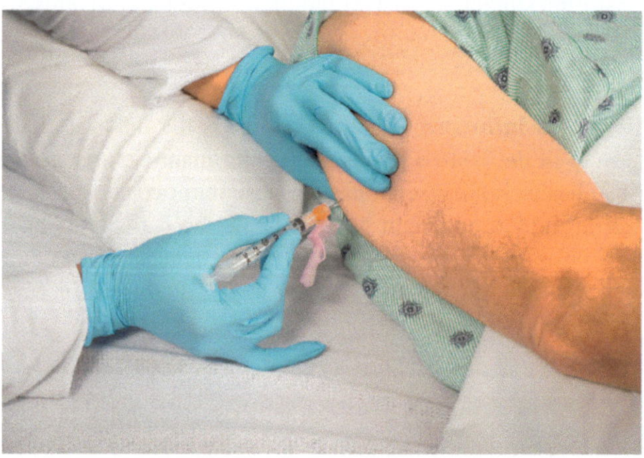

FIGURE 9.1 Subcutaneous injection.

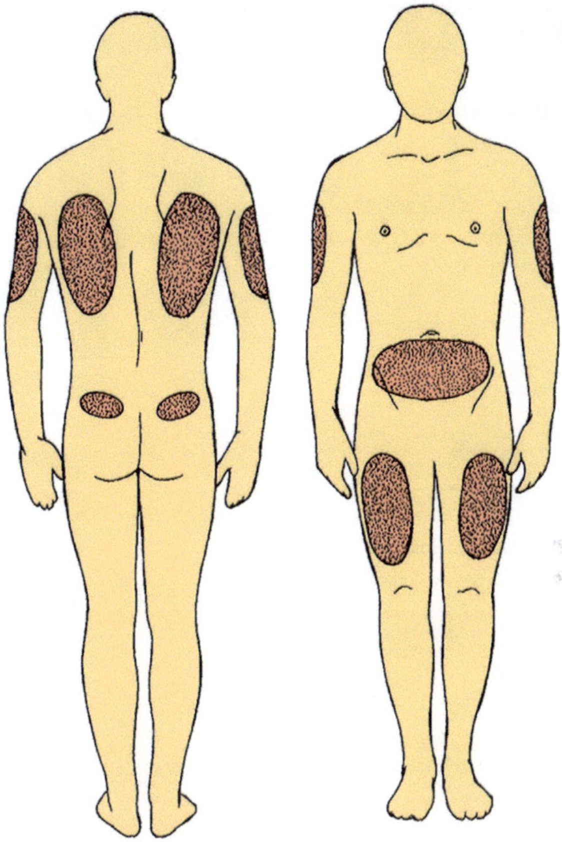

FIGURE 9.2 Sites used for subcutaneous injection.

For infants, the preferred site for IM injection is the **vastus lateralis muscle** (Figure 9.3). A needle gauge must be 22 to 25, with a length of 5/8 inch. The deltoid muscle is the preferred site in children 3 years and older.

Intradermal

The **intradermal route** is only widely used for allergy testing. Therefore this route is rarely used for vaccine administration. It is only used to administer Bacillus Calmette-Guérin (BCG) and some rabies vaccines (most given IM). It is essential to follow the manufacturer's guidelines for administration. The needle is held at a low angle (15 degrees). The needle is about 1/4 inch, with the entire bevel under the skin (Figure 9.4). The most common sites for intradermal vaccine administration are the inner surface of the forearm and the upper back, below the scapula. Because the skin is so thin, intradermal injections usually need to be delivered by trained health care professionals.

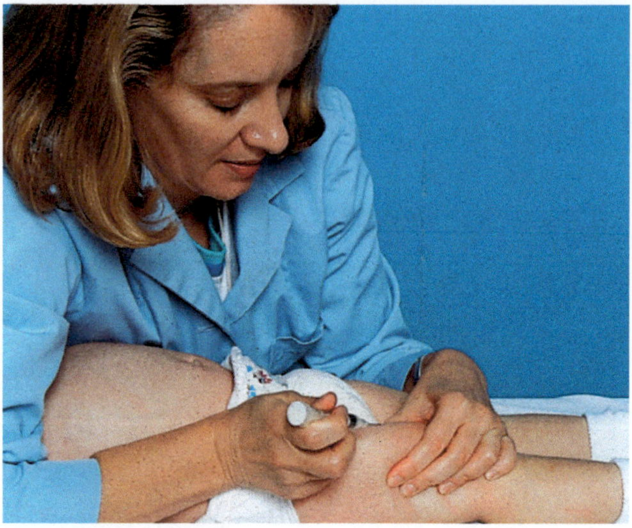

FIGURE 9.3 Intramuscular injection.

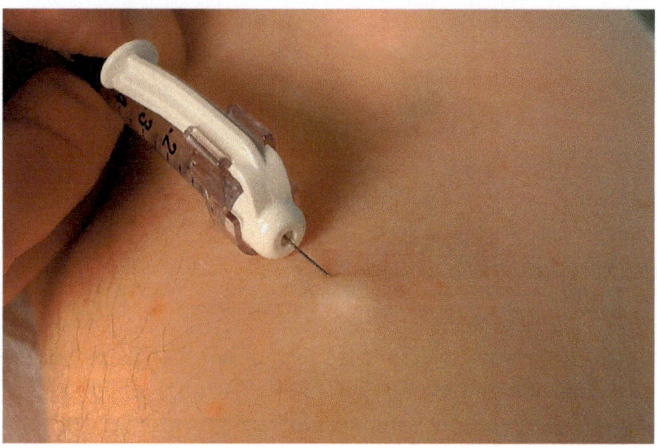

FIGURE 9.4 Intradermal injection.

You Should Remember

Regardless of the route, healthcare personnel must always perform hand hygiene before administering vaccines. Occupational Safety and Health Administration (OSHA) regulations usually do not require gloves to be worn unless the health professional involved is likely to come in contact with potentially infectious body fluids or has open hand lesions.

TEST YOUR KNOWLEDGE

1. What are examples of vaccines administered IM?
2. What are the most common sites of IM injections?

MULTIPLE-VACCINE ADMINISTRATION

If **multiple vaccines** must be administered, separate anatomical sites are used. If the same muscle group must be used, the injection sites must be separated by at least 1 inch. It is important to remember that oral vaccines are given first before any other types of vaccines. One reason for this is that, for example, infants will likely be less upset before injections and more likely to ingest the oral liquid. The more painful vaccines such as MMR, pneumococcal conjugate vaccine (PCV13, PCV15, or PCV20), and human papillomavirus should be administered last.

Examples of combination vaccines include diphtheria, tetanus, and pertussis (DTaP), trivalent inactivated polio vaccine (IPV) (three strains of the IPV), MMR, DTaP-*Haemophilus influenzae* type B (Hib), and Hib-hepatitis B.

DOCUMENTATION

The **National Childhood Vaccine Injury Act (NCVIA)** of 1986 was created to address public health concerns regarding the safety of vaccines and to reduce the liability to vaccine companies from adverse effect–related lawsuits so that vaccine production would not be slowed or stopped. Under this act, the first six items listed as follows must be documented in the patient's medical chart for each vaccination. Items 7 and 8 must be written based on best practice standards.

1. Date of administration
2. Manufacturer
3. Lot number
4. Name and title of vaccinator
5. Address of clinic/facility where the permanent record is located
6. Vaccine information statement: its date and the date given to the patient, or the family of the patient
7. Additional documentation includes vaccine type, route, dose volume, and site document vaccine refusal

After a vaccine is given, it must be reported to the patient's primary care provider and the state's **immunization information system** (IIS), if applicable. Any adverse events after the vaccine was given must also be documented and reported to the patient's primary care provider. Documentation of vaccination should be provided to the patient or guardian.

Many states have an **IIS**. Also known as an immunization registry, an IIS is a database that contains vaccination information for each child in a particular region, usually a state. The IIS is also used for adults. Vaccination information from multiple-vaccine providers can be entered into this central database. Providers can check the child's immunization status or last vaccination date for a series. Pharmacies that immunize children can participate in their state's IIS. To participate in the IIS plan, state instructions must be followed closely.

TEST YOUR KNOWLEDGE

1. How far apart on the body should multiple vaccines be administered?
2. What are examples of combination vaccines?
3. What six items *must* be documented in a patient's medical chart for every vaccination given?

VACCINATION SCHEDULES

To date, there has been extensive research on developing immunization schedules. Factors that must be considered include immune system development in children, maternal antibodies in infants, and the immunogenicity of vaccine antigens at different stages of development. Research on the time between doses and the timing of catch-up schedule dosing has also been considered. Vaccination schedules are updated regularly and posted on the CDC immunization schedule webpage. To read a vaccine schedule, start with the recommended plan for the patient's age. If the patient is behind on vaccines, refer to the catch-up schedule. Keep in mind which medical conditions and unique situations require additional vaccines. Also, consider medical conditions for which certain vaccines should be avoided.

Children From Birth Through 6 Years

Pediatric formulations for children 6 weeks through 6 years of age include DT (the generic formulation only, which does not include pertussis) and DTaP, which has various trade names from different manufacturers. Combination products that contain additional vaccine antigens are often used for infants. These include DTaP-hepatitis B-IPV and DTaP-IPV-Hib. Other products containing DTaP-IPV are approved for 4- to 6-year-old children for the fourth IPV dose and the fifth DTaP dose only. The CDC vaccination schedules for children 6 weeks through 6 years are shown in Figure 9.5.

Children 7 Years Through 17 Years

Children 7 or older and adults can receive the Td vaccine. Once again, this product does not include pertussis. Tdap is FDA approved for individuals 10

Your child needs vaccines as they grow!

2025 Recommended Immunizations for Birth Through 6 Years Old

Want to learn more?
Scan this QR code to find out which vaccines your child might need. Or visit **www2.cdc.gov/vaccines/childquiz/**

<table>
<tr><th>VACCINE OR PREVENTIVE ANTIBODY</th><th>BIRTH</th><th>1 MONTH</th><th>2 MONTHS</th><th>4 MONTHS</th><th>6 MONTHS</th><th>7 MONTHS</th><th>8 MONTHS</th><th>12 MONTHS</th><th>15 MONTHS</th><th>18 MONTHS</th><th>19 MONTHS</th><th>20–23 MONTHS</th><th>2-3 YEARS</th><th>4-6 YEARS</th></tr>
<tr><td>RSV antibody</td><td colspan="6">Depends on mother's RSV vaccine status</td><td colspan="6">Depends on child's health status</td><td></td><td></td><td></td></tr>
<tr><td>Hepatitis B</td><td>Dose 1</td><td colspan="2">Dose 2</td><td></td><td colspan="6">Dose 3</td><td></td><td></td><td></td><td></td></tr>
<tr><td>Rotavirus</td><td></td><td></td><td>Dose 1</td><td>Dose 2</td><td>Dose 3</td><td></td><td></td><td></td><td></td><td></td><td></td><td></td><td></td><td></td></tr>
<tr><td>DTaP</td><td></td><td></td><td>Dose 1</td><td>Dose 2</td><td>Dose 3</td><td></td><td></td><td></td><td colspan="2">Dose 4</td><td></td><td></td><td></td><td>Dose 5</td></tr>
<tr><td>Hib</td><td></td><td></td><td>Dose 1</td><td>Dose 2</td><td>Dose 3</td><td></td><td></td><td colspan="2">Dose 4</td><td></td><td></td><td></td><td></td><td></td></tr>
<tr><td>Pneumococcal</td><td></td><td></td><td>Dose 1</td><td>Dose 2</td><td>Dose 3</td><td></td><td></td><td colspan="2">Dose 4</td><td></td><td></td><td></td><td></td><td></td></tr>
<tr><td>Polio</td><td></td><td></td><td>Dose 1</td><td>Dose 2</td><td colspan="6">Dose 3</td><td></td><td></td><td></td><td>Dose 4</td></tr>
<tr><td>COVID-19</td><td></td><td></td><td></td><td></td><td colspan="10"></td></tr>
<tr><td>Influenza/Flu</td><td></td><td></td><td></td><td></td><td colspan="10">Every year. Two doses for some children</td></tr>
<tr><td>MMR</td><td></td><td></td><td></td><td></td><td></td><td></td><td></td><td colspan="2">Dose 1</td><td></td><td></td><td></td><td></td><td>Dose 2</td></tr>
<tr><td>Chickenpox</td><td></td><td></td><td></td><td></td><td></td><td></td><td></td><td colspan="2">Dose 1</td><td></td><td></td><td></td><td></td><td>Dose 2</td></tr>
<tr><td>Hepatitis A</td><td></td><td></td><td></td><td></td><td></td><td></td><td></td><td colspan="5">2 doses separated by 6 months</td><td></td><td></td></tr>
</table>

KEY

- ALL children should be immunized at this age
- SOME children should get this dose of vaccine or preventive antibody at this age
- Parents/caregivers should talk to their health care provider to decide if this vaccine is right for their child

Talk to your child's health care provider for more guidance if:

1. Your child has any medical condition that puts them at higher risk for infection.
2. Your child is traveling outside the United States. Visit **wwwnc.cdc.gov/travel** for more information.
3. Your child misses a vaccine recommended for their age.

CDC U.S. CENTERS FOR DISEASE CONTROL AND PREVENTION

FOR MORE INFORMATION
Call toll-free: 1-800-CDC-INFO (1-800-232-4636)
Or visit: www2.cdc.gov/vaccines/childquiz/

What diseases do these vaccines protect against?

BIRTH–6 YEARS OLD

VACCINE-PREVENTABLE DISEASE	DISEASE COMPLICATIONS
RSV (Respiratory syncytial virus) Contagious viral infection of the nose, throat, and sometimes lungs; spread through air and direct contact	Infection of the lungs (pneumonia) and small airways of the lungs; especially dangerous for infants and young children
Hepatitis B Contagious viral infection of the liver; spread through contact with infected body fluids such as blood or semen	Chronic liver infection, liver failure, liver cancer, death
Rotavirus Contagious viral infection of the gut; spread through the mouth from hands and food contaminated with stool	Severe diarrhea, dehydration, death
Diphtheria* Illness caused by a toxin produced by bacteria that infects the nose, throat, and sometimes skin	Swelling of the heart muscle, heart failure, coma, paralysis, death
Pertussis (Whooping Cough)* Contagious bacterial infection of the lungs and airway; spread through air and direct contact	Infection of the lungs (pneumonia), death; especially dangerous for babies
Tetanus (Lockjaw)* Bacterial infection of brain and nerves caused by spores found in soil and dust everywhere; spores enter the body through wounds or broken skin	Seizures, broken bones, difficulty breathing, death
Hib (Haemophilus influenzae type b) Contagious bacterial infection of the lungs, brain and spinal cord, or bloodstream; spread through air and direct contact	Depends on the part of the body infected, but can include brain damage, hearing loss, loss of arm or leg, death
Pneumococcal Bacterial infections of ears, sinuses, lungs, or bloodstream; spread through direct contact with respiratory droplets like saliva or mucus	Depends on the part of the body infected, but can include infection of the lungs (pneumonia), blood poisoning, infection of the lining of the brain and spinal cord, death
Polio Contagious viral infection of nerves and brain; spread through the mouth from stool on contaminated hands, food or liquid, and by air and direct contact	Paralysis, death
COVID-19 Contagious viral infection of the nose, throat, or lungs; may feel like a cold or flu. Spread through air and direct contact	Infection of the lungs (pneumonia); blood clots; liver, heart or kidney damage; long COVID; death
Influenza (Flu) Contagious viral infection of the nose, throat, and sometimes lungs; spread through air and direct contact	Infection of the lungs (pneumonia), sinus and ear infections, worsening of underlying heart or lung conditions, death
Measles (Rubeola)† Contagious viral infection that causes high fever, cough, red eyes, runny nose, and rash; spread through air and direct contact	Brain swelling, infection of the lungs (pneumonia), death
Mumps† Contagious viral infection that causes fever, tiredness, swollen cheeks, and tender swollen jaw; spread through air and direct contact	Brain swelling, painful and swollen testicles or ovaries, deafness, death
Rubella (German Measles)† Contagious viral infection that causes low-grade fever, sore throat, and rash; spread through air and direct contact	Very dangerous in pregnant women; can cause miscarriage or stillbirth, premature delivery, severe birth defects
Chickenpox (Varicella) Contagious viral infection that causes fever, headache, and an itchy, blistering rash; spread through air and direct contact	Infected sores, brain swelling, infection of the lungs (pneumonia), death
Hepatitis A Contagious viral infection of the liver; spread by contaminated food or drink or close contact with an infected person	Liver failure, death

*DTaP protects against tetanus, diphtheria, and pertussis †MMR protects against measles, mumps, and rubella

Last updated June 2025

FIGURE 9.5 CDC vaccination schedules for children 6 weeks through 6 years.

years of age and older. The primary vaccination series consists of five doses at 2, 4, 6, and 15 to 18 months and between 4 and 6 years of age. Booster doses are recommended at 11 to 12 years of age with Tdap and then every 10 years after that with Td. If the infant series was not given or was started late, the catch-up schedule specifies the dose timing and formulations to be used. Each of these vaccines is a 0.5-mL IM injection. The CDC vaccination schedules for children 7 years through 18 years are shown in Figure 9.6.

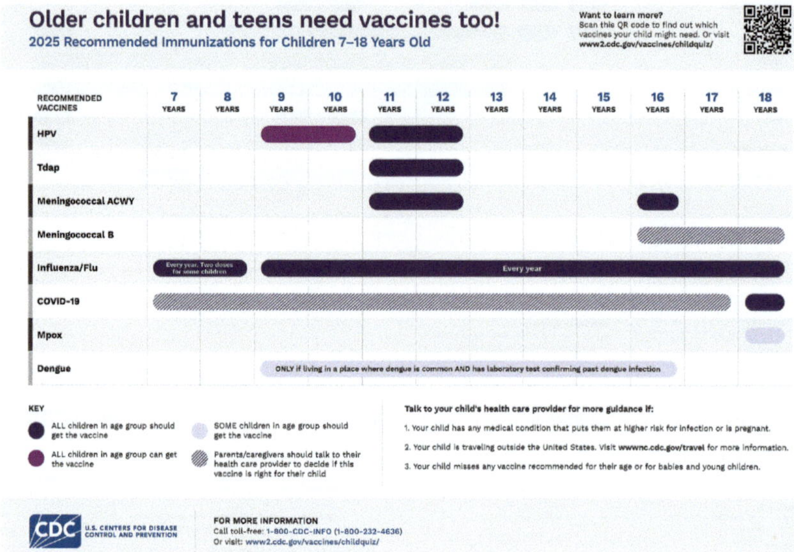

What diseases do these vaccines protect against?

7-18 YEARS OLD

VACCINE-PREVENTABLE DISEASE	DISEASE COMPLICATIONS	NUMBER OF VACCINE DOSES
HPV (Human papillomavirus) Contagious viral infection spread by close skin-to-skin touching, including during sex	Genital warts and many types of cancers later in life, including cancers of the cervix, vagina, penis, anus, and throat	2 or 3 doses
Tetanus (Lockjaw)* Infection caused by bacterial spores found in soil and dust everywhere; spores enter the body through wounds or broken skin	Seizures, broken bones, difficulty breathing, death	1 dose at age 11-12 years Additional doses if missed childhood doses 1 dose for dirty wounds
Diphtheria* Illness caused by a toxin produced by bacteria that infects the nose, throat, and sometimes skin	Swelling of the heart muscle, heart failure, coma, paralysis, death	1 dose at age 11-12 years Additional doses if missed childhood doses
Pertussis (Whooping Cough)* Contagious bacterial infection of the lungs and airway; spread through air and direct contact	Infection of the lungs (pneumonia), death; especially dangerous for babies	1 dose at age 11-12 years Additional doses if missed childhood doses 1 dose every pregnancy
Meningococcal** Contagious bacterial infection of the lining of the brain and spinal cord or the bloodstream; spread through air and direct contact	Loss of arm or leg, deafness, seizures, death	2 doses. Additional doses may be needed depending on medical condition or vaccine used.
Influenza (Flu) Contagious viral infection of the nose, throat, and sometimes lungs; spread through air and direct contact	Infection of the lungs (pneumonia), sinus and ear infections, worsening of underlying heart or lung conditions, death	1 dose each year 2 doses in some children aged 6months through 8 years
COVID-19 Contagious viral infection of the nose, throat, or lungs; may feel like a cold or flu. Spread through air and direct contact	Infection of the lungs (pneumonia); blood clots; liver, heart or kidney damage; long COVID; death	1 or more doses of the current COVID-19 vaccine depending on health status. For more information: **www.cdc.gov/covidschedule**
Mpox Contagious viral infection spread through close, often skin-to-skin contact, including sex; causes a painful rash, fever, headache, tiredness, cough, runny nose, sore throat, swollen lymph nodes	Infected sores, brain swelling, infection of the lungs (pneumonia), eye infection, blindness, death	2 doses
Dengue Viral infection spread by bite from infected mosquito; causes fever, headache, pain behind the eyes, rash, joint pain, body ache, nausea, loss of appetite, feeling tired, abdominal pain	Severe bleeding, seizures, shock, damage to the liver, heart, and lungs, death	3 doses

*Tdap protects against tetanus, diphtheria, and pertussis **Healthy adolescents: Meningococcal ACWY vaccine (2 doses); Meningococcal B vaccine (2 doses if needed).

FIGURE 9.6 CDC vaccination schedules for children 7 years through 17 years.

TEST YOUR KNOWLEDGE

1. What factors must be considered when vaccination schedules are developed, regardless of the patient's age?
2. What are the pediatric formulations for children 6 weeks through 6 years of age?
3. What is the primary vaccination series for Tdap?

Contraindications and Precautions

Any vaccine may be contraindicated in persons with proven immediate or **anaphylactic hypersensitivity** to any vaccine component (except egg allergy) or its container (such as latex). If additional doses are needed, this should be assessed by an allergist. A precaution is a condition that may increase the risk of an adverse reaction following immunization or compromise the vaccine's ability to produce immunity. Generally, vaccines are deferred when a precaution is present. However, there may be circumstances when the benefits of giving the vaccine outweigh potential risks or when reduced vaccine immunogenicity may significantly benefit an immunocompromised individual. Some precautions and contraindications depend on whether a vaccine is a live attenuated product or a nonlive product. Situations with specific contraindications or precautions include the following:

- **Gastroenteritis**
  - Delay oral typhoid, cholera, and travelers' diarrhea vaccines until the illness has resolved.
  - Defer rotavirus vaccine until the patient's condition improves unless deferral results in scheduling the first dose beyond the recommended age limit.
- **Inflammatory eye disease treated with steroids**
  - Defer first-generation smallpox vaccine, if a nonoutbreak situation, until the patient's condition resolves or the course of steroids is completed.
- **Measles**
  - Delay any vaccine that contains varicella for 6 weeks (a minimum of 4 weeks' delay can be applied if needed).
- **Medically attended wheezing** (in the 7 days before vaccination)
  - LAIV is contraindicated.
- **Tuberculosis, active, untreated**
  - A natural measles infection may exacerbate tuberculosis. However, there is no evidence that measles- or varicella-containing vaccines have this type of effect; MMR, MMR-varicella, varicella, and live zoster vaccines are contraindicated as a precautionary measure.

Mild illnesses, with or without fever (such as an upper respiratory tract infection or otitis media), do not increase the risk of adverse events after immunization or interfere with the response to vaccines. There are no associated contraindications or precautions, so these should not be used as a reason to withhold or delay immunization. The only exception is when nasal congestion is present, which could impede the delivery of LAIV to the nasopharyngeal mucosa. In these cases, the nonlive influenza vaccine can be offered.

A vaccine is contraindicated in a person with a documented history of confirmed anaphylaxis after the previous administration of the same vaccine. However, exceptions may apply (such as the Imvamune and mRNA COVID-19 vaccines). If there is uncertainty regarding the diagnosis of anaphylaxis or which vaccine (or vaccine component) may have triggered it, an expert must be consulted.

There are no contraindications or precautions associated with a history of a febrile seizure after a previous immunization. Children with a history of febrile seizures have no increased risk of developing any seizure disorder. Vaccines are generally safe for people with skin disorders. Vaccines should be administered to a nonaffected area of the skin for comfort. Some smallpox vaccines and BCG are exceptions to this. The Imvamune vaccine can be safely administered in people with eczema (atopic dermatitis). The BCG vaccine is contraindicated when there is extensive skin disease or burns.

Pertussis-containing vaccines should be delayed if a child has a suspected or known neurologic condition that is currently evolving. Examples include infantile spasms, progressive encephalopathy, and uncontrolled epilepsy. Once treatment has been started and the conditions have stabilized or resolved, the benefits and risks of vaccinating must be reconsidered. Suppose an exaggerated local reaction (such as excessive, painful swelling from the shoulder to the elbow) has occurred in the past after a diphtheria- or tetanus-containing vaccine. In that case, the patient should only receive a vaccine every 10 years. Additional emergency booster doses should not be given.

You Should Remember

There are no contraindications or precautions associated with a history of fainting after a previous immunization. The likelihood of fainting can be reduced by lowering stress in patients awaiting immunization. These measures include short waiting times, a comfortable room temperature, preparation of vaccines out of view of recipients, and privacy during the procedure. People should be immunized while seated or lying down.

You Should Remember

Every year, various medical boards and committees collaborate to develop recommendations for the routine use of vaccines in children and adolescents in the United States. Because a baby's immune system is not fully developed at birth, they face a greater risk of becoming infected and getting seriously ill from various diseases if they are not sufficiently vaccinated. Vaccination helps by building up their natural defenses.

You Should Remember

Egg allergy is one of the most common food allergies in childhood, with a prevalence of approximately 2%. It is often associated with eczema in infants and asthma in young children. However, allergic diseases are not a contraindication to immunization with egg protein–containing vaccines.

You Should Remember

Healthy preterm infants weighing 1500 grams or more at birth generally tolerate immunizations well, with rates of adverse events similar to the low rates also seen in full-term infants. Hospitalized premature infants should have continuous cardiac and respiratory monitoring for 48 hours after their first immunization.

TEST YOUR KNOWLEDGE

1. What is the definition of a vaccine "precaution"?
2. What vaccine precautions are taken for gastroenteritis?
3. When is a vaccine contraindicated for a specific person?

KEY TERMS

Immunization information system
Intradermal route
Intramuscular injections
Intussusception
Multiple vaccines
National Childhood Vaccine Injury Act
Oral vaccines
Subcutaneous injection
Vastus lateralis muscle

CASE STUDIES

Case Study 1

An oral rotavirus vaccine was accidentally administered to an infant by injection. The infant developed severe redness around the injection site, causing her to cry continuously. This indicated that there was likely some amount of pain also present. It was found that the nurse who had administered the injection was not fully trained and mistook the oral vaccine as injectable.

Critical Thinking Questions

1. What should healthcare workers required to administer vaccines do before every vaccination if an unfamiliar product is being used?
2. What are the contraindications of the rotavirus vaccine in infants?
3. How is the oral rotavirus vaccine intended to be correctly administered?

Case Study 2

A preterm male infant (born at 32 weeks of gestation) was given the BCG vaccine at 2 months. He received a full vaccine vial (10 times the usual dose) IM into his right thigh. The infant developed swelling in the right thigh, which worsened over time. An MRI of the right thigh showed an IM abscess in the vastus muscle. The spot was surgically drained. Afterward, the infant was treated with amoxicillin and clavulanic acid. The wound continued to discharge pus for almost 6 months, and a sinus formed that later healed, leaving a puckered scar.

Critical Thinking Questions

1. How is the BCG vaccine administered?
2. What are the contraindications of the BCG vaccine?
3. What does BCG stand for?

Case Study 3

A 1-year-old infant accidentally received a double dose of the same vaccine because an error was made in double-checking the generic components of two trade-name drugs: MMRII and Priorix. These trade-name drugs contain the live MMR vaccines. The error was correctly reported, and the family was apologized to.

Critical Thinking Questions

1. How are the MMRII and Priorix vaccines given?
2. What resources must be checked in order to determine which vaccines are needed for infants and when they are needed?
3. What is the correct way to report vaccine administration and any adverse events?

FURTHER READING

1. Abbas, A.K., Lichtman, A.H., Pillai, S., 2021. Cellular and Molecular Immunology, 10th Edition. Elsevier.
2. Alter, J., 2010. Vaccines (21st Century Skills Innovation Library). Cherry Lake Publishing.
3. Bansal, R., 2021. Antibodies and Their Role in Therapeutics (Biotechnology). Bansal.
4. Blaxill, M., Olmsted, D., 2015. Vaccines 2.0: The Careful Parent's Guide to Making Safe Vaccination Choices for Your Family. Skyhorse.
5. Cook, W., Klaas, K., 2020. Mayo Clinic Guide to Your Baby's First Years, 2nd Edition. Mayo Clinic Press.
6. Cowan, T., Fallon Morell, S., 2018. Vaccines, Autoimmunity, and the Changing Nature of Childhood Illness. Chelsea Green Publishing.
7. Doan, T., Lievano, F., Swanson-Mungerson, M., Viselli, S.M., 2021. Lippincott Illustrated Reviews: Immunology (Illustrated Reviews Series), 3rd Edition. Wolters Kluwer Health.

8. Feder, L., Hoang, L., 2017. The Parents' Concise Guide to Childhood Vaccinations – Revised and Updated (2nd) Edition – Practical Medical and Natural Ways to Protect Your Child. Hatherleigh Press.
9. Humphries, S., Bystrianyk, R., 2013. Dissolving Illusions – Disease, Vaccines, and the Forgotten History. CreateSpace Independent Publishing Platform.
10. Miller, N.Z., 2010. Vaccines, Autism and Childhood Disorders – Crucial Data That Could Save Your Child's Life. New Atlantean Press.
11. Miller, N.Z., 2016. Miller's Review of Critical Vaccine Studies: 400 Important Scientific Papers Summarized for Parents and Researchers. New Atlantean Press.
12. Morcan, J., Morcan, L., 2020. Vaccine Science Revisited – Are Childhood Immunizations As Safe As Claimed?. Sterling Gate Books.
13. Moskowitz, R., Holland, M., 2020. Vaccines: A Reappraisal. Skyhorse.
14. Murphy, K.M., Weaver, C., Berg, L., 2022. Janeway's Immunobiology, 10th Edition. W.W. Norton & Company.
15. Offit, P., Moser, C., 2011. Vaccines and Your Child: Separating Fact from Fiction. Columbia University Press.
16. Polinsky, P.V., Ginevra, D., 2022. Vaccines: A Graphic History (Medical Breakthroughs). Graphic Universe.
17. Rich, R.R., Fleisher, T.A., Schroeder Jr., H.W., Weyand, C.M., Corry, D.B., Puck, J.M., 2022. Clinical Immunology: Principles and Practice, 6th Edition. Elsevier.
18. Sears, R.W., 2011. The Vaccine Book: Making the Right Decision for Your Child (Sears Parenting Library). Little Brown, Spark.
19. Shope, T.R., Hashikawa, A.N., 2023. Managing Infectious Diseases in Child Care and Schools: A Quick Reference Guide, 6th Edition. American Academy of Pediatrics.
20. Thomas, P., Margulis, J., 2016. The Vaccine-Friendly Plan – Safe and Effective Approach to Immunity and Health – From Pregnancy Through Your Child's Teen Years. Ballantine Books.
21. Thompson, J., Camp, E., Boice, J., 2017. The Unvaccinated Child: A Treatment Guide for Parents and Caregivers. Vital Health Publishing, LLC.

Chapter 10

Adult Immunizations

Chapter Outline

Learning Objectives

After study of this chapter, readers should be able to:

1. Explain why it is recommended to get the flu vaccine annually.
2. Describe various types of diphtheria and tetanus vaccines.
3. Discuss the characteristics of shingles and their vaccines.
4. Identify human papillomavirus and its complications.
5. Explain the contraindications for the pneumococcal vaccine.
6. Describe a routine series of vaccines for hepatitis A and B.
7. Explain immunizations during pregnancy.
8. Discuss the COVID-19 vaccines.
9. Identify the signs and symptoms of Ebola.
10. Describe the monkeypox virus and its vaccine.

Vaccinology and Immunizations. http://doi.org/10.1016/B978-0-443-23915-1.00010-X

OVERVIEW

Vaccination is recommended throughout life to prevent vaccine-preventable diseases and their sequelae. The primary focus of vaccination programs has historically been directed to childhood immunizations. For adults, chronic diseases have been the primary focus of preventive and medical health care, though there has been increased emphasis on preventing infectious diseases. However, adult vaccination coverage remains low for most routinely recommended vaccines. Though adults are less susceptible to falling prey to traditional contagious pathogens, the probability of exposure to infectious agents has increased due to globalization and growing travel opportunities within and across countries. Thus there is an urgent need to address the problem of adult immunization. The adult immunization enterprise is more complex, encompassing various vaccines and a diverse target population. There needs to be coordinated public health infrastructure to support an adult immunization program as there is for children. Moreover, there is little coordination among adult healthcare providers regarding vaccine provision. Substantial improvement in adult vaccination is needed to reduce the health consequences of vaccine-preventable diseases among adults. Routine assessment of adult patient vaccination needs, recommendation, and offer of vaccines required for adults should be incorporated into the regular clinical care of adults. Despite the availability of vaccines, many adults remain unvaccinated because they are unaware of the need for adult vaccines or are misinformed about vaccines and the diseases they are designed to prevent.

INFLUENZA VACCINES

Influenza vaccines protect against influenza, or the flu, a contagious respiratory illness caused by viruses that infect the nose, throat, and sometimes the lungs. Influenza can cause mild to severe illness and sometimes lead to death. Immunization is the best way to protect against the flu. The vaccine prevents millions of illnesses and flu-related medical visits each year. For example, during 2019–20, the last flu season before the COVID-19 pandemic, flu vaccination prevented an estimated 7.5 million influenza illnesses, 3.7 million influenza-associated medical visits, 105,000 hospitalizations, and 6300 influenza-associated deaths. During seasons when flu vaccine viruses are similar to circulating flu viruses, the flu vaccine has been shown to reduce the risk of having to go to the doctor with flu by 40%–60%.

There are two main types of flu vaccine: the inactivated influenza vaccine delivered by intramuscular (IM) injection and the live attenuated influenza vaccine given as a nasal spray. The vaccines may be **trivalent vaccines** or **quadrivalent vaccines**. Children under 9 years of age who have never had an influenza vaccine need two doses, 4 weeks apart. Influenza viruses constantly mutate, so flu vaccines may be updated from one season to the next to protect against the viruses predicted for the upcoming flu season. However, because the protection offered by a flu vaccine declines over time, yearly vaccination is needed for the best protection.

The flu vaccines can protect against the four influenza viruses that research indicates will be most common during the upcoming season. Most flu vaccines are given IM with a needle, usually in the deltoid muscle, but there also is a nasal spray flu vaccine. Different flu vaccine manufacturers and multiple flu vaccines are licensed and recommended for use in the United States. For people younger than 65, the Centers for Disease Control and Prevention (CDC) recommends any licensed, age-appropriate flu vaccine over another during the 2022–23 flu season. Options for this age group include inactivated influenza vaccine, recombinant influenza vaccine, or live attenuated influenza vaccine, with no preference for any flu vaccine over another. Three flu vaccines are preferentially recommended for people 65 years and older over standard-dose, unadjuvanted flu vaccines. These are Fluzone high-dose quadrivalent flu vaccine, Flublok quadrivalent recombinant flu vaccine, and Fluad quadrivalent adjuvanted flu vaccine.

All flu vaccines for the 2022–23 season are quadrivalent, designed to protect against four flu viruses, including two influenza A viruses and two influenza B viruses. Common side effects from a flu shot include soreness, redness, swelling at the site of the injections, headache, fever, nausea, muscle aches, and fatigue. The flu shot, like other injections, can occasionally cause fainting. Life-threatening allergic reactions to flu shots are infrequent.

TETANUS, DIPHTHERIA, AND PERTUSSIS VACCINES

Diphtheria, tetanus, and pertussis are potentially severe bacterial diseases that can be safely prevented in adults and children with vaccines. For more details, see Chapter 8.

Diphtheria

Diphtheria is a bacterial pathogen. A toxin causes the disease symptoms. Diphtheria affects the mucous membranes of the mouth and throat. It causes a thick gray coating in the back of the throat, making it challenging to swallow and breathe. Other symptoms include fever, malaise, sore throat, and decreased appetite. The toxin may also result in myocarditis, coma, and death.

Tetanus

Tetanus is a disease caused by a toxin produced by the bacterium *Clostridium tetani*. Spores of the organism are found in soil and typically enter the body through a cut or wound. The spores grow and form toxins that cause muscle spasms and convulsions. The disease often starts with muscle spasms in the jaw, causing lockjaw, and then spreads to other muscles. Neonatal tetanus is a condition in newborns due to infection of the unhealed umbilical stump.

Pertussis

Pertussis, also called *whooping cough*, is a disease caused by a bacterium called *Bordetella pertussis*. Toxin and other molecules are produced by the bacteria that contribute to symptoms such as runny nose, sneezing, fever, and rapid-fire coughing, followed by a whooping noise as the patient inhales. Complications include bacterial pneumonia, seizures, encephalopathy, brain swelling from reduced oxygen supply to the brain, and death. Pertussis is contagious and transmitted through contact with respiratory droplets. Tetanus, diphtheria, and pertussis were discussed in greater detail in Chapter 8.

All adults who have never received a diphtheria-containing vaccine should get one Tdap shot. This can be given at any time and should be followed by a Td or Tdap shot every 10 years. Tdap vaccine is an acceptable alternative to the Td vaccine, including when a tetanus booster is indicated for wound management. Pregnant females should get one dose of the Tdap vaccine every pregnancy, preferably early in the third trimester. Several different types of vaccines can safely prevent diphtheria, tetanus, and pertussis:

- **DTaP** (diphtheria, tetanus, and acellular pertussis) vaccine, which is given to children
- **DT** (diphtheria and tetanus) vaccine, which is given to children
- **Tdap** (combined tetanus, diphtheria, and acellular pertussis) vaccine, which is given to adolescents and adults
- **Td** (tetanus and diphtheria) vaccine, which is given to adolescents and adults

You Should Remember

Abbreviations for vaccines can be confusing. With the tetanus, diphtheria, and pertussis vaccine, the capital letters DTaP indicate a higher antigen content. Younger children require a higher antigen content for the primary series. Therefore babies and young children are given DTaP, while older children will be given Tdap.

You Should Remember

If a person has had diphtheria or tetanus, they should still be immunized against it. If a person has had pertussis, immunity can be reduced over time. Vaccination is still recommended. The series does not need to be restarted if the vaccination schedule is interrupted.

You Should Remember

The CDC recommends a single dose of Tdap for healthcare personnel who have never received Tdap, regardless of the time since their most recent Td vaccination. After receiving one dose of Tdap, healthcare personnel should receive a dose of Td or Tdap every 10 years.

TEST YOUR KNOWLEDGE

1. What are the two main types of influenza vaccines?
2. What are the causes of diphtheria, tetanus, and pertussis?
3. Which diphtheria/tetanus/pertussis vaccinations are given to adults?

MEASLES, MUMPS, AND RUBELLA VACCINES

Measles is a disease caused by a virus. It is highly contagious through contact with respiratory droplets and aerosolized droplets. Measles causes high fever, cough, runny nose, eye redness, and rash. Complications from the disease include diarrhea, ear infections, pneumonia, **encephalitis**, seizures, and death (in 0.2% of cases).

Mumps is a viral illness that causes headaches, muscle aches, fever, decreased appetite, and malaise. A common symptom of the disease is swelling around the jawline from inflammation of the **salivary glands**. It can also cause inflammation of the testicles, meningitis, and encephalitis. Mumps is passed on through airborne transmission and direct contact with droplets or saliva.

Rubella, also known as **German measles**, is caused by a virus. It causes low-grade fever, malaise, swelling of lymph nodes, joint pain, and rash. It can cause congenital rubella syndrome in neonates from infection during pregnancy. Deafness is the most common effect, but other congenital disabilities, including eye, heart, and neurological abnormalities, can also occur. Rubella is spread through airborne and respiratory droplet transmission. See Chapter 8 for more discussion of measles, mumps, and rubella.

The measles, mumps, and rubella vaccine (MMR) is a live attenuated virus vaccine. A second live attenuated virus vaccine includes measles, mumps, rubella, and varicella antigens (MMRV). All children 12 months of age and older should receive the MMR vaccine (M-M-R II, by Merck). A second dose should be given at 4–6 years of age.

You Should Remember

Appropriate administration of the MMR vaccine confers immunity in 95% to 98% of recipients after the first dose and in 99% of recipients after the second dose. Adverse reactions can be reduced with properly dosed acetaminophen during vaccination or shortly afterward. The side effects are generally mild and predictable and, when they occur, are outweighed by the benefits associated with MMR immunity.

TEST YOUR KNOWLEDGE

1. What are the signs and symptoms of measles?
2. What congenital disabilities are related to rubella?
3. What are the available measles, mumps, and rubella vaccines?

VARICELLA VACCINE

The varicella-zoster virus causes varicella. There are two manifestations of the disease. The primary infection causes chickenpox; the recurrent infection causes herpes zoster or shingles. Chickenpox is characterized by a rash that begins on the head and progresses to the trunk and extremities. The rash has distinct lesions that change in appearance over time. The infection also can cause fever and malaise. Complications of the disease include secondary bacterial skin infection, aseptic meningitis, and encephalitis. Varicella was discussed in greater detail in Chapter 8.

The pediatric varicella vaccine product is a live attenuated viral vaccine. There is an individual varicella vaccine, or VAR (VARIVAX, Merck) and a combination product with MMR called MMRV (PROQUAD, Merck). The MMRV vaccine has more varicella antigens than the single-antigen varicella vaccine product. VAR is part of a routine immunization schedule, with the first dose given at 12–15 months of age. The booster dose is due at 4–6 years of age. For a "catch-up" schedule, the second dose can be given 3 months from the first if the child is younger than 13. If the child is 13 or older, two doses should be given 4 weeks after the first. Each dose of VAR and MMRV is 0.5 mL administered subcutaneously. MMRV can be used for children 12 months to 12 years old.

Contraindications include severe allergic reactions to previous doses of vaccine components, including neomycin and gelatin. Immunosuppression, febrile illness, pregnancy, and moderate or severe acute illness are contraindicated. The vaccine should be given later if the patient has recently received blood products. Avoid aspirin for 6 weeks after varicella vaccination due to the association of Reye syndrome with varicella.

ZOSTER RECOMBINANT VACCINE

Shingles is also called herpes zoster, a painful skin rash, usually with blisters (Figure 10.1) in addition to rash, fever, headache, chills, or upset stomach. Rarely, shingles can lead to complications such as pneumonia, hearing problems, blindness, encephalitis, or death. The risk of shingles increases with age. The most common complication of shingles is long-term nerve pain called **postherpetic neuralgia (PHN)**. It occurs in the areas where the shingles rash was and can last for months or years after the rash goes away. The pain from PHN can be severe and debilitating. Older adults with shingles are likely to develop PHN and have longer-lasting and more severe pain than younger people.

The varicella-zoster virus causes shingles, the same virus that causes chickenpox. After chickenpox, the virus stays in your body and can cause shingles later in life. Shingles cannot be passed from one person to another, but the virus that causes shingles can spread and cause chickenpox in someone who has never had the chickenpox vaccine.

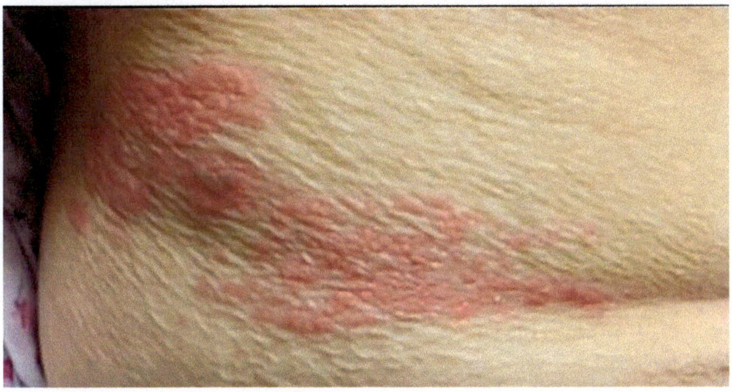

FIGURE 10.1 Shingles. *(From Wikimedia,* https://upload.wikimedia.org/wikipedia/commons/thumb/5/54/Herpes_Zoster_am_Hals.JPG/640px-Herpes_Zoster_am_Hals.JPG*)*

Two types of shingles vaccines are currently available: the live attenuated vaccine (Zostavax) and the recombinant adjuvant subunit vaccine (Shingrix). Shingrix is also recommended for adults 19 and older with weakened immune systems due to disease or therapy. People with weakened immune systems also have a higher risk of getting shingles and illness complications.

People who have had shingles and those who have received the varicella vaccine are recommended to get recombinant shingles. The vaccine is also recommended for people who have already received the live shingles vaccine. There is no live virus in the recombinant shingles vaccine. The shingles vaccine may be given at the same time as other vaccines. After injection of recombinant shingles vaccine, it may cause a sore arm with mild or moderate pain. Redness and swelling can also happen at the site of the injection. Tiredness, muscle pain, headache, shivering, fever, stomach pain, and nausea are common after recombinant shingles vaccine. These side effects may temporarily prevent a vaccinated person from doing regular activities. Though less common, people sometimes faint after vaccination. Symptoms of the side effects usually go away on their own in 2 to 3 days. However, it would be best if you still got the second dose of the vaccine. **Guillain-Barré syndrome** has been reported very rarely after the recombinant zoster vaccine. Adverse reactions should be reported to the Vaccine Adverse Event Reporting System. People with minor illnesses such as a cold may be vaccinated regardless.

You Should Remember

The shingles vaccine prevents people from getting shingles or PHN, a common complication of shingles. Healthy adults ages 50 and older should get the two-dose vaccine. Side effects are usually mild but include pain, redness, and swelling at the injection site.

TEST YOUR KNOWLEDGE

1. What are the signs and symptoms of chickenpox?
2. When is the varicella vaccine administered?
3. What are the available types of shingles vaccines?

HUMAN PAPILLOMAVIRUS VACCINE

Human papillomavirus (HPV) is a small double-stranded DNA virus that commonly infects humans. The oncogenic characteristics of HPV derive from the oncoproteins E6 and E7 that act in inhibiting p53 and pRB tumor suppressors. About 5% of all cancers worldwide are attributable mainly to high-risk ones, including HPV types 16, 18, 31, 33, 35, 39, 45, 51, 52, 56, 58, and 59. Infection with HPV is common after sexual activity begins, but most do not cause symptoms or disease and are cleared within 12–24 months postinfection. Only a tiny fraction of those infections that persist or progress to a preneoplastic lesion result in cancer. The persistence of HPV infection is needed to start the oncogenic process. Clearance of infection is typical in young adults. Viral load and viral type are the primary cofactors progressing infection to cervical intraepithelial lesions and cancer. Smoking, hormonal exposure, and human immunodeficiency virus (HIV) are additional exposures that increase the risk of progression to cancer. The adverse health effects of HPV infections can be primarily controlled through vaccination and screening (see Chapter 8).

HPV is the most common sexually transmitted infection in the United States. There were about 43 million HPV infections in 2018, mostly in people in their late teenage years and early 20s. There are many different types of HPV. Some cause health conditions such as genital warts and cancers. However, HPV vaccines can prevent these conditions from developing. HPV can be spread through all sexual intercourse and even close skin-to-skin touching. About 85% of people will get an HPV infection in their lifetime.

The minimum interval is 5 months between the first and second doses. If a double dose is administered after a shorter interval, a third dose should be used at least 5 months after the first dose and 12 weeks after the second. If the vaccination schedule is interrupted, vaccine doses do not need to be repeated (no maximum interval). Immunogenicity studies have shown that two doses of HPV vaccine given to 9- to 14-year-olds at least 6 months apart provided as good or better than three doses given to older adolescents or young adults.

A three-dose schedule is recommended for people who get the first dose between 10 and 12 years of age. In a three-dose series, the second dose should be given 1 to 2 months after the first dose, and the third should be given 6 months after the first dose. The minimum intervals are 4 weeks between the first and second doses, 12 weeks between the second and third doses, and 5 months between the first and third doses. If a vaccine dose is administered after a shorter interval, it should be readministered after another minimum interval has elapsed since the most recent amount. If the vaccination schedule is interrupted, vaccine doses do not need to be repeated (no maximum interval).

HPV immunizations are generally safe in individuals with HIV except for live virus vaccines in people with low CD4 counts. In those individuals with HIV who have advanced immunosuppression, live vaccines can cause a potentially life-threatening disseminated infection because of the live pathogen in the vaccine.

You Should Remember

The CDC recommends three doses of HPV vaccine (at 0, 1–2, and 6 months apart) for people ages 9 to 26 years if they have certain immunocompromising conditions. People with lower immune responses such as HIV infection, cancer, transplantation, autoimmune disease, or taking immunosuppressant medications, should receive three doses to ensure maximum benefit. However, children with asthma, diabetes, and other conditions that do not suppress the immune response to vaccination can receive a two-dose schedule.

TEST YOUR KNOWLEDGE

1. How common is HPV infection?
2. What is the dosage schedule for the HPV vaccine?
3. How many doses of the HPV vaccine are recommended for people between ages 9 and 26 if they have certain immunocompromising conditions?

PNEUMOCOCCAL VACCINES

Pneumococcal disease is an infection caused by the bacterium known as *Streptococcus pneumoniae*, which can cause pneumonia, **bacteremia**, and meningitis. Pneumococcal pneumonia is prevalent in children under age 2 and adults over 65. Pneumococcal meningitis is the leading cause of bacterial meningitis in patients with sickle cell disease and HIV infection in the United States. People most likely to be infected include those of African American heritage, Alaskan Natives, and Native Americans. For more details, see Chapter 8.

Three pneumococcal vaccines are available: the 13-valent PCV13 (PREVNAR 13), the 20-valent conjugate vaccine (PREVNAR 20), and the 23-valent polysaccharide PPSV23.

The 13 capsular polysaccharides in this vaccine are conjugated to a modified diphtheria toxin, CRM197, to improve the immune response. PCV13 is part of the routine vaccination schedule of infants. Intramuscular injections of 0.5 mL per dose are given at 2, 4, and 6 months of age. A booster dose at 12–15 months of age is also provided. The catch-up schedule should be followed for unvaccinated children 7 months and older. Please pay special attention to the dosing interval with each age group as it changes.

PREVNAR 20 offers the broadest serotype coverage of any pediatric pneumococcal conjugate vaccine, helping to protect against all 20 serotypes contained in the vaccine. Administer PREVNAR 20 as a four-dose series at 2, 4, 6, and 12 through 15 months of age (and at least 2 months after the third dose). The first dose may be given as early as 6 weeks of age. The PREVNAR 20 vaccine is injected only IM. Each injection contains a 0.5-mL dose using a sterile needle attached to the supplied prefilled syringe.

The PPSV23 vaccine contains a polysaccharide capsule component of 23 different serotypes of the bacteria. Because it is a polysaccharide vaccine, it is less effective in young children. PPSV23 is a 0.5-mL dose given primarily through IM injection. It should only be given to children 2 years and older with certain medical conditions outlined in the vaccination schedule. A single dose is given to patients with chronic diseases and standard immune systems. A second dose of PPSV23 will be given 5 years after the first dose for children with specific immunocompromising needs. PCV13 is a conjugate vaccine.

Contraindications for pneumococcal vaccine include severe allergic reactions to vaccine components, or following a prior dose of vaccine, and moderate or severe acute illness. Patients with **asplenia** or a spleen dysfunction, with sickle cell disease, are immunocompromised, have HIV, have a **cochlear implant**, or have a cerebrospinal fluid leak are at increased risk for pneumococcal disease.

You Should Remember

Pneumococcal pneumonia causes an estimated 150,000 hospitalizations each year in the United States. Pneumococcal meningitis and bacteremia killed approximately 3250 people in the United States in 2019. The case fatality rate of pneumococcal meningitis is about 8% among children and 22% among adults.

TEST YOUR KNOWLEDGE

1. Which diseases does *S. pneumoniae* cause?
2. What pneumococcal vaccines are currently available?
3. What are the contraindications for pneumococcal vaccines?

RESPIRATORY SYNCYTIAL VIRUS VACCINES

Respiratory syncytial virus (RSV) is a common respiratory virus that usually causes mild symptoms similar to colds. The virus is generally spread through direct contact, such as via droplets from another person's cough or sneeze that then contact another person's eyes, nose, or mouth. It can also be spread by touching a surface upon which the virus is present, such as a doorknob, and then touching the face before washing the hands.

RSV can cause illness in people of all ages but is more severe in infants and older adults, especially if they have chronic medical conditions (heart or lung disease or weakened immune systems). Older adults in nursing homes or long-term care facilities have the most severe illnesses and complications. Symptoms include a runny nose, decreased appetite, coughing, sneezing, fever, and wheezing. While most people recover in 1 or 2 weeks, the condition can become severe and cause shortness of breath and low oxygen levels. RSV may lead to worsening medical conditions such as asthma, chronic obstructive pulmonary disease, or congestive heart failure. Older adults and infants who become very ill with RSV may need to be hospitalized. The condition can be fatal.

The RSV vaccine can prevent lower respiratory tract disease caused by RSV. The CDC recommends that adults 60 years or older receive one dose of the RSV vaccine, based on discussions between the patient and healthcare provider. Studies are ongoing as to whether revaccination may be needed for some patients. The RSV vaccine can be given at the same time as other vaccines. The vaccine provider must be told if the patient has had an allergic reaction after a previous dose of the vaccine or if there are any present severe, life-threatening allergies. People with a cold or another minor illness can still receive the vaccine. Those who are moderately or severely ill should wait until they recover before getting the RSV vaccine.

You Should Remember

The first FDA approval for an RSV vaccine in the United States occurred on May 3, 2023. It was called Arexvy, approved for preventing lower respiratory tract disease caused by RSV in individuals 60 and older. The developing company was GlaxoSmithKline (GSK). The FDA then approved Abrysvo, Pfizer's vaccine for the same group of people, on May 31, 2023.

HEPATITIS A VACCINE

Hepatitis A (HepA) is caused by a virus that enters the mouth and replicates in the liver. It causes fever, abdominal pain, malaise (tiredness), nausea, and jaundice (about 4 weeks later). Symptoms occur more often in older children and adults. It is transmitted through the fecal-oral route from contact with an infected person or from ingestion of food or water that has been contaminated. Some affected people have no symptoms and are unaware that they are infected. The incubation period between 2 weeks and 6 months after exposure. There may be fatigue, fever, loss of appetite, nausea, vomiting, abdominal pain, light-colored stools, dark urine, **jaundice**, and joint pain. Symptoms of chronic viral hepatitis may require decades to develop.

There are approximately 20,000 HepA infections per year in the United States. There is an effective vaccine available. Outbreaks are related to contaminated food or person-to-person transmission. It is spread when the virus is ingested, even in tiny amounts, through close personal contact with an infected person or contaminated food or drink. HepA is common in many countries, especially those with poor sanitation. It can last from a few weeks to several months.

The HepA vaccine is an inactivated whole-virus vaccine. It is recommended as part of routine immunizations for all children starting at 1 year of age. The series is two doses, with the second dose given at least 6 months after the first. The HepA vaccine is to be administered by IM injection. There are different doses and formulations for children and adults. Two brands are licensed in the United States for children: VAQTA (Merck) and HAVRIX (Merck). Pediatric formulations are approved for children 12 months to 18 years. The pediatric formulations are 0.5 mL per dose; adult formulations are 1 mL per dose. Contraindications and precautions include severe allergic reactions to components (including neomycin) and moderate to severe illness.

Children 1 year or older should be vaccinated against HepA. Follow the guidance of immunization schedules for other high-risk groups and situations requiring HepA vaccination. The first year HepA was routinely recommended as part of the childhood immunization schedule was 2006. Therefore children born before 2005 may not have been vaccinated as part of their routine immunization schedule. HepA vaccine can prevent disease after exposure in individuals 12 months through 40 years of age.

HEPATITIS B VACCINE

Hepatitis B (HepB) is a viral infection of the liver. The condition can be acute or chronic. Chronic disease can result in cirrhosis (scarring of liver cells), liver failure, and liver cancer. HepB virus can be found in bodily fluids, with the highest concentrations of the virus in blood and serous fluids (body fluids resembling serum). Primary transmission mechanisms are perinatal (mother to baby), sexual contact, and exposure to contaminated needles. In infants infected through perinatal transmission, 90% will become chronically infected with HepB without postexposure prophylaxis. HepB vaccine is the only vaccine given to babies at birth. HepB is a recombinant vaccine that is administered via IM injection.

HepB causes about 14,000 new annual infections. Still, about 880,000 adults in the United States are estimated to have chronic HepB. It mainly spreads when infected blood, semen, or certain other body fluids, even in tiny amounts, contact an uninfected person. This may be through childbirth, sexual intercourse, sharing contaminated items, direct contact with open sores, and poor infection control in healthcare facilities. About 66% of infected people are unaware of their condition. In 2020, the rate of new cases was about 12 times higher in Asian Pacific Islanders than in non-Hispanic Caucasians. HepB is one of the leading causes of liver cancer. HepB can range from a mild illness over a few weeks to a serious lifelong condition.

HepB products are available in single-dose vials and prefilled syringes. The HepB vaccine is recommended within 24 hours of birth for all medically stable infants with a birth weight of at least 2 kg if the mother is HepB surface antigen negative. If the baby's birth weight is less than 2 kg, the dose can be given at 1 month of age on discharge from the hospital. If the mother is HepB surface antigen positive or unknown, the vaccine should be offered without regard to birth weight and within 12 hours of birth. HepB is the only vaccine that can be administered at birth. In the routine series of three doses of HepB vaccine, the first dose is typically given within 24 hours, the second dose is given 1–2 months after the first dose, and the third dose is given between 6 months and 18 months. Four doses are permitted if a combination product is used for subsequent doses. Contraindications and precautions include severe allergic reactions to components (yeast protein, latex in prefilled syringes packaging) and moderate to severe illness. HepA and HepB were also discussed in Chapter 8.

You Should Remember

The HepB vaccine is recommended for all infants, all children or adolescents younger than 19 years of age who have not been vaccinated, all adults aged 19 through 59 years, and adults aged 60 years or older with risk factors for HepB infection.

You Should Remember

All adequately vaccinated individuals have shown evidence of immunity to HepB in the form of persisting anti-HB response to a vaccine challenge. Nonetheless, several countries administer booster doses to specific risk groups. Boosters may be used to provide protective immunity against benign breakthrough infection. During regular testing for anti-HB, when the titer falls below 10 mIU/mL, a booster injection is advised for immunocompromised patients. Long-term monitoring should continue to confirm the absence of clinically significant breakthrough episodes of HepB and to determine whether a carrier state develops after 15 years. Nonresponders to a primary course should continue to be studied.

TEST YOUR KNOWLEDGE

1. What is the cause of HepA?
2. What does a chronic HepB infection result in?
3. For which groups of adults is the HepB vaccine recommended?

MENINGOCOCCAL VACCINES

Meningococcal disease refers to any illness caused by bacteria called *Neisseria meningitidis*. These illnesses are often severe and deadly and include infections of the lining of the brain and spinal cord (meningitis) and bloodstream. For more information, see Chapter 8. Several types of meningococcal vaccines exist, such as serogroups A, C, W, and Y (MenACWY). The routine vaccination begins with one dose of MenACWY at 11 to 12 years of age, followed by a booster at 16 to 18. MenACWY is required at a younger age for patients with certain medical conditions or high-risk situations, such as HIV infection, persistent complement component deficiency, and the use of complement inhibitor drugs. Two vaccines are available that protect against serogroups A, C, W, and Y. MenACWY-D (MENACTRA, by Sanofi Pasteur) contains polysaccharide components conjugated to diphtheria toxoid. It can be given in persistent complement component deficiency, a specific type of immune system disorder, and for travelers in particular regions to children as young as 9 months. However, patients 9 to 23 months with certain conditions (such as asplenia, sickle cell disease, or HIV infection) should not receive this vaccine until 2 years of age. MenACWY-D is available in single-dose vials that do not require reconstitution.

MenACWY-CRM (MENVEO, by GSK) contains polysaccharide components conjugated to a protein called CRM197. Children with certain high-risk conditions (including HIV) should be vaccinated following the appropriate immunization schedule as early as 2 months old. MenACWY-CRM is supplied in two vials per dose. One vial contains liquid MenCYW-135 components; the other contains freeze-dried MenA components. These vials must be mixed before administration. Contraindications for meningococcal vaccines include severe allergic reactions to components of the immunization or moderate/severe illness.

IMMUNIZATIONS DURING PREGNANCY

Certain vaccines are safe and recommended for females before, during, and after pregnancy to help keep them and their babies healthy. The antibodies mothers develop in response to these vaccines protect them, cross the placenta, and help protect their babies from serious diseases early in life. Vaccinating during pregnancy also helps protect a mother from transmitting certain conditions to her newborn. The CDC recommends that pregnant females get two vaccines during every pregnancy: the inactivated flu vaccine (the injection, not the live nasal flu vaccine) and the Tdap vaccine. Pregnant females should get the Tdap vaccine between 27 and 36 weeks of each pregnancy. This vaccine is recommended during every pregnancy, regardless of how long it has been since you previously received the Tdap vaccine. It is safe for females to receive most vaccines right after giving birth, even while breastfeeding. Pregnant females should not get HPV, MMR, live flu (nasal), varicella, yellow fever, typhoid fever, and Japanese encephalitis vaccines (see also Chapter 12).

SPECIAL-USE VACCINES

There are some specific vaccines that healthcare professionals should focus on. This chapter will discuss only the COVID-19, Ebola, tuberculosis (TB), and anthrax vaccines.

COVID-19 Vaccines

COVID-19 was a global outbreak of coronavirus in 2019. It is an infectious disease caused by the severe acute respiratory syndrome coronavirus 2 (SARS-CoV-2). The first cases of novel coronavirus were detected in China in December 2019, with the virus spreading rapidly to other countries worldwide. The scientists focused on one "prototype" coronavirus and created a vaccine. That vaccine could then be customized to fight different coronaviruses.

Using their prototype coronavirus, the researchers studied the spike protein, which appears on the surface of coronaviruses. These spikes let the coronavirus latch onto cells in our bodies. When the body's immune system sees the spike protein, it makes antibodies to protect it from infection. This makes it a promising vaccine target. Traditionally, researchers would try putting the spike protein in the vaccine. When injected, the vaccine would stimulate a person's immune system to protect them from a particular coronavirus. During a pandemic, the team knew it would take too long to make large amounts of a specific spike protein. Therefore they studied a faster way to get a spike protein into the body. This new approach injects mRNA instructions for the spike protein into a person's muscle. The muscle cells then make the spike protein. And then, the body's immune system causes the needed antibodies to protect itself. The COVID-19 outbreak was also discussed in Chapter 1.

The NIHVaccine Research Center worked with a company called Moderna to use this information to customize their prototype approach to the severe acute respiratory syndrome coronavirus 2 spike protein quickly. By early February, a COVID-19 vaccine candidate had been designed and manufactured. This vaccine is called mRNA-1273. By March 16, 2020, this vaccine had entered the first phase of clinical trials. Other vaccines, including a similar one from Pfizer and BioNTech SE, entered clinical trials not long after. On December 18, 2020, after demonstrating 94% efficacy, the FDA authorized the NIH-Moderna vaccine for emergency use. Just days earlier, the similar Pfizer/BioNTech vaccine had become the first COVID-19 vaccine to be approved for use in the United States.

There are also four approved vaccines in the United States: Pfizer-BioNTech, Moderna mRNA COVID-19, Novavax subunit COVID-19, and Johnson & Johnson's COVID-19 vaccines. All of these vaccines are injected IM in the deltoid muscle. The advantages of getting COVID-19 vaccines include a lower risk of severe illness, hospitalization, and death from COVID-19 than people who are unvaccinated or have only received the primary series. Updated COVID-19 boosters can help restore decreased protection since the previous vaccination. The updated boosters provide added protection against the recent **Omicron subvariants** that are more contagious than the previous ones. The CDC will continue to provide updates as we learn more.

The adverse effects include severe allergic reactions, myocarditis, and pericarditis associated with mRNA COVID-19 vaccination, mostly among males ages 12 to 39. These rare risks may be further reduced with a longer interval between the first and second doses. Cases of myocarditis and pericarditis have also been reported in people who received the Novavax COVID-19 vaccine. There is a potential cause-and-effect relationship between the Johnson & Johnson/Janssen COVID-19 vaccine and a rare and severe adverse event: blood clots with low platelets (**thrombocytopenia syndrome**).

You Should Remember

COVID-19 vaccines have undergone—and will continue to experience—the most intensive safety monitoring in US history. Evidence from the hundreds of millions of COVID-19 vaccines already administered in the United States and the billions of vaccines administered globally demonstrate that they are safe and effective.

TEST YOUR KNOWLEDGE

1. Which vaccinations are recommended during pregnancy?
2. What were the three recommendations for the first COVID-19 vaccines?
3. What are the four approved COVID-19 vaccines in the United States?

EBOLA VACCINE

Ebola is a severe and often deadly disease caused by a virus. Symptoms include fever, diarrhea, vomiting, bleeding, and often death. Ebola can occur in humans and other primates (gorillas, monkeys, and chimpanzees). The Ebola outbreak in West Africa began in March 2014 and was the largest hemorrhagic viral epidemic in history. Almost 40% of the people who developed Ebola in this outbreak died. There is no known cure for Ebola. Experimental treatments have been used, but none have been thoroughly tested to see if they work well and are safe.

The Ebola vaccine is a live virus vaccine administered IM. The vaccine contains a weakened strain of the vesicular stomatitis virus (VSV) that has been altered to include a gene from the Ebola virus (EBOV). There are currently two approved Ebola vaccines: a single-dose adenovirus 5 serotype (Ad5)/EBOV vaccine in China and a two-dose recombinant VSV (rVSV)/Ad5 vaccine approved in the Russian Federation "for emergency use." In addition, there are two investigational vaccines, the rVSV/Zaire Ebola virus (ZEBOV) vaccine made by Merck and the Ad26 ZEBOV/modified vaccinia Ankara-Bavarian Nordic (MVA-BN)-Filo vaccine. ERVEBO (Ebola Zaire vaccine) is approved by the FDA for preventing disease caused by the EBOV (species *Zaire ebolavirus*) in individuals 18 years of age and older as a single-dose administration. ERVEBO is a replication-competent, live attenuated recombinant VSV vaccine manufactured by Merck. Becoming infected with EBOV from the vaccine is impossible because it only contains a gene from the EBOV, not the whole virus. Specifically, it includes a gene for the EBOV glycoprotein that replaces the gene for the native VSV glycoprotein.

The vaccine is given as a single-dose vaccine. It is safe and protective against the EBOV (species *Z. ebolavirus*) only, which has caused the most significant and deadly Ebola outbreaks to date. This is the first FDA-approved vaccine for an ebolavirus. Side effects of the Ebola vaccine include headache, fever, muscle pain, fatigue, nausea, skin rash (including blisters), and abnormal sweating. The Ebola vaccine is contraindicated in people with weakened immune systems, pregnant or breastfeeding females, and children younger than 1 year old.

TUBERCULOSIS VACCINE

TB is an infectious disease that most often affects the lungs and is caused by bacteria. It spreads through the air when infected people cough, sneeze, or spit. About a quarter of the global population is estimated to have been infected with TB bacteria. About 5% to 10% of people infected with TB will eventually get symptoms and develop TB. Those who are infected but not (yet) ill with the disease cannot transmit it. TB is usually treated with antibiotics and can be fatal without treatment. In certain countries, the Bacille Calmette-Guérin (BCG) vaccine is given to babies or small children to prevent TB.

TB mainly affects adults in their most productive years. However, all age groups are at risk. Over 80% of cases and deaths are in low- and middle-income countries. TB occurs in every part of the world. In 2021, the most significant number of new TB cases occurred in WHO's South-East Asian region (46%), followed by the African Region (23%) and the Western Pacific (18%). Around 87% of new TB cases occurred in the 30 high-TB-burden countries, with more than two-thirds of the global total in Bangladesh, China, the Democratic Republic of the Congo, India, Indonesia, Nigeria, Pakistan, and the Philippines.

The BCG vaccine is not given as part of the routine vaccination schedule; it is provided only when a child or adult is thought to have an increased risk of contracting TB. The BCG vaccine should only be given once in a lifetime. The vaccine is most effective in infants and children aged under 16. BCG vaccination is rarely given to anyone over 16 because there is little evidence that it works well in adults. However, it is given to adults aged 16 to 35 who are at risk of TB through their work, such as some healthcare workers, veterinary staff, and abattoir workers.

You Should Remember

Many people born outside of the United States have been vaccinated against BCG. People previously vaccinated with BCG may receive a TB skin test to assess a TB infection. Vaccination with BCG may cause a positive reaction to a TB skin test. A positive response to a TB skin test may be due to BCG vaccination or infection with TB bacteria.

TEST YOUR KNOWLEDGE

1. What are the features of the EBOV vaccine?
2. How is TB spread?
3. Which adults may need to receive the BCG vaccine?

ANTHRAX VACCINE

Anthrax is a severe infectious disease. It is caused by gram-positive, rod-shaped bacteria known as *Bacillus anthracis*, which occurs naturally in soil and often affects animals worldwide. There are four types of anthrax: cutaneous (involving the skin), inhalation (affecting the lungs), gastrointestinal (affecting the digestive system), and injection (affecting the skin or other body parts).

Anthrax can cause illness if humans come into contact with infected animals or contaminated animal products, resulting in severe disease. However, anthrax is not contagious among humans. Infection occurs when anthrax spores enter the body and are activated. The bacteria can then multiply and spread, producing toxins. This may occur if humans breathe in the spores or consume contaminated food or water, or if the spores enter a wound. Anthrax is less common in the United States than in Central and South America, sub-Saharan Africa, central and southwestern Asia, southern and eastern Europe, and the Caribbean. It can cause blisters or bumps, inflammation, ulcerations, fever, chills, chest discomfort, shortness of breath, confusion, dizziness, coughing, nausea, vomiting, stomach pain, headache, extreme sweating, fatigue, body aches, sore throat, painful swallowing, hoarseness, diarrhea, flushing of the face, red eyes, fainting, and abscesses.

The anthrax vaccine is not currently recommended for the general population anywhere globally. However, because anthrax spores were sent via the mail with criminal intent in the United States following September 11, 2001, any presumed incident related to bioterrorism in the future would almost immediately cause a reevaluation of the current recommendations. In all likelihood, revised recommendations for receipt of the anthrax vaccine would only target groups at high risk of exposure based on the situation. The risk for exposure to anthrax in the United States is low. Currently, the anthrax vaccine is only recommended in the United States for military personnel, lab personnel, and handlers of animals or animal products who are at the highest risk for exposure to anthrax spores. The vaccine is given as a series of five shots. After the first shot, the vaccine is given 4 weeks, 6 months, 12 months, and 18 months later, annually or every 3 years after that, depending on risk.

The anthrax vaccine is approved by the FDA and recommended for adults 18 through 65 years of age who are at risk of exposure to anthrax bacteria, including certain laboratory workers who work with *B. anthracis*, people who handle potentially infected animals or their carcasses, some military personnel (determined by the Department of Defense), and some emergency and other responders whose response activities might lead to exposure.

The CDC recommends 5 IM doses for preexposure vaccination at 0, 1, 6, 12, and 18 months, followed by annual boosters. For postexposure immunization, the CDC recommends three subcutaneous doses at 0, 2, and 4 weeks in conjunction with a 60-day course of appropriate antimicrobial agents at the preferred injection site for muscle in the upper arm. The selected site for subcutaneous injections is the fatty tissue over the deltoid muscle. Use a needle length appropriate for the age and size of the recipient. The vaccine is made by taking a strain of the bacterium and growing it in the laboratory. The bacteria release several harmful toxins into the surrounding broth. These toxins are responsible for disease in those infected with the anthrax bacteria. The toxins are then inactivated with formaldehyde, so they can no longer cause disease. The anthrax bacteria are filtered out of the vaccine. Therefore the anthrax vaccine is similar to the "acellular" pertussis vaccine.

You Should Remember

The safety and efficacy of administering the anthrax vaccine during the same visit as other licensed vaccines have not been evaluated. If an anthrax vaccine is to be given during the same visit as another injectable vaccine, the vaccines should be administered at different injection sites if possible. Each vaccine should be issued with a separate syringe.

TEST YOUR KNOWLEDGE

1. What are the four types of anthrax?
2. In the United States, which individuals are recommended to receive the anthrax vaccine?
3. What is the dosing regimen for the anthrax vaccine?

Monkeypox Vaccine

The **monkeypox** (mpox) virus is an *Orthopoxvirus* that causes **mpox**, a disease with symptoms similar to smallpox, although less severe. While smallpox was eradicated in 1980, mpox continues to occur in countries of central and west Africa. Since May 2022, cases have been reported from countries without previously documented mpox transmission outside the African region. Two distinct clades of the mpox virus have been identified: clade I (formerly known as the Congo Basin [central African] clade) and clade II (the former West African clade).

Mpox is a zoonosis, a disease transmitted from animals to humans, with cases often found close to tropical rainforests where some animals carry the virus. Evidence of mpox virus infection has been found in animals, including squirrels, Gambian pouched rats, dormice, different species of monkeys, and others. The disease can also spread from humans to humans. It can be transmitted through contact with bodily fluids, skin lesions, or internal mucosal surfaces, such as in the mouth or throat, respiratory droplets, and contaminated objects. People with mpox often get a rash that may be located on the head, hands, feet, chest, face, or mouth or near the genitals, including the penis, testicles, labia, vagina, and anus (Figure 10.2). The incubation period is 3–17 days. During this time, a person does not have symptoms and may feel fine.

JYNNEOS is the only vaccine that is FDA approved to prevent mpox disease. JYNNEOS is also approved for the prevention of smallpox disease. It is a live virus vaccine that contains modified vaccinia Ankara-Bavarian Nordic, a weakened, nonreplicating orthopoxvirus. JYNNEOS may be safely used in significantly immunocompromised individuals who may not be candidates or

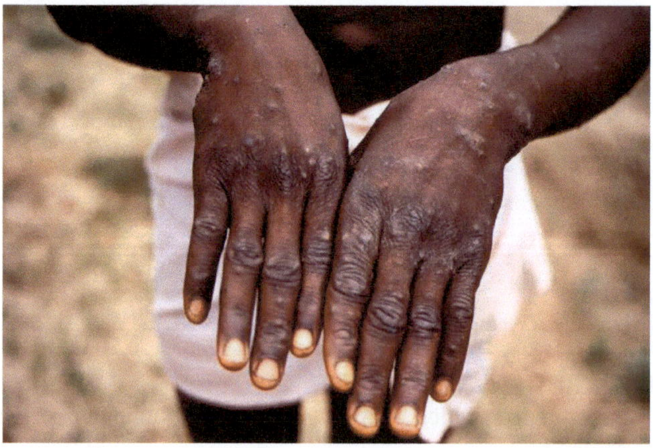

FIGURE 10.2 Mpox rash.

recommended to receive certain live vaccines. JYNNEOS is approved for use in individuals 18 years of age and older who are determined to be at high risk for smallpox or mpox infection. JYNNEOS is approved for administration subcutaneously (beneath the skin) as a two-dose series, 4 weeks apart. JYNNEOS was initially developed for use in the event of a smallpox bioterrorist attack in specific populations (immunocompromised individuals) as an alternative to ACAM2000, which had specific severe reactions.

JYNNEOS is a two-dose vaccine that protects against mpox and smallpox infections. Two doses of the vaccine are needed for the best protection. The second dose is given 4 weeks after the first dose. Vaccinated people should continue avoiding close skin-to-skin contact with anyone with mpox.

You should not get the vaccine if you have a severe allergic reaction such as anaphylaxis after getting the first dose of the JYNNEOS vaccine. Extra caution must be taken if you are allergic to any vaccine. You can still be vaccinated with JYNNEOS, but the provider may need to monitor you for 30 minutes afterward for signs of an allergic reaction. There should be a conversation with the provider if you are allergic to gentamicin, ciprofloxacin, chicken protein, or egg protein.

The vaccination is given intradermally in the forearm, upper back below the shoulder blade, or the skin of the shoulder above the deltoid muscle. It can also be given subcutaneously under the skin on the back of the upper arm. If you ever have keloid scars or are under age 18, the vaccine should be given subcutaneously. Getting the vaccine intradermally or subcutaneously appears to be equally effective against mpox. The second dose should be given 28 days after the first dose or as soon as possible.

You Should Remember

A person with mpox can spread it to others from when symptoms start until the rash has fully healed and a fresh layer of skin has formed. As of February 2023, new data show that some people can spread mpox to others from 1 to 4 days before their symptoms appear. It is unclear how many people this affected during the current outbreak. There is currently no evidence showing that people who never develop symptoms have spread the virus to someone else.

You Should Remember

ACAM2000 is not approved or authorized for emergency use against mpox. ACAM2000 may be used against mpox under the FDA's expanded access investigational new drug mechanism, which requires informed consent and additional investigational new drug requirements.

TEST YOUR KNOWLEDGE

1. What are the two distinct types (clades) of the mpox virus?
2. How is mpox spread between humans?
3. For which group of people is the JYNNEOS vaccine approved?

KEY TERMS

Asplenia
Bacteremia
Cochlear implant
German measles
Guillain-Barré syndrome
Jaundice
Monkeypox
Postherpetic neuralgia
Quadrivalent vaccines
Salivary glands
Shingles
Thrombocytopenia syndrome
Trivalent vaccines

CASE STUDIES

Case Study 1

A 2-year-old child developed multiple facial lesions, followed by a fever. His mother took him to the emergency department, where the lesions were swabbed. Varicella was confirmed. The child was given acyclovir, and symptoms started to subside within a few days.

Critical Thinking Questions

1. What are the potential complications of varicella (chickenpox)?
2. At what age(s) should a child receive the varicella vaccine?
3. What are the contraindications of the varicella vaccine?

Case Study 2

A 28-year-old female was diagnosed with cervical cancer, which caused chronic pelvic pain and bleeding after intercourse. She had never received the HPV vaccine. Her treatment included weekly chemotherapy sessions, daily radiation, and internal radiation placement treatments. Though she survived the cancer, her procedures resulted in her being infertile. The patient now does much work advocating for the importance of early HPV vaccination.

Critical Thinking Questions

1. What factors make it more likely that HPV infection will progress to cancer?
2. What is the vaccination schedule for HPV?
3. What precautions are taken regarding HPV vaccination if a person has HIV?

Case Study 3

A 30-year-old pregnant female developed a cough, fever, night sweats, weight loss, and hemoptysis. She had never received the BCG vaccination. Chest auscultation revealed crepitations through both lungs, and a chest X-ray and CT scan revealed nodules that indicated the patient had TB. Blood and sputum samples were taken. After delivering a healthy baby girl, cultures were taken from the placenta and the patient's cerebrospinal fluid. TB was confirmed. The patient was given ceftriaxone, azithromycin, and the combination HREZ therapy (isoniazid, rifampicin, ethambutol, and pyrazinamide). Over time, the patient fully recovered, and her baby was treated with isoniazid, rifampicin, and pyrazinamide/pyridoxine.

Critical Thinking Questions

1. What is the description of TB, and how does it spread?
2. Where in the world does TB occur the most?
3. At what age should the BCG vaccine be given?

FURTHER READING

1. Balaji, R., 2023. Validation of a Candidate Vaccine for Pulmonary Tuberculosis. Balaji.
2. Findlay, H., 2022. Influenza Virus: Therapeutics and Vaccines. States Academic Press.
3. Franco, E.L., 2011. Human Papillomavirus Vaccines. Future Medicine, Inc.
4. Green, A.V., 2022. Monkeypox Vaccines as We Have Never Known Before The Monkeypox Virus and What You Should Understand. Green.
5. Hernandez, J.C., 2022. Influenza Vaccine: History, Prevention, and Treatment. Hernandez.
6. Lenox, D.A., 2022. Pneumococcal Vaccine: How To Protect Yourself From Pneumococcal Disease. Lennox.
7. Miller, N.Z., 2016. Miller's Review of Critical Vaccine Studies: 400 Important Scientific Papers Summarized for Parents and Researchers. Skyhorse.
8. Moskowitz, R., Holland, M., 2020. Vaccines: A Reappraisal. Skyhorse.
9. O'Leary, M.R., O'Leary, D.S., 2018. The Texas Meningitis Epidemic (1911-1913): Origin of the Meningococcal Vaccine. iUniverse.
10. Rappuoli, R., Vozza, L., 2022. Vaccines in the Global Era: How To Deal Safely and Effectively With the Pandemics of Our Time. WSPC.
11. Rees, A.R., 2022. A New History of Vaccines for Infectious Diseases: Immunization – Chance and Necessity. Academic Press.
12. Schama, S., 2023. Foreign Bodies: Pandemics, Vaccines, and the Health of Nations. Ecco.
13. Thomas, P., Margulis, J., 2016. The Vaccine-Friendly Plan: Dr. Paul's Safe and Effective Approach to Immunity and Health-from Pregnancy Through Your Child's Teen Years. Ballantine Books.
14. USAF Counterproliferation Center, and Penny Hill Press Inc, 2016. The Anthrax Vaccine Debate: A Medical Review for Commanders. CreateSpace Independent Publishing Platform.
15. Wadman, M., 2017. The Vaccine Race: Science, Politics, and the Human Costs of Defeating Disease. Viking.
16. Watson, C.P.N., Gershon, A.A., Oxman, M.N., 2017. Herpes Zoster: Postherpetic Neuralgia and Other Complications: Focus on Treatment and Prevention. Adis.

Chapter 11

Immunology in Older Adults

Chapter Outline

Learning Objectives

After study of this chapter, readers should be able to:

1. Describe the process of immunosenescence during aging.
2. Give some examples of autoimmune disorders in older adults.
3. Describe the significant proinflammatory markers.
4. Identify the role of nutritional approaches in reversing immunosenescence.
5. Describe the effects of zinc deficiency on the thymus gland.
6. Explain immune cell changes in older adults.
7. Describe the selenoproteins in older adults.
8. Explain the role of vitamin E in boosting immunity.
9. Describe the effect of vitamin D on the pathophysiology of COVID-19 disease in older adults.
10. Explain strategies for enhancing vaccine effectiveness in older adults.

OVERVIEW

Aging is a complex process affecting various physiological functions, including the development and maintenance of the immune system. Aging of the immune system, or immunosenescence, is multifaceted and impairs both

Vaccinology and Immunizations. http://doi.org/10.1016/B978-0-443-23915-1.00011-1

innate and adaptive responses. It is characterized by changes in T-cell subsets, cellular-and molecular-level alterations, and thymic atrophy. Overall, immunosenescence attenuates the host's ability to mount a robust or effective immune response. Consequently, resistance to pathogens is impaired, and older adults are 2–10 times more likely to die of infection than younger adults. Immunosenescence and concurrent health problems involving the lungs and heart increase the risk of complications and death from viral infections in older adults. Influenza is the fifth leading cause of death among people aged 50 years and older, and this group is a significant target of vaccination campaigns. However, as a result of immunosenescence, when vaccinated, seniors experience a lower antibody response than that observed in young, healthy people. Experts estimate that the detrimental effects of aging on response to vaccination will continue to increase in importance as a public health concern in the 21st century. Immunosenescence also results in a loss of the ability to recognize "self" and "foreign" antigens and is accompanied by increased autoantibody production and autoimmune disorders.

IMMUNOSENESCENCE

Senescence is a normal physiological process in which organ function slowly changes with age. When it concerns the immune system, it is termed *immunosenescence*. Consequently, immunosenescence is a process of immune dysfunction that occurs with age and includes the remodeling of lymphoid organs, leading to changes in the immune function of older people. Many factors, including aging, chronic inflammation, and changes in the microenvironment, regulate the process of immunosenescence. Moreover, an important distinguishing feature is that the thymus gradually atrophies and degenerates with age, decreasing T-cell output. This process is considered a manifestation of immunosenescence. Therefore understanding how to restore thymus function and the production of T cells provides an effective strategy for immunosenescence intervention.

Additionally, inflammation related to advanced age will produce a **senescence-associated secretory phenotype** involving the immune system. Furthermore, intrinsic factors in immune system cells and potential extrinsic factors often overlooked can cause immunosenescence. Its complexity supports the idea that it will lead to a compromised immune response, leading to various diseases closely related to the development of infections, autoimmune diseases, and malignant tumors.

The method of immunosenescence can alter the immune response, thus leading to the occurrence of various diseases such as malignant tumors and infections. Many factors can activate the immunosenescence process, resulting in an age-related decrease in T-cell output and loss of a cell's power of division and growth. Consistent with this concept, identifying hallmarks and characteristics associated with immunosenescence is essential for exploring its impact and significance.

During aging, the **cytotoxic activity** of immune cells, interferon-gamma, **granzyme B**, and **perforin** decreases. Additionally, the body's metabolism changes as the immune system ages, showing increased **glycolysis** and decreased **mitochondria** function.

Another hallmark of senescent T cells is **telomere** shortening caused by the continuous replication of T cells and decreased expression of the human telomerase RNA component. It should be noted that in the process of immunosenescence, the activating receptor expression of natural killer (NK) cells is reduced.

IMMUNE CELL CHANGES IN OLDER ADULTS

The body may heal more slowly in older adults. There are fewer immune cells in the body to bring about healing. The immune system's ability to detect and correct cell defects also declines. This can increase the risk of infections, autoimmune disorders, and cancer. Older adults are more susceptible to a variety of conditions. The immune system cannot distinguish the self from the non self-antigens, causing **autoimmune disorders**. There are over 100 known autoimmune disorders, including, but not limited to, **psoriasis**, rheumatoid arthritis (RA), lupus, **celiac disease**, and **inflammatory bowel disease**. According to the National Institute of Environmental Health Sciences, as many as 23.5 million people in the United States have an autoimmune disorder. However, the onset of most autoimmune diseases occurs in individuals younger than 60. **Giant cell arteritis** is the most common autoimmune condition that most commonly occurs in older adults. It causes inflammation of the arteries, affecting the head and neck. Symptoms include headaches and changes in vision.

Anatomical and functional changes often occur in aged lymphatic vessels. The aging-associated remodeling of the vascular wall is characterized by decreased muscle cells and enlarged lymphatic diameter, which lead to contractile dysfunction. Aging-related hyperpermeability, resulting from reduced **glycocalyx** and intercellular junctions, contributes to bacterial escape in aged lymphatic vasculature. Meanwhile, aging induces the basal activation of perilymphatic mast cells, restricting the recruitment of immune cells and affecting the reactions to acute inflammation. Thus aging is a significant risk factor for decreased pump activity, increased permeability, and delayed immune response in the lymphatic system. Understanding the mechanisms underlying lymphatic aging is crucial for treating vascular diseases in older adults.

TEST YOUR KNOWLEDGE

1. What are the definitions of senescence and immunosenescence?
2. Which factors can activate the immunosenescence process?
3. What are examples of autoimmune disorders related to immunosenescence?

CANCERS IN OLDER ADULTS

Roughly 50% of cancer cases occur in people aged 65 years or older. Older people are often diagnosed later and might receive less intensive treatment, affecting the outcome. In addition, cancer in older adults might be associated with biological differences in tumor and microenvironment behavior, a domain that has been poorly studied so far. Several studies indicate notable changes in tumor-infiltrating immune cells in tumors of older versus younger people. More research is needed and might lead to a better understanding of the biology of aging and malignancy. This knowledge could provide new perspectives for more personalized cancer treatments, eventually improving the global outcomes of older patients with cancer.

Aging is a paramount risk factor for most cancers, explaining the dramatic increase in the number of older adults with cancer. Some of the most frequently diagnosed malignancies in older adults are lung, breast, prostate, pancreatic, bladder, and skin cancers. Over time, an individual may continually be exposed to the effects of harmful environmental factors such as ultraviolet light and chemical toxins, as well as harmful lifestyle factors such as smoking, being overweight, and consuming an unhealthy diet. These cumulative exposures can trigger cellular DNA mutations that could lead to cancer development.

Some challenges associated with treating cancer in older adults may not be present when treating younger patients. For instance, older adults are more likely to have a preexisting health issue such as hypertension or diabetes mellitus. Another concern is that older adults often do not have the same level of independence as their younger counterparts due to limited mobility or an inability to care for themselves. Furthermore, an individual's support system may dwindle over the years, leading to feelings of loneliness and isolation—and perhaps a heightened sense of mortality if they were close to others who battled and succumbed to cancer. All of these factors can complicate cancer treatment.

Nevertheless, *novel cancer treatments* targeting older adult patients are being prioritized due to the increasing aging population. **Immunotherapy** in malignant tumor treatment has significantly changed the prospects of cancer treatment and improved the survival of patients with cancer. However, immunotherapy results in older adults and young patients could be more consistent, likely due to different types, stages of tumor development, and accompanying diseases. Several types of immunotherapy are used to treat cancer. These include:

- **Immune checkpoint inhibitors** are a type of immunotherapy drug that blocks immune checkpoints. These checkpoints are a normal part of the immune system and keep immune responses to cancer cells from being too strong. These drugs allow immune cells to respond more strongly to cancer by blocking them.

- **T-cell transfer therapy** is a treatment that boosts the natural ability of your T-cells to fight cancer. In this treatment, immune cells are taken from the tumor. Those most active against the cancer are selected or changed in the lab to attack the cancer cells better, grown in large batches, and put back into the body through a needle in a vein. T-cell transfer therapy may also be called adaptive therapy, immunotherapy, or immune cell therapy.
- **Monoclonal antibodies** are immune system proteins created in the lab designed to bind to specific targets on cancer cells. Some monoclonal antibodies mark cancer cells so that the immune system will better see and destroy them. Such monoclonal antibodies are a type of immunotherapy. Monoclonal antibodies may also be called therapeutic antibodies.
- **Treatment vaccines** work against cancer by boosting the immune system's response to cancer cells. Treatment vaccines are different from the ones that help prevent disease.

Immunotherapy has been used to treat a variety of cancers. Although age is one of the most significant risk factors for **tumorigenesis**, more studies are needed considering the high incidence of tumors in older people. Immunotherapy may be used for brain, breast, cervical, bladder, and colorectal cancer.

You Should Remember

As a universal biological phenomenon, aging is an inevitable trend during the lifespan and closely affects the immune system. The immune system can protect the human body from internal or external pathogens. It interacts with neural, circulatory, and other methods.

TEST YOUR KNOWLEDGE

1. What are some of the most frequently diagnosed malignancies in older adults?
2. How has immunotherapy influenced the treatment of cancers in older adults?
3. How do immune checkpoint inhibitors work?

PROINFLAMMATORY MARKERS

Blood tests to assess the presence of **inflammatory markers** can detect inflammation caused by many diseases, including infections, autoimmune conditions, and cancers. The tests do not identify what is causing the inflammation: it might be as simple as a viral infection or as severe as cancer. The significant proinflammatory markers, including cytokines and interleukins (ILs) are responsible for early responses. Others include C-reactive protein (CRP), erythrocyte sedimentation rate, procalcitonin, serum amyloid A, ceruloplasmin, hepcidin, and haptoglobin.

Cytokines are any of several substances, such as interferon, IL, and growth factors, secreted by specific immune system cells and affecting other cells.

ILs are cytokines that were first thought to be expressed by leukocytes alone but have later been found to be produced by many other body cells. They play essential roles in the activation and differentiation of immune cells, as well as proliferation, maturation, migration, and adhesion.

The liver produces CRP. The level of CRP rises when there is inflammation throughout the body. It is one of a group of proteins called acute-phase reactants that go up in response to inflammation. The levels of acute-phase reactants increase in response to specific inflammatory proteins (cytokines). These proteins are produced by white blood cells during inflammation. CRP tests help detect infection, chronic inflammatory disease such as RA or lupus, and risk of heart disease.

Procalcitonin is a biomarker released in response to bacterial infections and can differentiate the etiology of infectious processes. It can be employed as a tool to guide appropriate antibiotic therapy and thus has a role in antibiotic stewardship.

Serum amyloid A is a highly conserved acute-phase protein released in response to inflammation or infection. Production of acute-phase serum amyloid A is stimulated by proinflammatory cytokines such as IL-6, IL-1, **tumor necrosis factor**, and interferon-γ.

Ceruloplasmin is a serum ferroxidase responsible for 95% of copper transport in the blood. It is well known for its role in the pathogenesis of **Wilson disease** and regulating iron metabolism. Also, it is a positive acute-phase reactant, meaning its levels will increase in inflammatory conditions or cell injury. Copper is a trace element that acts as a cofactor for multiple enzymes in critical cellular reactions, for instance, **cytochromes**, which participate in the electron transport chain and redox catalysis. Recent studies have shown that alterations of ceruloplasmin protein and copper homeostasis are associated with Alzheimer disease.

Hepcidin is a hormone that regulates how the body uses iron. It controls how much iron is available for essential body functions such as making **hemoglobin** and red blood cells. It also limits the amount of available iron for the body to use, so the cells do not experience iron overload.

Haptoglobin is a protein made by the liver. It attaches to a specific type of hemoglobin. Hemoglobin is a protein in the red blood cells that carries oxygen from the lungs to the rest of the body. Most hemoglobin is inside red blood cells, but small amounts circulate in the bloodstream.

TEST YOUR KNOWLEDGE

1. What are examples of proinflammatory markers?
2. What are ILs?
3. When do levels of CRP rise?

NUTRITIONAL FACTORS

Prominent nutritional approaches are used to delay or reverse immunosenescence and improve the aged host's resistance to infection. Besides genetics, environmental factors significantly impact the immune system's composition and function. Nutrition is a well-recognized, modifiable factor in this regard. Nutritional interventions are a practical, logistically feasible, and cost-effective approach to tackling immunosenescence and its associated diseases. Compelling evidence suggests that a suboptimal status of essential nutrients contributes to the immunological defects observed with aging.

Furthermore, evidence indicates that increased intake of some nutrients above the recommended levels is needed to maintain the immune system's proper function and reduce the incidence of infection in older adults. Also, various nonnutrient dietary components have been shown to affect immune cell function, though with varying qualitative and quantitative efficacy. Nutritional interventions may involve macronutrients (e.g., dietary lipids) and micronutrients (e.g., vitamin E and zinc), functional foods such as probiotics, and total calorie control. Some studies, such as those on vitamin E and zinc, provide information regarding nutrients' effectiveness in older people.

Effects of Vitamin C

Vitamin C plays a crucial role in seniors' health, helping to protect against free radical damage and strengthen the immune system. It improves human resistance system components such as antimicrobial and NK-cell activities, lymphocyte proliferation, chemotaxis, and delayed-type hypersensitivity. Vitamin C stimulates neutrophil migration to the site of infection and enhances phagocytosis, oxidant generation, and microbial killing. At the same time, it protects host tissue from excessive damage by improving neutrophil apoptosis and clearance by macrophages and decreasing neutrophil necrosis. Vitamin C deficiency is associated with increased susceptibility to infections, a less robust immune response, poor wound healing, and an increased risk of pneumonia.

Vitamin C is an antioxidant essential for producing collagen and carnitine and is crucial to our immune response. Research has shown that certain cells in the immune system, such as phagocytes and T cells, accumulate vitamin C and rely on it to perform their task. A deficiency in vitamin C means we have less resistance against specific pathogens. The beneficial effects of vitamin C supplementation include the following:

- Improving outcomes in older adults who have acute respiratory infections
- Reducing recurrent acute respiratory distress syndrome
- Reducing the severity and duration of the common cold
- Reducing the length of hospital stay and symptoms in older adult patients with pneumonia

- Reducing the time of mechanical ventilation in patients in the intensive care unit
- Preventing the common cold in people who are vitamin C deficient
- Preventing the incidence of pneumonia in people who are vitamin C deficient

Effects of Vitamin D

Vitamin D is a group of **lipophilic hormones** with pleiotropic actions. The vitamin has been traditionally related to bone metabolism. However, several studies in the last decade have suggested its role in sarcopenia, cardiovascular and neurological diseases, insulin resistance and diabetes, malignancies, and autoimmune diseases and infections. In the pandemic era, by considering the response of the different branches of the immune system to SARS-CoV-2 infection, there can be various analyses, including the pleiotropic effects of vitamin D and how its multimodal modulatory effect on the immune system can affect the pathophysiology of COVID-19 disease. There can also be analyses of the possible relationship between the well-known circannual fluctuations in blood levels of this hormone and the epidemiological trend of this infection, particularly in the older adult population.

The biologically active form of vitamin D, calcitriol, can influence the innate and adaptive arms of the immune response. In several studies, calcifediol levels have been inversely correlated with upper respiratory tract infections, and this activity is related to its role in innate immunity. Cathelicidin is one of the main underlying mechanisms because this peptide increases the phagocytic and germicidal activity, acting as a chemoattractant for neutrophils and monocytes, representing the first barrier in the respiratory epithelium to pathogenic invasion.

Furthermore, vitamin D exerts a predominantly inhibitory action on the adaptive immune response, and it influences either cell-mediated or humoral immunity through suppression of B-cell proliferation, immunoglobulin production, or plasma cell differentiation. This role is played by promoting the shift from a type 1 to a type 2 immune response. In particular, the suppression of Th1 response is due to inhibiting T-cell proliferation, proinflammatory cytokine production, and macrophage activation. Finally, T cells also play a fundamental role in viral infectious diseases. CD4 T cells support B-cell antibody production and coordinate the activity of the other immunological cells. CD8 T lymphocytes remove infected cells and reduce viral load. For all these reasons, vitamin D_3 could have a protective role against lung damage produced by COVID-19 by modulating tissue sensitivity to **angiotensin II**.

You Should Remember

Serum calcifediol levels, as suggested by the inverse correlation with upper respiratory tract infections, play a role in the innate immune response. Because of its chemoattractant action for neutrophils and monocytes, cathelicidin represents the first barrier in the respiratory epithelium to pathogenic invasion.

TEST YOUR KNOWLEDGE

1. How crucial is vitamin C in the diets of older adults?
2. What are some of the effects of vitamin D?
3. How does vitamin D affect the adaptive immune response?

Effects of Vitamin E

Vitamin E, a very effective chain-breaking, lipid-soluble antioxidant in the membrane of all cells, is particularly enriched in the membrane of immune cells, which protects them from oxidative damage related to high metabolic activity in these cells. Vitamin E is considered one of the most effective nutrients for enhancing immune function. Several animal and human studies have indicated that vitamin E deficiency impairs both humoral and cell-mediated immune functions. Conversely, supplementation with vitamin E above recommended levels, especially in older people, has enhanced immune response, possibly associated with increased resistance against several pathogens. Vitamin E is a generic term for all tocopherols and tocotrienols that exhibit the biological activity of α-tocopherol.

Older adults have an increased incidence of infection and prolonged infection recovery times. These complications result in high mortality rates among older people, and one of the underlying causes might be their compromised immune response. Thus it is anticipated that supplementing older adults with vitamin E would be a valuable strategy to enhance a human host's resistance to infection by improving immune function.

Effects of Zinc

Zinc is a trace element essential for the growth and development of all organisms, and its impact on the immune system has been a topic of intensive study. The importance of zinc to immune function has been well documented in studies on zinc-deficient humans. Zinc deficiency affects multiple immune cell types in innate and adaptive immunity. For instance, zinc deficiency is known to cause thymus involution and reduction in Th1 cells, leading to an imbalance of Th1/Th2. Further, this deficiency causes a decrease in an array of immune functions such as lymphocyte proliferation, IL-2 production, antibody response, NK-cell activity, and certain parts of neutrophils. One of the best-demonstrated examples is **acrodermatitis enteropathica**, a rare, inheritable metabolic disorder in which zinc deficiency is caused by zinc-specific malabsorption. Patients of this disease have thymic atrophy, lymphopenia, and intercurrent infection due to impaired cell-mediated immune function, which can be reversed by zinc supplementation. These zinc-related impairments in immune function are similar to those observed in older people. Not surprisingly, zinc-deficient subjects are more susceptible to various pathogens than older people.

In contrast to the relatively straightforward association of zinc deficiency with impaired immune function, zinc supplementation's beneficial effects on immune response have yet to be consistently demonstrated, particularly in human studies. In animal models, zinc supplementation can reverse thymic involution, as shown by increased thymosin activity, thymus weight, and the absolute number of T cells in thymocytes. Therefore zinc deficiency induces immunological changes similar to those observed in older people. Many older adults have low serum zinc levels due to inadequate intake, impaired metabolism, infection, and inflammation.

Effects of Selenium

The body needs selenium (Se) for the immune system to work correctly. It can help boost white blood cells, improving the body's ability to fight illness and infection. Adequate levels of Se are essential for initiating immunity, but they also regulate excessive immune responses and chronic inflammation. Se is a vital trace element for controlling immune functions through the redox-regulating activity of selenoproteins (e.g., glutathione peroxidase), protecting immune cells from oxidative stress. However, Se has biological bimodal action in cancer, depending on the concentration. At nutritional low doses, Se, depending on its form, may act as an antioxidant, protecting against oxidative stress and supporting cell survival and growth. Thus it plays a chemopreventive role, while at supranutritional higher pharmacological doses, Se acts as a pro-oxidant, inducing redox signaling and cell death. To date, many studies have been conducted on the benefits of Se intake in reducing the risk of cancer incidence at the nutritional level, indicating that Se likely functions as an immunostimulatory, such as reversing the immunosuppression in the tumor microenvironment towards antitumor immunity by activating immune cells and releasing proinflammatory cytokines such as interferon-gamma.

Se is an essential component of various enzymes and proteins, called **selenoproteins**, that help to make DNA and protect against cell damage and infections; these proteins are also involved in reproduction and the metabolism of thyroid hormones. Se-containing antioxidants protect against DNA damage and mutations. It is also essential for the immune defense and helps destroy abnormal cells. Se also regulates inflammatory processes that often occur in connection with cancers. It stops free radical damage before premature wrinkles have a chance to form. It also helps to protect cell membranes against ultraviolet damage, inflammation, and pigmentation.

You Should Remember

Se is needed for the proper functioning of the immune system. It appears to be an essential nutrient in counteracting the development of virulence and inhibiting HIV progression to AIDS. An elevated Se intake may be associated with reduced cancer risk. Deficiency is accompanied by loss of immunocompetence, probably linked with Se being found in significant amounts in immune tissues such as the liver, spleen, and lymph nodes. Both cell-mediated immunity and B-cell function can be impaired.

TEST YOUR KNOWLEDGE

1. How effective is vitamin E for enhancing immune function?
2. What conditions may develop due to a zinc deficiency?
3. How does Se protect against cancer?

ENHANCING VACCINE EFFECTIVENESS

A falling birth rate, increasing life expectancy, and dramatic demographic changes result in an ever-aging population. Aging is accompanied by increased susceptibility to bacterial and viral infections indicative of a decline in immunity. It also has implications for vaccination programs, and there is clear evidence that the reduction in adaptive immunity results in dramatically reduced vaccine responses and vaccine longevity in older adults.

The immune system in older adults is particularly susceptible to infectious diseases and displays reduced response to vaccination. The world population is rapidly aging, and preventing infectious diseases in older adults has become a significant public health issue. To this end, developing novel vaccines especially suited to raising protective immunity in the aging population is necessary. Approaches in this direction include high-dose vaccines, booster vaccinations, different immunization routes, time of day of vaccine administration, exercise, the mitigating effects of stress, and the use of new adjuvants. These approaches, still empirical, must be supported by intensive research to unravel the biological and molecular mechanisms underlying immunosenescence. Only this knowledge will allow us to design systems for immune rejuvenation and more effective vaccines for protecting older people.

You Should Remember

Data from a recent study that examined morning versus afternoon influenza vaccine administration in older adults showed that males (but not females) who were vaccinated in the morning mounted a better peak antibody response to the influenza strain. This indicates that hormonal and cytokine diurnal rhythms may influence the magnitude of response to some vaccines.

KEY TERMS

Acrodermatitis enteropathica
Autoimmune disorders
Celiac disease
Ceruloplasmin
Cytotoxic activity
Giant cell arteritis
Glycocalyx
Glycolysis
Granzyme B
Haptoglobin
Hemoglobin
Hepcidin
Inflammatory bowel disease
Inflammatory markers
Immune checkpoint inhibitors
Mitochondria
Monoclonal antibodies
Psoriasis
Selenoproteins

Senescence
Senescence-associated secretory phenotype
T-cell transfer therapy
Treatment vaccines
Tumorigenesis
Tumor necrosis factor
Wilson disease

CASE STUDIES

Case Study 1

A 76-year-old female, initially diagnosed with generalized osteoarthritis, was reexamined after developing inflammation in her wrists and knees. She had become unable to dress herself, lost 5 pounds within 1 month, and had repeated falls. The physical examination resulted in suspicion of RA, and laboratory studies revealed an elevated erythrocyte sedimentation rate, increased CRP level, and anticitrullinated peptide antibodies. Hand radiographs showed periarticular osteoporosis. A diagnosis of RA was made. Treatments involved methotrexate, prednisone, and a biologic agent. Along with physical therapy, the patient's condition stabilized.

Critical Thinking Questions

1. What causes autoimmune disorders, and how many of them are there?
2. Which tests can be used to determine if RA is present in an individual?
3. How can immune cell changes in older adults influence the development of a disease such as RA?

Case Study 2

A 72-year-old male presented with many right-sided lung nodules discovered via CT scan. There were also lymph nodes and bone metastases. Pathological examination revealed a moderately differentiated lung adenocarcinoma of stage IV. Due to the patient's immunohistochemistry and gene test results, the patient had no alternative options for targeted therapy. A combination of pembrolizumab (a type of immunotherapy) and chemotherapy was recommended, but the patient refused the chemotherapy portion of the treatment.

Further genetic tests revealed that pembrolizumab monotherapy may prove to be successful. The patient's condition began to stabilize with this therapy. The patient continued to improve over 3 ½ years of treatment, and the cancer was completely stabilized.

Critical Thinking Questions

1. How common are cancers in older adults, and what factors affect their outcome?
2. What are some of the most frequently diagnosed malignancies in older adults?
3. How has immunotherapy improved cancer treatments?

FURTHER READING

1. Abbas, A.K., Lichtman, A.H., Pillai, S., 2021. Cellular and Molecular Immunology, 10th Edition. Elsevier.
2. Abbas, A.K., Lichtman, A.H., Pillai, S., 2023. Basic Immunology Functions and Disorders of the Immune System, 7th Edition. Elsevier.
3. Bueno, V., Lord, J.M., Jackson, T.A., 2016. The Ageing Immune System and Health. Springer.
4. Bueno, V., Pawelec, G., 2021. Healthy Longevity and Immune System (Healthy Ageing and Longevity, 16). Springer.
5. Chiu, H., Shulman, K., 2017. Mental Health and Illness of the Elderly (Mental Health and Illness Worldwide). Springer.
6. Coico, R., Sunshine, G., 2015. Immunology: A Short Course, 7th Edition. Wiley Blackwell.
7. Dettmer, P., 2021. Immune: A Journey into the Mysterious System That Keeps You Alive. Random House.
8. Doan, T., Lievano, F., Swanson-Mungerson, M., Viselli, S., 2021. Immunology, 3rd Edition. Lippincott/Wolters Kluwer. (Illustrated Reviews)
9. Delves, P.J., Martin, S.J., Burton, D.R., Roitt, I.M., 2017. Roitt's Essential Immunology, 13th Edition. Wiley Blackwell. (Essentials)
10. DiNicolantonio, J., Land, S., 2021. The Immunity Fix – Strengthen Your Immune System, Fight Off Infections, Reverse Chronic Disease, and Live a Healthier Life. Land.
11. Epstein, T.E.G., Nyenhuis, S.M., 2019. Treatment of Asthma in Older Adults: A Comprehensive, Evidence-Based Guide. Springer.
12. Filmore, S., 2021. Boost Immune System: For the Elderly. Filmore.
13. Greene, J., 2019. The Immunity Code – The New Paradigm for Immune Centric Health and Radical Anti-Aging. Joel Greene.
14. Hawley, L., Ziegler, R.J., Clarke, B.L., 2013. BRS Microbiology and Immunology (Board Review Series), 6th Edition. Wolters Kluwer/Lippincott, Williams, & Wilkins.
15. Kabelitz, D., Bhat, J., 2020. Epigenetics of the Immune System (Translational Epigenetics Book 16). Academic Press.
16. Kau, A.L., Monroy, J.M., Polk, B.I., Rigell, C.J., 2021. The Washington Manual: Allergy, Asthma, and Immunology – Subspecialty Consult, 3rd Edition. Wolters Kluwer.
17. Kennedy, H.L., 2023. Aging and Health for the U.S. Elderly – A Health Primer for Ages 60 to 90 Years. University of Missouri Press.
18. Kippola, P., Hyman, M., 2019. Beat Autoimmune – The 6 Keys to Reverse Your Condition and Reclaim Your Health. Kensington.
19. Lipman, F., Claro, D., 2020. The New Rules of Aging Well: A Simple Program for Immune Resilience, Strength, and Vitality. Artisan.
20. Male, D., 2021. Immunology: An Illustrated Outline, 6th Edition. CRC Press.
21. Male, D., Stokes Peebles Jr., R., Male, V., 2020. Immunology, 9th Edition. Elsevier.
22. Marotta, F., 2023. Gut Microbiota in Aging and Chronic Diseases (Healthy Ageing and Longevity Book 17). Springer.
23. Miles, E.A., Calder, P., Childs, C.E., 2020. Diet and Immune Function (Nutrients). Mdpi AG.
24. Miller, H., 2023. Healthy Aging and Immune System. American Medical Publishers.
25. Murphy, K.M., Weaver, C., Berg, L., 2022. Janeway's Immunobiology, 10th Edition. W.W. Norton & Company.
26. Musi, N., Hornsby, P., 2021. Handbook of the Biology of Aging (Handbooks of Aging). Academic Press.

27. Parham, P., 2021. The Immune System, 5th Edition. W.W. Norton and Company.
28. Punt, J., Stranford, S., Jones, P., Owen, J., 2018. Kuby Immunology, 8th Edition. W.H. Freeman.
29. Ruebush, M., 2023. Immunology & Microbiology Essentials (Medical School Companion). Ruebush.
30. Sompayrac, L.M., 2019. How the Immune System Works (The How It Works Series), 6th Edition. Wiley Blackwell.
31. Turgeon, M.L., 2021. Immunology & Serology in Laboratory Medicine, 7th Edition. Mosby.

Chapter 12

Vaccines for Travelers

Chapter Outline

Learning Objectives

After study of this chapter, readers should be able to:

1. Describe the signs and symptoms of typhoid fever.
2. Explain the steps for travelers in the prevention of typhoid fever.
3. Discuss the characteristics of the yellow fever vaccine.
4. Identify the time and dose of the meningococcal vaccine.
5. Describe Japanese encephalitis and the effectiveness of its vaccine.
6. Identify the contraindications of the cholera vaccine.
7. Describe the two types of rabies vaccines.
8. Describe the route or routes of the meningococcal conjugate vaccine.
9. Identify the contraindications of rabies vaccines.
10. Describe the timelines for different vaccinations for travelers.

OVERVIEW

Vaccines protect travelers from serious diseases. Depending on where you travel, a traveler may come in contact with rare diseases in the United States, like yellow fever. Some vaccines may also be required for travelers to certain places. Some countries require proof of vaccination for certain diseases, like COVID–19 or yellow fever. Traveling in developing countries and rural areas may require more vaccines for tourists. If a traveler is pregnant or has an ongoing

Vaccinology and Immunizations. http://doi.org/10.1016/B978-0-443-23915-1.00021-4

illness or weakened immune system, they may need additional vaccines. It is essential to be up to date on routine vaccinations. While measles is rare in the United States, it is more common in parts of Asia and Africa. Depending on the travel location and the disease's prevalence in that area, vaccination against one or more of the following diseases may be recommended before the trip.

COVID-19 VACCINE FOR TRAVELERS

Starting May 12, 2023, non-citizen non-immigrant air passengers no longer needed to show proof of being fully vaccinated with an accepted COVID-19 vaccine to board a flight to the United States. The CDC's Amended Order Implementing the Presidential Proclamation on the Safe Resumption of Global Travel During the COVID-19 Pandemic expired when the Presidential Proclamation Advancing the Safe Resumption of Global Travel During the COVID-19 Pandemic came about. For more detail, see Chapters 3 and 10.

TYPHOID FEVER VACCINE

Typhoid fever is a life-threatening infection caused by the bacterium Salmonella typhi. It is usually spread through contaminated food or water, and patients carry the bacteria in their bloodstream and intestinal tract.

Signs and symptoms include prolonged high fever, fatigue, headache, nausea, abdominal pain, decreased appetite, and constipation or diarrhea. Some patients may develop rashes. Severe cases can lead to serious complications or death. Vomiting and diarrhea are more common in children. Typhoid fever is confirmed via blood testing. Though improved living conditions and antibiotics have significantly reduced typhoid fever cases and deaths in industrialized countries, the disease remains a public health problem in developing areas of African, Eastern Mediterranean, Southeast Asian, and Western Pacific regions. As of 2019, there were 9 million estimated cases of typhoid fever annually, resulting in about 110,000 deaths annually. Risks are higher in populations that lack access to safe water and adequate sanitation. Children are at the highest risk.

Typhoid can be treated with antibiotics. Antimicrobial resistance is common, however, with more complicated and expensive treatments needed in the most affected regions. After symptoms subside, individuals may still carry typhoid bacteria and can spread it to others by shedding bacteria in their feces.

There are two vaccines available for typhoid fever that are quite different. Typhoid vaccine live oral Ty21a (VIVOTIF, Swiss PaxVax) is an oral live attenuated vaccine for persons six years and older. The dose of vaccine is one capsule by mouth every other day for four doses. Doses should be administered with cool water 1 hour before and 2 hours after a meal. The capsules are stored in a refrigerator. The regimen should be completed at least one week before travel. A booster is needed every five years if there is continued exposure.

Typhoid conjugate vaccine is administered as one injectable dose in children from 6 months and adults up to 65 years. Two other vaccines have been used for many years, including travelers in older children and adults at risk of contracting typhoid. These vaccines do not provide long-lasting immunity; repeat or booster doses are required. They are also not approved for children younger than two years of age. The first is an injectable vaccine based on the purified antigen for people aged two years and older. The WHO prequalified two typhoid conjugate vaccines in 2017 and are being introduced into childhood immunization programs in typhoid-endemic countries. Typhoid vaccines lose effectiveness over time. The injectable vaccine requires a booster every two years, and the oral vaccine requires an advocate every five years.

While traveling, the following recommendations should be followed to stop the spread of typhoid:

- Ensure that food is cooked correctly and served while hot
- Avoid raw milk and any related products – drink only pasteurized or boiled milk
- Avoid ice unless it is made from safe water
- If the quality of drinking water is questionable, it should be boiled or disinfected with a slow-release disinfectant designed for this purpose.
- Hands should be washed often with soap and thorough scrubbing, especially after contact with pets or farm animals or after using the bathroom.
- Fruits and vegetables must be washed carefully – especially if they are to be eaten while raw; if possible, they should be peeled before eating.

The typhoid vaccine should not be given to those with a confirmed anaphylactic reaction within 72 hours of a previous dose of the same vaccine.

You Should Remember

Typhoid fever is a life-threatening illness caused by **Salmonella typhi** and can affect anyone, though travelers visiting developing countries are at the highest risk. The infection is spread directly from person to person or through contaminated food or water. The available vaccines provide some protection for people traveling to areas where the disease is common, and it is also recommended for those living in a household with a person who is a typhoid fever carrier.

TEST YOUR KNOWLEDGE

1. What are the signs and symptoms of typhoid fever?
2. What are the two available vaccines for typhoid fever?
3. What recommendations should be followed to stop the spread of typhoid fever?

YELLOW FEVER VACCINE

Yellow fever is an acute viral hemorrhagic disease transmitted by infected mosquitoes. It is referred to as "yellow" because patients often develop **jaundice**. Signs and symptoms include high fever, headache, muscle pain, nausea, vomiting, and fatigue. Some patients become severely ill, which may result in death within 7 to 10 days. There is no existing treatment. Yellow fever is endemic in tropical areas of Africa, Central America, and South America. Large epidemics occur when infected people introduce the virus into heavily populated areas with high mosquito density or where there is little to no immunity because of a lack of vaccination. Infected mosquitoes of the **Aedes aegypti** species can transmit the virus between individuals (see Fig. 12.1).

Yellow fever vaccine is a live virus vaccine made from the 17D strain of the virus. It is recommended for persons nine months or older who travel to high-risk areas. The yellow fever vaccine in the U.S. is the 17D-204 strain vaccine, YF-VAX (manufactured by Sanofi Pasteur). YF-VAX supplies had been depleted at one point in 2017. The alternative 17D-204 product, STAMARIL, produced in France by Sanofi Pasteur, is available at specific locations around the U.S. under an expanded access investigational new drug (IND) program. Both products, STAMARIL and YF-VAX, are produced in chick embryos.

These vaccines are highly effective, safe, and affordable. Only one dose is needed for most travelers. Certain groups, such as persons who have received a bone marrow transplant after original vaccination, pregnant women, and HIV-infected women, may require additional doses due to decreased response. The vaccine is 0.5 mL in volume and is administered through subcutaneous (SC) or intramuscular (IM) injections. The yellow fever vaccine is contraindicated in

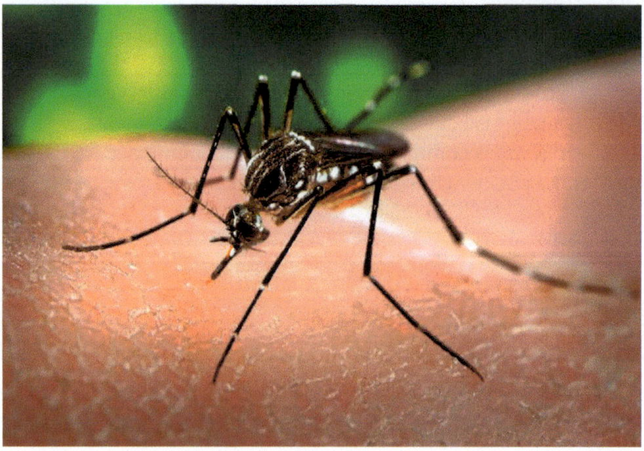

FIGURE 12.1 Mosquitoes of the Aedes aegypti species.

patients with a history of severe allergies. It should also be avoided in children less than six months of age or with symptomatic HIV infection. Some countries mandate yellow fever vaccination before entry. The vaccine must be given at least ten days before travel.

You Should Remember

If the toxic phase of yellow fever develops, a high fever will be present. The liver and kidneys are most affected, and jaundice, dark urine, and abdominal pain with vomiting are often present. Bleeding can occur from the mouth, nose, eyes, or stomach. About half of the patients who enter this toxic phase die within 7 to 10 days.

TEST YOUR KNOWLEDGE

1. Why is yellow fever named as such?
2. Where is yellow fever endemic?
3. Though most people only need one dose of the vaccine, which individuals may need multiple doses?

HEPATITIS A VACCINE

Hepatitis A is highly common in many other countries outside of the United States. Travelers from Central or South America, Mexico, Asia (except Japan), Africa, and Eastern Europe should get the hepatitis A vaccine. Babies aged six months and older should get the hepatitis A vaccine before traveling outside of the U.S.

International travelers to certain countries where hepatitis A is prevalent should receive the vaccination. Infants 6-11 months old in this category should receive one dose of HepA before departure and be revaccinated with two additional doses following a routine schedule (this is an off-label use of HepA vaccine for children under 12 months of age). For more information about hepatitis A, see Chapter 10.

MENINGOCOCCAL VACCINE

Meningococcal disease can cause a severe infection of the blood and the tissues around the spinal cord and brain. Neisseria meningitidis bacteria, or meningococci, are spread through saliva or spit and close or ongoing contact. If traveling to a high-risk area, you should be vaccinated against meningococcal meningitis with a MenACWY vaccine, also known as the quadrivalent meningococcal meningitis vaccine. Only one dose should be given IM 2 to 3 weeks before travel.

Travelers going to Saudi Arabia to participate in the Hajj or Umrah religious observances are required to get the meningococcal conjugate vaccine. The vaccine can protect individuals for five years. Travelers should receive vaccines

7–10 days before travel to enable time for protective antibody levels to develop. The vaccine should be given intramuscularly or subcutaneously based on manufacturer's recommendations.

JAPANESE VIRAL ENCEPHALITIS VACCINE

Japanese encephalitis is a viral brain infection spread through mosquito bites. It is most common in rural areas in Southeast Asia, the Pacific islands, and the Far East. The virus is found in pigs and birds and is passed to mosquitoes when they bite infected animals. It cannot be spread from person to person. Most people infected by the Japanese encephalitis virus have either no or mild, short-lived symptoms, often mistaken for flu. Around 1 in every 250 people infected with Japanese encephalitis develop more severe symptoms as the infection spreads to the brain. This usually happens 5 to 15 days after infection. Up to 1 in every three people who develop these more severe symptoms will die due to the disease. In those who survive, these symptoms tend to improve slowly.

The Japanese encephalitis vaccine is more than 90% effective. The duration of protection with the vaccine is unclear, but its effectiveness decreases over time. Doses are given either IM or SC. There are several types of inactivated vaccines and one type of live attenuated vaccine currently used in the world – inactivated mouse brain–derived vaccines, inactivated Vero-cell–derived vaccines, primary hamster kidney (PHK) cell–derived, purified vaccines, and live attenuated vaccines.

The **inactivated vaccine** (manufactured as IXIARO) is the only JE vaccine licensed and available in the United States. This vaccine was approved in March 2009 for use in people aged 17 years and older and in May 2013 for use in children two months through 16 years of age. Other JE vaccines are manufactured and used in other countries but are not licensed in the United States. IXIARO is given as a two-dose series, with the doses spaced 28 days apart. Adults aged 18–65 can get the second dose as early as seven days after the first dose. The last dose should be given at least one week before travel. A booster dose (third dose) should be given if a person has received the two-dose primary vaccination series one year or more previously and there is a continued risk for JE virus infection or potential for reexposure. For adults and children aged three years or older, each dose of IXIARO is 0.5 mL. For children aged two months through 2 years, each dose is 0.25 mL.

There is currently no cure for Japanese encephalitis. Treatment involves supporting the body's functions to fight off the infection. An infected person must usually be admitted to the hospital for fluids, oxygen, and medication to treat symptoms. A severe allergic reaction after a previous dose of IXIARO, after any other JE vaccine, or after any component of IXIARO is a contraindication to further doses. The vaccine contains **protamine sulfate**, a compound known to cause allergic reactions in some people. Administration of IXIARO to pregnant women usually should be deferred. However, pregnant women who must travel to an area with high infection risk should be vaccinated when the disease risk outweighs the theoretical risk of immunization.

You Should Remember

Japanese encephalitis is a flavivirus related to dengue, yellow fever, and West Nile viruses. Mosquitoes spread it and are the primary cause of viral encephalitis in many Asian countries. Twenty-four countries in the World Health Organization's Southeast Asia and Western Pacific regions have endemic transmission of the virus, exposing over 3 billion people to risks of infection.

TEST YOUR KNOWLEDGE

1. How often does a Japanese encephalitis infection become serious?
2. Which Japanese encephalitis vaccine is licensed in the United States?
3. What does treatment for Japanese encephalitis usually require?

CHOLERA VACCINE

Cholera is a diarrheal illness caused by the toxins produced by Vibrio cholerae. The cholera vaccine available in the U.S. (Vaxchora®, by Paxvax) is an oral dosage form that should be taken at least ten days before travel. This vaccine is not approved for children. The CDC recommends vaccination for people traveling to or living in areas of active cholera transmission.

Vaxchora® (lyophilized CVD 103-HgR) is a single-dose, oral vaccine FDA-approved in the United States for use in people aged 2 to 64 who are traveling to an area of active cholera transmission. Vaxchora® should be taken at least ten days before travel to a place of active cholera transmission. The vaccine manufacturer reports that Vaxchora® reduces the chance of moderate and severe diarrhea in people by 90% at ten days and 80% three months after. How long protection lasts beyond 3 to 6 months after vaccination is unknown.

The cholera vaccine should be postponed in the presence of any acute illness. A history of severe systemic reaction or allergic response following a prior dose of cholera vaccine is a contraindication to further use. Pregnant women are vulnerable to complications of cholera. Killed oral cholera vaccines are not recommended for pregnant women, though there is no evidence of harmful effects during pregnancy.

RABIES VACCINE

Rabies is a fatal disease that mandates proper prophylaxis after rabies virus exposure to prevent death. It is caused by lyssavirus, which affects the brain and spinal cord. The virus is typically transmitted to humans through the bite of an infected animal. The condition causes pain and numbness, fever, weakness, and headache. These symptoms may last for days. Symptoms then progress to cerebral dysfunction, anxiety, confusion, agitation, hydrophobia, spasms, coma, and death. The rabies vaccine is recommended before travel to certain countries as **pre-exposure prophylaxis**. It is also recommended as post-exposure prophylaxis after contact with or a bite from certain animals.

There are two rabies vaccines available. The first is a human diploid cell culture vaccine (HDCV) manufactured by Sanofi. The second is the PCECV vaccine (RabAvert®, Bavarian Nordic), produced in chick embryo cell culture. These vaccines protect against human rabies and are nerve tissue and cell culture vaccines. WHO recommends replacing nerve tissue vaccines with more efficacious, safer vaccines developed through cell culture as soon as possible.

Pre-exposure prophylaxis is getting rabies vaccine doses before exposure to the rabies virus. This can help protect a person against unrecognized rabies exposures or when rabies post-exposure prophylaxis may be delayed. A 2-dose pre-exposure prophylaxis schedule has replaced the 3-dose program to watch for up to 3 years. High-risk groups requiring pre-exposure prophylaxis are veterinarians and their staff, animal handlers, rabies researchers, certain laboratory workers, and people who may be in contact regularly with the rabies virus or animals that may carry it. The vaccination series for postexposure prevention in persons previously vaccinated is two doses at 0 and 3 days.

The **post-exposure prophylaxis** (PEP) regimen involves the administration of human rabies immune globulin (HRIG), which is given only once, and a series of four 1.0 mL rabies vaccinations. The first vaccination is given on the first day of treatment (designated Day 0), and three additional rabies vaccinations are given on Days 3, 7, and 14. Immunocompromised persons receive a fifth vaccination on Day 28 and should be tested for seroconversion 7 to 14 days following completion of the PEP regimen.

Human rabies immune globulin (HRIG) is infiltrated around the bite(s) site and provides rapid passive immune protection with a half-life of approximately 21 days. It is administered only once, on the first day of the PEP regimen. A maximum of the recommended dosage of HRIG should be given because excessive HRIG can partially suppress the active production of antibodies. If the HRIG was not administered on Day 0, it may be administered up to and including Day 7 of the PEP regimen. Beyond Day 7, HRIG is not indicated, as the patient's antibody response to the vaccine occurs in that timeframe. The recommended dosage of HRIG is 20 IU/kg body weight for all ages, including children. Infiltrate as much of the HRIG as possible into and around the bite wound. Administer the remaining HRIG IM at a site distant from the first vaccination site, generally in the quadriceps or deltoids. If there is no wound, such as following a bat-in-the-bedroom exposure, administer the entire HRIG dose IM in the deltoid or quadriceps muscles.

Previously vaccinated individuals are those who have completed a pre-exposure or post-exposure regimen of HDCV or PCECV or who have received a different vaccine outside of the U.S. Following an exposure, previously vaccinated persons are given two 1.0 mL doses of vaccine IM in the deltoid area on Days 0 and 3. No HRIG is administered. If the patient's previous pre- or post-exposure vaccination regimen was administered before 1985, then the person is considered unvaccinated. Administer the full rabies PEP regimen, including HRIG.

Once the decision to initiate rabies PEP has been made, the PEP regimen should be started as soon as possible. Every effort should be made to adhere to the recommended PEP regimen schedule, especially the first two days of treatment, Days 0 and 3. After Day 3 of the regimen, deviations of a few days are acceptable. For most minor delays or interruptions, the vaccination schedule can be shifted and resumed as though the patient were on schedule. For example, if a patient misses the dose scheduled for Day 7 and presents for vaccination on Day 10, the Day 7 dose should be administered that day, and the final dose should be given one week later on Day 17.

For both products, each dose is 1 mL given by IM injection in the deltoid muscle in adults and older children and vastus lateralis in infants and small children. The gluteal area should never be used for rabies vaccine injections because administration in this area can result in lower antibody titers. Doses of rabies vaccine administered in the gluteal site should not be counted as valid doses and should be repeated.

Contraindications for pre-exposure prophylaxis vaccine include a history of anaphylaxis. However, due to the fatality of rabies, there are no contraindications to post-exposure prophylaxis.

You Should Remember

Rabies occurs in many countries worldwide and causes tens of thousands of deaths every year – mainly in Asia and Africa. The majority of deaths consist of children. Dogs are the primary source of human rabies deaths. Globally, rabies causes estimated economic costs of more than $8.6 billion per year, yet it can be prevented by vaccinating dogs and cats and preventing dog bites.

TEST YOUR KNOWLEDGE

1. What are the signs and symptoms of rabies?
2. Which high-risk groups require preexposure prophylaxis against rabies?
3. How are the rabies vaccines administered?

KEY TERMS

Aedes aegypti
Jaundice
Post-exposure prophylaxis
Pre-exposure prophylaxis
Protamine sulfate
Salmonella typhi
Yellow fever

CASE STUDIES

Case Study 1

A 48-year-old woman vacationed in The Gambia, a country that does not require travelers to have a yellow fever vaccine. About a week after arriving, the woman developed a high fever, chills, headache, and muscle pain. She was hospitalized with jaundice, severe weakness, and anuria when she returned home. Tests revealed her to be positive for yellow fever. She soon began bleeding from her bowel and developed hypovolemic shock. She was intubated and placed on ventilation. Blood transfusions were performed, but the patient became comatose and died seven days later.

Critical Thinking Questions

1. How do large epidemics of yellow fever occur?
2. For whom is the yellow fever vaccine recommended?
3. How is the yellow fever vaccine administered?

Case Study 2

A 1-year-old baby boy from South Asia was hospitalized for a high fever, cough, runny nose, and a widespread skin rash. The child was lethargic, refused to breastfeed, and had decreased urine output. Tests revealed him to have meningitis, and physicians realized that the meningococcal vaccine in his area is not a routine part of the childhood immunization schedule. The baby was treated with IV fluids, acetaminophen, IV antibiotics, and vasopressors. He also received transfusions of red blood cells and plasma. He slowly recovered and was eventually discharged. After one week, the boy's parents brought him in for a checkup, and the symptoms had resolved.

Critical Thinking Questions

1. What can meningococcal disease cause?
2. How are Neisseria meningitidis bacteria spread?
3. When should the two meningococcal vaccines be administered before traveling?

Case Study 3

A 34-year-old man vacationed in China and returned home to the United States, where he developed a headache that worsened until he became confused, had slurred speech, and could not walk without assistance. In the local emergency department, he started hallucinating. He also had a high fever, neck stiffness, ataxia, and increased muscle tone. A brain MRI revealed hyperintensities in the deep gray nuclei and possible subacute infarcts in the right thalamus and midbrain. Tests revealed him to be positive for Japanese encephalitis. The patient was treated with broad-spectrum antibacterial agents and acyclovir. He slowly improved and was discharged within two weeks, recovering completely.

Critical Thinking Questions

1. How is Japanese encephalitis spread from animals to humans?
2. What are the available types of Japanese encephalitis vaccines?
3. How is the Japanese encephalitis vaccine administered?

FURTHER READING

1. Davis, C.E., 2012. The International Traveler's Guide to Avoiding Infections. Johns Hopkins University Press., Book 1
2. Davis, E., 2008. Vaccine Alternatives – How to Prevent and Treat Illness Using Natural Remedies – An Essential Guide for Patients, Parents, Travelers, and Healthcare Workers. R&H Publishing.
3. Ertl, H.C.J., 2020. Rabies and Rabies Vaccines. Springer.
4. Gullberg, R.M. (2021). Health Advice & Immunizations for Travelers – Intended for International Travelers & Travel Clinics. Gullberg.
5. Ikidde, U., 2017. Essential Family and Travellers' Health – Health Advice Everyone Should Know. WriterMotive.
6. Jong, E.C., Sanford, C., 2008. The Travel and Tropical Medicine Manual, 4th Edition. Saunders/Elsevier.
7. Mackenzie, J.S., Barrett, A.D.T., Deubel, V., 2012. Japanese Encephalitis and West Nile Viruses Current Topics in Microbiology and Immunology. Springer., Book 267)
8. Nalin, D. (2022). Cholera Control in 2021: Bioecology, Immunology, Current and Future Vaccines and Treatment Options (Tropical Medicine and Infectious Disease). MDPI.
9. O'Leary, M.R., O'Leary, D.S., 2018. The Texas Meningitis Epidemic (1911-1913): Origin of the Meningococcal Vaccine. iUniverse.
10. Rappuoli, R., Vozza, L., 2022. Vaccines in the Global Era: How to Deal Safely and Effectively With the Pandemics Of Our Time. World Scientific Publishing Company.

Answer Key to Critical Thinking Questions in Case Studies

CHAPTER 1: THE IMMUNE SYSTEM

There is no case studies for the print or ebook for the following chapters 1, 5 & 6.

CHAPTER 2: INTEGRATIVE IMMUNOLOGY

Clinical Case Study 1

1. Rocky Mountain spotted fever (RMSF) is an infection caused by the bite of an infected tick. It affects over 2000 people annually in the United States and usually occurs from April until September. It can occur anytime during the year when the weather is warm.
2. A classic case of RMSF involves a rash that appears 2–4 days after the onset of fever as small, flat, pink macules on the wrists, forearms, and ankles and spreads to the trunk and sometimes the palms and soles.
3. RMSF is among the most severe of human infectious diseases, with a mortality of 20%–25% unless treated with an appropriate antibiotic.

Clinical Case Study 2

1. Fungal infections usually affect the skin, hair, nails, or mucous membranes, but they can also infect the lungs or other parts of the body. Fungal infections are more common in places on the body that trap moisture or have much friction.
2. People are at higher risk for disease, especially severe ones if they have poor circulation or diabetes or a weakened immune system from cancer or cancer treatment, immunosuppressant medications, and HIV/AIDS.
3. **Histoplasma** is the fungus that causes histoplasmosis and can infect your lungs, brain, or other body parts.

Vaccinology and Immunizations. https://doi.org/10.1016/B978-0-443-23915-1.00017-2

CHAPTER 3: HISTORY OF VACCINES

Clinical Case Study 1

1. The rabies virus is transmitted through direct contact with saliva from an infected animal. Humans usually get rabies from the bite of a rabid animal. Less often, transmission occurs from scratches, abrasions, or open wounds exposed to infectious saliva or other material from an infected animal.
2. The incubation period for rabies can last for weeks to months, based on the location of the exposure site, the type of rabies virus, and any existing immunity.
3. The first actual treatment for rabies occurred in the 1880s because of the work of Louis Pasteur in developing the vaccine. In 1885, a young boy was attacked by a rabid dog. Pasteur inoculated the boy 13 times over 11 days, and the boy completely recovered.

Clinical Case Study 2

1. The first recorded cases of hepatitis B (HepB) are believed to be those following the administration of the smallpox vaccine, which was given to shipyard workers in Germany in 1883.
2. A plasma-derived HepB vaccine was first licensed in the United States in 1982. Recombinant HepB vaccines replaced the plasma-derived vaccine in 1986, and the plasma-derived type is no longer used in the United States
3. The rate of reported acute HBV infections declined by about 90% since recommendations for vaccination were first issued.

Clinical Case Study 3

1. Tuberculosis (TB) is caused by the bacterium known as *Mycobacterium tuberculosis*, which usually attacks the lungs.
2. TB can affect many body organs such as the lungs, kidneys, spine, skin, brain, and the urinary tract or genital organs.
3. Miliary TB is a potentially fatal form of disseminated disease due to the hematogenous spread of tubercle bacilli to the lungs and other organs. It causes millet seed–sized tuberculous foci to form, each 1 to 2 mm in size. There is simultaneous involvement of two or more noncontinuous organ sites of the body or infection of the blood, bone marrow, or liver. The classical hallmark is mottling seen in chest radiographs.

Clinical Case Study 4

1. Pneumococcal disease is an infection caused by the bacterium known as *Streptococcus pneumoniae*, which can cause pneumonia, bacteremia, or meningitis. Pneumococcal pneumonia is the most common type of bacterial pneumonia.

2. Severe pneumococcal infections are more common in children under age 2 and adults over age 65, persons with sickle cell disease or HIV infection, and those with poorly functioning or removed spleens.
3. The first vaccine licensed for use in the United States became available in 1977 and was a polyvalent pneumococcal vaccine. The first conjugate pneumococcal vaccine was approved in 2000.

Clinical Case Study 5

1. The highest risks for developing severe COVID-19 disease are older people, those who are obese, and those with underlying chronic medical conditions, including cardiovascular disease, diabetes mellitus, chronic respiratory disease, and cancer.
2. The history of COVID-19 began in December 2019 when patients in Wuhan, China, started experiencing symptoms of a pneumonia-like illness that did not respond well to standard treatments. The first death from the disease occurred in January 2020 in China.
3. By April 4, 2020, more than 1 million cases of COVID-19 were confirmed worldwide, which was more than a 10-fold increase in less than 1 month. This fact means that only about 4 months have passed to reach this many cases—a rapidly developing pandemic.

CHAPTER 4: VACCINE PREPARATION AND CLASSIFICATIONS

Clinical Case Study 1

1. In a phase II trial, the vaccine being developed is given to 100 to 300 volunteers to further assess its safety and ability to generate an immune response. Participants have the same characteristics (such as age, gender, or physical health) as those for whom the vaccine is intended. There are usually multiple trials to evaluate various age groups and different vaccine formulations. A group that did not get the vaccine is generally included as a control group to determine whether the changes in the vaccinated group are attributed to the vaccine or have happened by chance.
2. In a phase III trial, the vaccine being developed is given to 1000 to 3000 volunteers and compared to a similar group of people who did not get the vaccine but received a control product to determine if it is effective against the disease it is designed to protect against and to study its safety in a much larger group of people. Most of the time, phase III trials are conducted across multiple countries and sites within a country to ensure that the findings of the vaccine performance will apply to many different populations.
3. During phase II and III trials, the volunteers and scientists conducting the study are kept from knowing which volunteers had received the vaccine being tested or the control product. This is called "blinding." It is necessary

to ensure that neither the volunteers nor the scientists are influenced in assessing the vaccine's safety or effectiveness. After the trial and all the results are finalized, the volunteers and trial scientists are informed who received the vaccine and the control product.

Clinical Case Study 2

1. The general stages of vaccine development include research and discovery, proof of concept, testing, manufacturing, approving, recommending the vaccine for use, and monitoring safety after approval.
2. A biological license application, submitted to the FDA as the new vaccine is being approved, includes preclinical and clinical data, details about the manufacturing process, and information about the manufacturing facility.
3. A control product is also known as a *placebo*, a substance with no therapeutic effect used in the *control group* of subjects. This is the group that is not receiving the actual vaccine being tested.

Clinical Case Study 3

1. Vaccine safety research ensures that the benefits of vaccines approved in the United States outweigh the risks, defines which groups should not receive certain vaccines, describes adverse events and side effects reported after vaccination, and evaluates whether reported side effects and adverse events can be directly linked to a vaccine.
2. In a phase I trial, the vaccine being developed is given to a few volunteers (20 to 100) to determine its safety, confirm that it generates an immune response, and find the proper dosage. Generally in this phase, vaccines are tested on young, healthy adult volunteers. Information is gathered on the vaccine's safety and side effects and how well the vaccine works to cause an immune response.

Clinical Case Study 4

1. Vaccine effectiveness studies utilize sources of vaccine history data to minimize bias. These include medical records, state and jurisdiction vaccine registries, and vaccination cards. Factors influencing vaccine effectiveness include age, underlying medical conditions such as diabetes mellitus and cancer, and history of prior infection.
2. Vaccine development usually begins in a university, medical center, or small biotech company research laboratory. Grants from the government or private foundations most often fund scientists in these laboratories. These scientists often spend years researching the effectiveness of their ideas, developing reagents and tests to measure their success, and, finally, using animals for testing. Sometimes, pictures are tested on small animals such as mice, rats, or rabbits, and then on larger animals such as monkeys.

CHAPTER 5: THE PROCESS OF VACCINE APPROVAL

There are no Clinical Cases in this chapter.

CHAPTER 6: PREVENTION AND ERADICATION OF INFECTIOUS DISEASES

There are no Clinical Cases in this chapter.

CHAPTER 7: VACCINE SAFETY AND ERRORS

Clinical Case Study 1

1. Pooled vaccination error prevalence was calculated to be 1.15 per 10,000 vaccine doses. The most commonly reported vaccination errors were "wrong vaccine administered" and "off-schedule administration."
2. Most of the time, these errors go unreported or, even worse, may need to be recognized.
3. Vaccination errors usually do not cause direct harm to patients, but subtherapeutic doses, incorrect vaccines, or expired vaccines can make patients more susceptible to disease.

Clinical Case Study 2

1. The most commonly reported vaccine errors include wrong vaccine, dose, age, and expired, contaminated, or deteriorated vaccine administration.
2. Healthcare professionals must, every time that they give an immunization, write down the lot number of the vaccine and the expiration date of the vaccine.
3. Vaccine administration errors can have many consequences, including inadequate immunological protection, possible injury to the patient, cost, inconvenience, and reduced confidence in the healthcare delivery system.

CHAPTER 8: PREVENTABLE CHILDHOOD INFECTIONS

Clinical Case Study 1

1. The causative pathogen for pertussis is *Bordetella pertussis*, a gram-negative bacterium.
2. The paroxysmal stage of pertussis is the second of three phases. After 10–14 days, this starts with increased cough severity and frequency. Repeated consecutive forceful coughs during expiration are followed by a fast and deep inspiration known as *the whoop*. Copious viscid mucus can be expelled or bubble from the nostrils during or after the paroxysmal stage. Vomiting is common. Infants may choke, with or without cyanosis, more often than whooping.

3. Early treatment of pertussis most effectively reduces symptom severity during the disease course. For seriously ill infants, hospitalization with respiratory isolation should be undertaken and continued until antibiotics have been administered for 5 days. Suction to remove excess throat mucus can be lifesaving. Some infants require oxygen, tracheostomy, or nasotracheal intubation. To avoid disturbances, the seriously ill infant is kept in a dark, quiet room with minimal disruptions. Patients treated at home must be isolated—especially from susceptible infants—for 4 weeks or more until symptoms have subsided. In the catarrhal stage, antibiotics may lessen symptoms, but once paroxysms are established, they are only used to limit disease spread. Preferred antibiotics include azithromycin, erythromycin, clarithromycin, and trimethoprim-sulfamethoxazole. Antibiotics are also used for bacterial complications such as bronchopneumonia or otitis media.

Clinical Case Study 2

1. Risk factors for meningococcal disease include infants younger than 1 year old, adolescents and young adults aged 16 through 23, college students living in residence halls, and people with certain medical conditions that affect the immune system, such as HIV.
2. Acute bacterial meningitis must be treated immediately with IV antibiotics and sometimes corticosteroids. This helps to ensure recovery and reduce the risk of complications such as brain edema and seizures. The antibiotic or combination depends on the type of bacteria causing the infection.
3. Antibiotic prophylaxis for close contact with patients with meningococcal disease includes rifampin, ciprofloxacin, or ceftriaxone. If these are contraindicated, a single dose of azithromycin can be an alternative. There are two types of meningococcal vaccines licensed in the United States: meningococcal conjugate (MenACWY) vaccines and serogroup B meningococcal (MenB) vaccines. These vaccines help protect against all three serogroups (B, C, and Y) of *Neisseria meningitidis* bacteria, most seen in the United States.

Clinical Case Study 3

1. The human papillomavirus (HPV) is the most common sexually transmitted infection in the United States. There are more than 43 million HPV infections annually in the United States, often among people in their late teens or early 20s. Within 10 years after the HPV vaccine was introduced, the prevalence of HPV types 6, 11, 16, and 18 has decreased to 86% among females aged 14–19 and 71% among females aged 20–24.
2. Cervical cancers are caused mainly by HPV-16 and HPV-18.
3. Removing samples of abnormal areas is critical because treatment is based on the severity of the abnormality. If the biopsy shows dysplasia or cancer, treatment is started.

CHAPTER 9: PEDIATRIC IMMUNIZATIONS

Clinical Case Study 1

1. Patients should be assessed for vaccine contraindications and precautions before vaccine administration. A screening questionnaire is used that should be filled out by each patient or guardian before the vaccine is given. Screening questionnaires ask about past and current illnesses or health conditions that could be a reason not to give a vaccine. The questionnaires also have questions about allergies, the use of medications or blood products that could interfere with the vaccine's effect, and past reactions to vaccines. The answers to these questions must be evaluated before any vaccine administration.
2. The rotavirus vaccine is contraindicated in infants with a history of intussusception or uncorrected congenital malformation of the gastrointestinal tract that would predispose to intussusception.
3. The oral rotavirus vaccine is administered as drops into the mouth.

Clinical Case Study 2

1. The intradermal route is used to administer the BCG vaccine. The needle is held at a low angle (15 degrees). The needle is about 1/4 inch, with the entire bevel under the skin.
2. The BCG vaccine is contraindicated when there is extensive skin disease or burns.
3. BCG stands for Bacillus Calmette-Guérin.

Clinical Case Study 3

1. The MMRII and Priorix vaccines are given subcutaneously.
2. The CDC's vaccination schedule for children between 6 weeks and 6 years must be checked to determine which vaccines are needed for infants and when they are required.
3. After a vaccine is given, it must be reported to the patient's primary care provider and the state's immunization information systems, if applicable. Any adverse events after the vaccine was given must also be documented and reported to the patient's primary care provider. Documentation of vaccination should be provided to the patient or guardian.

CHAPTER 10: ADULT IMMUNIZATIONS

Clinical Case Study 1

1. Varicella (chickenpox) complications include secondary bacterial infections of the skin, pneumonia, aseptic meningitis, and encephalitis.

2. Varicella vaccine is part of a routine immunization schedule, with the first dose given at 12–15 months of age. The booster dose is due at 4–6 years of age. For a "catch-up" schedule, the second dose can be given 3 months from the first. If the child is 13 or older, a double dose should be given four weeks after the first dose.
3. Contraindications include severe allergic reactions to previous doses or vaccine components, including neomycin and gelatin. Immunosuppression, febrile illness, pregnancy, and moderate or severe acute illness are contraindicated. The vaccine should be given later if the patient has recently received blood products. Avoid aspirin for 6 weeks after varicella vaccination due to the association of Reye syndrome with varicella.

Clinical Case Study 2

1. Viral load and viral type are the primary cofactors for progressing from infection to cervical intraepithelial lesions and cancer. Smoking, hormonal exposure, and HIV are additional exposures that increase the risk of progression to cancer.
2. Vaccinating all 11- to 12-year-olds can protect them long before exposure. The CDC recommends two doses of HPV vaccine for all adolescents at age 11 or 12 years. A two-dose schedule is recommended for people who get the first dose before their 15th birthday. In a two-dose series, the second dose should be given 6–12 months after the first dose. A three-dose schedule is recommended for people who get the first dose between 10 and 12 years of age. In a three-dose series, the second dose should be given 1 to 2 months after the first dose, and the third should be given 6 months after the first dose. The minimum intervals are 4 weeks between the first and second doses, 12 weeks between the second and third doses, and 5 months between the first and third doses.
3. Immunizations are generally safe in individuals with HIV except for live virus vaccines in people with low CD4 counts. In those individuals with HIV who have advanced immunosuppression, live vaccines can cause a potentially life-threatening disseminated infection because of the live pathogen in the vaccine.

Clinical Case Study 3

1. TB is an infectious disease that most often affects the lungs and is caused by bacteria. It spreads through the air when infected people cough, sneeze, or spit. About a quarter of the global population is estimated to have been infected with TB bacteria. About 5%–10% of people infected with TB will eventually get symptoms and develop TB.

2. TB occurs in every part of the world. In 2021, the most significant number of new TB cases occurred in WHO's South-East Asian region (46%), followed by the African region (23%) and the Western Pacific (18%). Around 87% of new TB cases occurred in the 30 high-TB-burden countries, with more than two-thirds of the global total in Bangladesh, China, the Democratic Republic of the Congo, India, Indonesia, Nigeria, Pakistan, and the Philippines.
3. The BCG vaccine is not a routine vaccination schedule. It is given only when a child or adult is thought to have an increased risk of contracting TB. The BCG vaccine should only be provided once in a lifetime. The vaccine is most effective in infants and children aged under 16. BCG vaccination is rarely given to anyone over 16 because there is little evidence that it works well. However, it is given to adults aged 16 to 35 who are at risk of TB through work, such as some healthcare workers, veterinary staff, and abattoir workers.

CHAPTER 11: IMMUNOLOGY IN OLDER ADULTS

Clinical Case Study 1

1. The immune system cannot distinguish the self from the non–self-antigens, causing autoimmune disorders. There are over 100 known autoimmune disorders, including, but not limited to, psoriasis, rheumatoid arthritis, lupus, celiac disease, and inflammatory bowel disease.
2. C-reactive protein tests determine infection, chronic inflammatory disease such as rheumatoid arthritis or lupus, and risk of heart disease.
3. The body may heal more slowly in older adults. There are fewer immune cells in the body to bring about healing. The immune system's ability to detect and correct cell defects also declines. This can increase the risk of infections, autoimmune disorders (including rheumatoid arthritis), and cancer.

Clinical Case Study 2

1. Roughly 50% of cancer cases occur in people aged 65 years or older. Older people are often diagnosed later and might receive less intensive treatment, affecting the outcome. In addition, an older age might be associated with biological differences in tumor and microenvironment behavior, a domain that has been poorly studied so far.
2. Some of the most frequently diagnosed malignancies in older adults are lung, breast, prostate, pancreatic, bladder, and skin cancers.
3. Immunotherapy in malignant tumor treatment has significantly changed the prospects of cancer treatment and improved the survival of patients with cancer.

CHAPTER 12: VACCINES FOR TRAVELERS

Clinical Case Study 1

1. Large epidemics of yellow fever occur when infected people introduce the virus into heavily populated areas with high mosquito density or where there is little to no immunity because of a lack of vaccination.
2. The yellow fever vaccine is recommended for persons 9 months and older traveling to or living in high-risk areas.
3. The yellow fever vaccine is 0.5 mL in volume and is administered through subcutaneous or IM injection.

Clinical Case Study 2

1. Meningococcal disease can cause a severe infection of the blood and the tissues around the spinal cord and brain.
2. *N. meningitidis* bacteria, or meningococci, are spread through saliva or spit and close or ongoing contact.
3. The MenACWY vaccine, or quadrivalent meningococcal meningitis vaccine, is a single injection that should be given 2 to 3 weeks before travel. The meningococcal conjugate vaccine can protect individuals for 5 years and should be given 7–10 days before travel to enable time for protective antibody levels to develop.

Clinical Case Study 3

1. The Japanese encephalitis virus is found in pigs and birds and is passed to mosquitoes when they bite infected animals. People get the virus when infected mosquitoes then bite them. It cannot be spread from person to person.
2. There are several types of inactivated vaccines and a kind of live attenuated vaccine currently used in the world to prevent Japanese encephalitis: inactivated mouse brain–derived, inactivated Vero cell–derived, primary hamster kidney cell–derived, purified, and live attenuated vaccines.
3. The inactivated vaccine against Japanese encephalitis, IXIARO, is given as a two-dose series, with the doses spaced 28 days apart. Adults aged 18–65 can get the second dose as early as 7 days after the first dose. The last amount should be given at least 1 week before travel. A booster dose (third dose) should be given if a person has received the two-dose primary vaccination series 1 year or more previously and there is a continued risk for Japanese encephalitis virus infection or potential for reexposure. For adults and children aged 3 years or older, each dose of IXIARO is 0.5 mL. For children aged 2 months through 2 years, each amount is 0.25 mL.

Glossary

Accidental cell death: An uncontrolled process caused by severe injury, such as chemical or mechanical damage.

Acetylcholine: A neurotransmitter that plays a role in memory, learning, attention, arousal, and involuntary muscle movement.

Acid mantle: An excellent, slightly acidic film on the surface of human skin, acting as a barrier to bacteria, viruses, and other potential contaminants that might penetrate the skin.

Acquired immune deficiency syndrome: A disease due to infection with the human immunodeficiency virus.

Acrodermatitis enteropathica: An inherited form of zinc deficiency caused by a defect in zinc absorption.

Active humoral immunity: Any form of immunity that occurs due to the formation of an adaptive immune response from the body's immune system.

Acute respiratory distress syndrome: A life-threatening lung injury that causes dangerously low oxygen levels in the blood.

Adaptive immune system: The immunity involves specific immune cells and antibodies to attack and destroy foreign invaders.

Adenoid: A mass of lymphatic tissue located behind the nasal cavity in the roof of the nasopharynx, where the nose blends into the throat.

Adrenal catecholamine: Hormones made by your adrenal glands, two small glands located above the kidneys. These hormones are released into the body in response to physical or emotional stress. The main types of catecholamines are dopamine, norepinephrine, and epinephrine. Epinephrine is also known as adrenaline.

Adverse events: A harmful outcome when a patient receives medical care.

Adverse reactions: An unexpected or unintended effect suspected to be caused by a medicine. All medicines can cause adverse reactions in some people. Adverse reactions can range from headaches and upset stomach to severe ones such as liver or kidney injury.

Aedes aegypti: The vector involved in urban transmission of yellow fever where only humans are the amplifying host.

African sleeping sickness: Also called sleeping sickness, it is caused by a parasite. People can get this parasite when an infected Tsetse fly bites them.

Agglutination: A reaction in which particles (as red blood cells or bacteria) suspended in a liquid collect into clumps and which occurs primarily as a serological response to a specific antibody.

Allogenic cells: Refer to transferring cells, tissues, or organs from one individual of the same species to another.

Alveolar macrophages: Also known as dust cells, these are white blood cells and the first line of defense against invading respiratory pathogens.

Amoebic dysentery: An infection of the intestines caused by a parasitic amoeba *Entamoeba histolytica*. It can cause frequent stools with blood or mucus, stomach pain, and fever.

Ancestor cells: Precursor cells are a generic term for cells that cannot renew. However, they have been found to generate tissue stem cells in some cases, thus contributing to the formation of tissues.

Anorexia: An eating disorder and severe mental health condition where people are of low weight due to limiting how much they eat and drink.

Anthrax: A severe infectious disease caused by a gram-positive, rod-shaped bacterium known as *Bacillus anthracis*. It occurs naturally in soil and commonly affects domestic and wild animals worldwide. People can get sick with anthrax if they come in contact with infected animals or contaminated animal products.

Antibodies: A protein component of the immune system that circulates in the blood, recognizes foreign substances such as bacteria and viruses, and neutralizes them.

Antibody titer: A laboratory test that measures the level of antibodies in a blood sample.

Antigen-antibody complexes: The complex formed by the binding of an antibody to an antigen. Antigen-antibody complexes initiate immune responses. They are also known as immune complexes.

Antigen-binding sites: The basic structure of the immunoglobulin molecule is the antigen-binding, or antibody-combining, area formed by a portion of the heavy and light chains. Every immunoglobulin molecule has at least two of these sites, which are identical.

Antigen-presenting cells: A large group of various cells that trigger the cellular immune response by processing an antigen and exposing it in a form recognizable by T cells in the process known as antigen presentation.

Antigen-specific T cells: T cells are human T cells that have been activated by a specific antigen derived from viruses, bacteria, tumor cells, and, in the case of autoimmune disease, peptides derived from normal tissues.

Antigenic determinants: Regions of proteins that can trigger a cellular immune response mediated by T or B cells.

Antigens: Any substance that causes the immune system to produce antibodies against it.

Apoptosis: The process of programmed cell death.

Arthralgia: Pain in a joint.

Aseptic meningitis: An inflammation of the meninges due to various etiologies with negative cerebrospinal fluid bacterial cultures.

Aspergilloma: A fungus ball or mycetoma composed of *Aspergillus* hyphae, cellular debris, and mucus. It is a noninvasive type of chronic pulmonary aspergillosis.

Asphyxia: A condition arising when the body is deprived of oxygen, causing unconsciousness or death due to suffocation.

Asplenia: The absence of a spleen.

Astrocytes: Release and respond to pro- and antiinflammatory signals such as cytokines and chemokines.

Auditory tube: A bony and cartilaginous tube connecting the middle ear with the nasopharynx and equalizing air pressure on both sides of the tympanic membrane. It is also called acoustic tube and pharyngotympanic tube.

Autoimmune disorders: An illness that causes the immune system to produce antibodies that attack normal body tissues.

Bacteremia: The presence of bacteria in the bloodstream.

Basophils: A white blood cell that works closely with your immune system to defend your body from allergens, pathogens, and parasites. Basophils release enzymes to improve blood flow and prevent blood clots.

Binary fission: A type of asexual reproduction where a parent cell divides, resulting in two identical cells, each having the potential to grow to the size of the original cell.

Biological license application: Requests permission to introduce or deliver a biologic product into interstate commerce.

Biomarker: A biological molecule found in blood, other body fluids, or tissues that indicates a normal or abnormal process, condition, or disease. It can be used to determine how effectively the body responds to treatment for a specific condition. Also known as a molecular marker or signature molecule.

Biometry: The development and application of statistical methods to many biological topics.

Biotechnology: The use of advances in molecular biology for applications in human health.

Blastomyces: The fungi that cause blastomycosis, commonly infecting the bones, skin, and lungs.

Blood-brain barrier: This allows the vessels in the CNS to tightly regulate the movement of ions, molecules, and cells between the blood and the brain.

Bone marrow: A spongy substance found in the center of the bones. It manufactures bone marrow stem cells and other substances, producing blood cells.

Bovine colostrum: The milk cows produce for the first several days following birthing.

Breakbone fever: Also called dengue fever, this is an acute infectious mosquito-borne fever that is temporarily incapacitating but rarely fatal.

Budding: An asexual mode of producing new organisms. In this process, a new organism is developed from a small part of the parent's body.

Bulbar paralysis: A set of conditions that can occur due to damage to the lower cranial nerves. Clinical features of bulbar palsy range from difficulty swallowing and a lack of a gag reflex to an inability to articulate words and excessive drooling. A brainstem stroke or tumor most commonly causes bulbar palsy.

***Candida albicans*:** A fungal infection caused by a yeast. Some species of *Candida* can cause disease in people; the most common is *Candida albicans*. *Candida* usually lives on the skin and inside the body, such as the mouth, throat, gut, and vagina, without causing problems.

Candidiasis: A fungal infection caused by a yeast (fungus) called *Candida*.

Capsid: The protein shell of a virus.

Celiac disease: A severe autoimmune disease that occurs in genetically predisposed people where ingesting gluten leads to damage in the small intestine.

Cellular immunity: An immune response that does not involve antibodies. Instead, cell-mediated immunity is the activation of phagocytes, antigen-specific cytotoxic T lymphocytes, and the release of various cytokines in response to an antigen.

Central immune tolerance: The protein shell of a virus enclosing its genetic material.

Cephalic tetanus: A rare form of tetanus defined as trismus plus paralysis of one or more cranial nerves. The most frequently involved cranial nerve is the seventh.

Ceruloplasmin: A protein that is made in the liver. It stores and carries copper from the liver into the bloodstream and to the parts of the body that need it.

Chemokinesis: The response of a cell to a chemical that causes the cell to change its movement by speeding it up, slowing it down, or changing its direction. The molecules that achieve these results are called chemokines.

Chemotaxis: The directed migration of a cell in response to a chemical stimulus such as a growth factor.

Chiggers: The common name for species of the Trombiculid family of mites. Bites from the larva of these mites can cause local pruritus and irritation. This is called trombiculiasis.

Chlamydiae: Obligate, intracellular, nonmotile, gram-negative bacteria with a unique biphasic developmental cycle.

Cholera: An acute diarrheal illness caused by infection of the intestine with *Vibrio cholerae* bacteria.

Chromoblastomycosis: A chronic granulomatous infection of the skin and subcutaneous tissue caused by several different dematiaceous fungi and resulting in the formation of slow-growing warty plaques and cauliflower-like lesions that may ulcerate.

Coccidioidomycosis: Also called valley fever, this is caused by a fungus that grows in the soil and dirt in some areas of California and the southwestern United States.

Cochlear implant: An electronic device that improves hearing. It can be an option for people with severe hearing loss from inner ear damage who cannot hear well with hearing aids.

Cognitive tests: Checks for problems with mental function. It involves answering simple questions and performing simple tests.

Colposcopy: A diagnostic procedure that allows a physician to check the cervix and the wall of the vagina for abnormal tissue.

Commensal bacteria: Types of bacteria that live on or within a host organism in a manner where the host is neither harmed nor benefited. Essentially, it is a symbiosis—but only beneficial for one party.

Community immunity: Also known as herd immunity, this refers to "Protection from an infectious disease that occurs when many people in a community are vaccinated against it." This means that vaccination protects the vaccinated person and also the whole community.

Complement activation: Attracting and activating inflammatory cells and also known as complement cascade, it is a part of the immune system that enhances the ability of cells to clear microbes and damaged cells from an organism.

Complement: A large number of distinct plasma proteins that react with one another to opsonize pathogens and induce a series of inflammatory responses that help to fight infection.

Complete antigens: One that both induces an immune response and reacts with its products, whereas an incomplete antigen or hapten is unable to induce an immune response alone but can react with its products, for example, antibodies.

Congenital rubella syndrome: An infant illness that results from maternal infection with rubella virus during pregnancy. When rubella infection occurs during early pregnancy, serious consequences—such as miscarriages, stillbirths, and a constellation of severe congenital disabilities in infants—can result.

Conjugate vaccines: A subunit vaccine that combines a weak antigen with a potent antigen as a carrier so that the immune system responds more strongly to the weak antigen.

Constant region: Determines the mechanism used to destroy the antigen.

Coryza: An acute inflammation of the mucous membrane of the nasal cavities.

Cyanosis: A bluish color of mucous membranes or skin.

Cross-reacting antigens: Measures the extent to which different antigens appear similar to the immune system.

Cryptococcus: A pulmonary or disseminated infection acquired by inhalation of soil contaminated with the encapsulated yeasts *Cryptococcus neoformans*.

Cytokines: Small secreted proteins released by cells that specifically affect cell interactions and communications.

Cytotoxic activity: A substance or process can damage cells or cause them to die.

Cytotoxic T cells: A type of immune cell. They destroy cells infected with viruses. Another name for cytotoxic T cells is killer T cells. Cytotoxic T cells are one of the three main types of cells developed in the thymus.

Defensin: A family of potent antibiotics made within the body by neutrophils and macrophages.

Delirium tremens: A severe form of alcohol withdrawal. It involves sudden and severe mental or nervous system changes.

Delta hepatitis: A liver infection caused by the hepatitis D virus. It only occurs in people infected with the hepatitis B virus.

Demyelination: A loss of myelin with relative preservation of axons.

Dendritic cells: Professional antigen-presenting cells that inform the fight against invasive pathogens while enforcing tolerance to self and harmless environmental antigens.

Dengue: A viral infection that spreads from mosquitoes to people. It is more common in tropical and subtropical climates.

Dermcidin: An antimicrobial peptide secreted by sweat glands that attacks any bacteria on the skin.

Diapedesis: The passage of blood cells through capillary walls into the tissues.

Diffuse lymphoid tissue: Localized collections of lymphocytes are common in the lamina propria of the alimentary and respiratory tracts.

DiGeorge syndrome: DiGeorge syndrome is a genetic condition caused by a missing piece of chromosome 22. The disease, present from birth, can cause many lifelong problems, including heart defects and learning difficulties.

Diphtheria: A severe infection caused by strains of *Corynebacterium diphtheriae* that make toxins.

Dust cells: A type of macrophage, a professional phagocyte, found in the airways and at the level of the alveoli in the lungs but separated from their walls.

Dysphagia: Difficulty swallowing food or liquids.

Ebola: Also known as Ebola virus disease and Ebola hemorrhagic fever, this is a viral hemorrhagic fever in humans and other primates, caused by ebolaviruses.

Ecchymosis: A flat blue or purple patch measuring 1 cm or more in diameter.

Ecological niche: The position of a species within an ecosystem, describing both the conditions necessary for the persistence of the species and its ecological role in the ecosystem.

Elek test: An *in vitro* virulence test performed on specimens of *C. diphtheriae*, the bacteria that causes diphtheria. It is used to test for the toxigenicity of *C. diphtheriae* strains. The test uses immunodiffusion.

Emergency use authorization: The authority allows the FDA to help strengthen the nation's public health protections against chemical, biological, radiological, and nuclear threats.

Encephalitis: An inflammation of the brain.

Endogenous antigens: Exist on cells inside the body. They tell the immune system they are either friendly ("self") or harmful. These include cells infected with bacteria or a virus that mark themselves to be destroyed by the immune system.

Endogenous: Having an internal cause or origin.

Endotoxemia: The presence of endotoxin within the blood.

Enterocyte: Intestinal absorptive cells are simple columnar epithelial cells that line the inner surface of the small and large intestines.

Eosinophils: White blood cells that primarily attack parasitic infections but also are involved with allergies and asthma.

Epstein-Barr virus: Also known as human herpesvirus 4, this is a member of the herpes virus family. It is one of the most common human viruses.

Eukaryote: A cell that contains membrane-bound structures, it is the basis for every multicellular organism, including animals, plants, and humans, as well as some unicellular organisms such as protozoa.

Eumycetoma: A chronic deep fungal infection of the skin and subcutaneous tissue.

Evanescent: Tending to disappear quickly or for a relatively short duration.

Exogenous antigens: Foreign substances that can enter the body through the nose, mouth, or cuts in the skin. These include viruses, bacteria, pollen, parasites, and fungi.

Exotoxin: A soluble poisonous substance produced during the growth of a microorganism and released into the surrounding medium.

Expiration date: The time during which the product is known to remain stable, which means it retains its strength, quality, and purity when it is stored according to its labeled storage conditions.

Fc receptors: Bind to antibodies attached to infected cells or invading pathogens.

Ferroptosis: A type of cell death caused by iron-mediated peroxidation of cellular lipids that leads to tissue dysfunction in several human cells.

Fibroblast: A type of cell that contributes to the formation of connective tissue, a fibrous cellular material that supports and connects other tissues or organs in the body. Fibroblasts secrete collagen proteins that help maintain the structural framework of tissues.

Flaccid paralysis: A neurological condition characterized by weakness or paralysis and reduced muscle tone without other apparent cause (e.g., trauma).

Genital warts: A common sexually transmitted infection caused by human papillomavirus that causes small growths in and around the genitals and rectum.

Genome: The entire set of DNA instructions found in a cell. In humans, the genome consists of 23 pairs of chromosomes in the cell's nucleus and a small chromosome in the cell's mitochondria. A genome contains all the information needed for an individual to develop and function.

German measles: Rubella is a contagious disease caused by a virus. Most people who get rubella usually have a mild illness with symptoms that can include a low-grade fever, sore throat, and a rash that starts on the face and spreads to the rest of the body.

Giant cell arteritis: A disorder that causes inflammation of the arteries, usually in the scalp, neck, and arms.

Gliosis: A process leading to scars in the central nervous system that involves the production of a dense fibrous network of neuroglia in areas of damage.

Glottis: The vocal apparatus of the larynx consists of the true vocal folds (vocal cords) and the opening between the vocal cords.

Glycocalyx: A dense, gel-like meshwork that surrounds the cell, constituting a physical barrier for any object to enter the cell. For example, the glycocalyx was identified to play an essential role in preventing the entry of pathogens into the cell.

Glycolysis: The process in which glucose is broken down to produce energy.

Gram stain: One of the most crucial staining techniques in microbiology to classify bacterial species into two large groups: gram-positive bacteria and gram-negative bacteria.

Granulomatous: A genetic disorder in which white blood cells called phagocytes cannot kill certain bacteria and fungi.

Granzyme(s): A family of cytotoxic proteases, they are critical players in cytotoxic T-lymphocyte elimination of target cells.

Guillain-Barré syndrome: A rare condition in which a person's immune system attacks the peripheral nerves. People of all ages can be affected, but it is more common in adults and males. Most people recover fully from even the most severe cases of Guillain-Barré syndrome.

Habitat: A place where an organism makes its home. A habitat meets all the environmental conditions an organism needs to survive.

Hallucination: A false perception of objects or events involving the senses, such as sight, sound, smell, touch, and taste.

Hapten: A small molecule that, when combined with a larger carrier such as a protein, can produce antibodies that bind specifically to it.

Haptoglobin: A protein made by the liver, which attaches to a specific type of hemoglobin.

Haptokinesis: Slow or diminished movement of body musculature.

Haptotaxis: The motility of cells up a gradient of substrate-bound molecules. There is a wide variety of procedures to set up this gradient *in vitro* to study haptotaxis.

Helminths: Parasitic worms that cause a wide variety of infectious diseases. They are large microparasites; adults can generally be seen with the naked eye.

Hemoglobin: The protein contained in red blood cells that is responsible for the delivery of oxygen to the tissues.

Hemoptysis: The discharge of blood or blood-stained mucus through the mouth from the bronchi, larynx, trachea, or lungs.

Hepatitis B surface antigen (HBsAg): The most useful screening tests for chronic HBV infection or immunity to HBV. HBsAg is present in most chronically infected persons. Lack of anti-HBs in an unvaccinated HBsAg-negative person indicates susceptibility to HBV infection.

Hepcidin: A peptide hormone produced in the liver that plays a crucial role in iron homeostasis.

Histoplasma: An infection caused by a fungus called *Histoplasma*. The fungus lives in the environment, particularly in soil containing large bird or bat droppings.

Homeostasis: The state of balance within all physical systems needed for a body to function correctly and survive is homeostasis. In a state of homeostasis, body levels constantly adjust to changes outside and inside the body.

Human papillomavirus infection: A viral infection commonly causes skin or mucous membrane growths (warts).

Humoral immunity: The production of antibody molecules in response to an antigen.

Hydrophobia: An extreme dread or fear of water, mainly associated with painful involuntary throat spasms from a rabies infection.

Hyphae: A long, branching, filamentous structure of a fungus.

Hypothalamus: An area of the brain that produces hormones that control body temperature, hunger, and heart rate.

Hypoxia: A state in which oxygen is not available in sufficient amounts at the tissue level to maintain adequate homeostasis; this can result from inadequate oxygen delivery to the tissues due to low blood supply or low oxygen content in the blood.

Immune checkpoint inhibitors: A type of immunotherapy involving blocking immune checkpoint proteins from binding with partner proteins.

Immune deficiencies: Usually result from the use of a medication or a severe, long-lasting disorder (such as cancer) but occasionally are inherited. People usually have frequent, unusual, or unusually severe or prolonged infections and may develop an autoimmune disease or cancer.

Immune escape variants: Helps the virus to evade the human immune system and cause infection and reinfection to the human.

Immunization information system: Confidential, population-based, computerized databases that record all immunization doses administered by participating providers to persons residing within a given geopolitical area.

Immunization protocols: Approved steps and methods by which vaccines are administered.

Immunogenicity: The ability of cells/tissues to provoke an immune response is generally considered an undesirable physiological response.

Immunoglobulins: Also known as antibodies, glycoprotein molecules are produced by plasma cells (white blood cells).

Immunologic tolerance: A complex series of mechanisms that impair the immune system to mount responses against self-antigens.

Immunological memory: The ability of the immune system to respond more rapidly and effectively to pathogens encountered previously and reflects the preexistence of a clonally expanded population of antigen-specific lymphocytes.

Immunological tolerance: The process by which immune cells are made unresponsive to self-antigens to prevent damage to healthy tissues.

Immunometabolism: The interface between immunology and metabolism.

Immunosenescence: A process of immune dysfunction that occurs with age and includes remodeling of lymphoid organs, leading to changes in the immune function of older people,

***In vitro* experiments:** Medical procedures, tests, and experiments outside a living organism.

Inactivated vaccines: Composed of dead or inactivated viruses and bacteria and therefore differ from live but attenuated vaccines.

Incubation period: The time it takes for an infection to develop after a person has been exposed to a disease-causing organism (such as bacteria, viruses, or fungi). The incubation period ends when the first signs or symptoms of the disease appear.

Infectious hepatitis: A contagious liver disease caused by the hepatitis A virus.

Inflammatory bowel disease: A term for two conditions (Crohn disease and ulcerative colitis) characterized by chronic gastrointestinal tract inflammation.

Inflammatory markers: Blood tests detect inflammation in the body caused by many diseases. This can include infections, autoimmune conditions, and cancers.

Infrastructure: The basic physical systems of a business, region, or nation often involve public goods or production processes. Infrastructure includes transportation, sewage, communication networks, water, and school systems.

Ingredient: Any substance that is used in the manufacture of a cannabis product and is intended to be present in the product's final form.

Innate immune cells: A nonspecific mechanism for fighting against infections. This immune response is rapid, occurring minutes or hours after aggression, and is mediated by numerous cells, including phagocytes, mast cells, basophils, eosinophils, and the complement system.

Innate immunity: The body's first line of defense against germs entering the body.

Institute for Safe Medication Practices: The global authority, a nonprofit organization that educates the healthcare community and consumers about safe medication practices.

Interferons: A group of signaling proteins made and released by host cells in response to the presence of several viruses.

Interleukins: Proteins produced by various cells in the inflammatory response to infections. The immune system triggers their production in response to pathogens or cytokines.

Intestinal crypts: A sterile invagination composed of goblet and stem cells, which can secrete mucus and antimicrobial peptides such as cryptdins.

Intracellular degradation: A highly regulated process. Rates of protein degradation. Increase or decrease under many physiological and pathological conditions.

Intradermal route: Injections into the dermis, just below the epidermis. The intradermal injection route has the longest absorption time of all parenteral routes.

Intramuscular injection: Installing medications into the depth of specifically selected muscles.

Intussusception: A severe condition in which part of the intestine slides into an adjacent portion of the intestine.

Investigational new drug: A drug or biological drug that has not been approved for general use by the FDA. It is used in a clinical trial to investigate its safety and efficacy.

Jamestown Canyon virus: Spread to people by infected mosquitoes. The virus is found throughout the United States, but most cases are reported from the upper Midwest. Cases occur from late spring through midfall.

Japanese encephalitis: A brain infection caused by the Japanese encephalitis virus. While most conditions result in little or no symptoms, occasional inflammation of the brain occurs.

Jaundice: Yellowish pigmentation of the skin, tissues, and body fluids caused by the deposition of bile pigments.

Kawasaki disease: A rare heart condition that causes a high fever and inflammation of the blood vessels. It usually affects children under the age of 5.

Keratin: A protein that helps form hair, nails, and the epidermis. It helps support the skin, heal wounds, and keep nails and hair healthy. There are 54 kinds of keratin in the body.

Keratinized tissue: Also known as keratinized mucosa, refers to the band of tissue surrounding the teeth at the point where they meet the gums.

Kidney failure: When kidneys have stopped working well enough to survive without dialysis or a kidney transplant.

Koplik spots: The peculiar spots present on the buccal mucosa and are considered a diagnostic of measles.

Kupffer cells: Specialized macrophages in the liver, particularly at the lining of liver sinusoids.

La Crosse encephalitis: A viral illness transmitted to people through the bite of an infected mosquito.

Lamina propria: Loose connective tissue in a mucosa. It supports the delicate mucosal epithelium, allows the epithelium to move freely to deeper structures, and provides for immune defense.

Langerhans cells: Reside in the epidermis as a dense network of immune system sentinels. They determine the appropriate adaptive immune response (inflammation or tolerance) by interpreting the microenvironmental context in which they encounter foreign substances.

Leukemia: A type of cancer found in the blood and bone marrow and caused by the rapid production of abnormal white blood cells.

Leukocytosis: An increase in white cells in the blood, especially during an infection.

Leukopenia: A condition with an abnormally reduced amount of white blood cells.

Lichen planus: A condition of the skin, hair, nails, mouth, and genitals. The cause of lichen planus is unknown. It is thought to be related to the immune system or an abnormal response of the immune system to certain medicines.

Lingual tonsil: Located on the posterior surface of the tongue, which also places them near the opening of the oral cavity into the pharynx.

Lipolysis: The process of breaking down lipids.

Live attenuated vaccines: A disease-causing virus or bacterium weakened in a laboratory, so it cannot cause disease. Live attenuated viruses are often used as vaccines because, although weakened, they can stimulate a robust immune response.

Lot number: An identification number assigned to a particular quantity or lot of material from a single manufacturer.

Lyme disease: A bacterial infection spread to humans by infected ticks. It is also known as Lyme borreliosis. Ticks are tiny spiderlike creatures found in woodland and moorland areas.

Lymph nodes: Small structures that filter foreign substances such as cancer cells and infections.

Lymphocytes: A type of white blood cell part of the immune system. There are two main types of lymphocytes: B cells and T cells. The B cells produce antibodies to attack invading bacteria, viruses, and toxins.

Lymphoid follicles: A regular component of gut-associated lymphatic tissue. They are aggregates of lymphocytes surrounding germinal centers that straddle the muscularis mucosae.

Lymphoma: A broad term for cancer that begins in cells of the lymph system. The two main types are Hodgkin lymphoma and non-Hodgkin lymphoma. Hodgkin lymphoma can often be cured. The prognosis of non-Hodgkin lymphoma depends on the specific type.

Macrophages: Specialized cells involved in detecting, phagocytosis, and destroying bacteria and other harmful organisms.

Malaria: A severe and sometimes fatal disease caused by a parasite that commonly infects a specific type of mosquito that feeds on humans.

Malnutrition: A lack of proper nutrition caused by needing more to eat, not eating enough of the right things, or being unable to use the food that one does eat.

Margination: Accumulation and adhesion of leukocytes to the epithelial cells of blood vessel walls at the site of injury in the early stages of inflammation.

Mastitis: An inflammation of breast tissue that sometimes involves an infection.

Measles: A highly contagious, severe airborne disease caused by a virus that can lead to severe complications and death.

Medication administration record: Keep track of every dose the individual you support takes or misses for whatever reason. A medication administration record includes vital information about the individual's medication, including the medication name, amount taken, special instructions, and date and time.

Megakaryocytes: A large bone marrow cell with a lobated nucleus that produces blood platelets (thrombocytes) necessary for normal clotting.

Memory T cells: Antigen-specific T cells that remain long term after an infection has been eliminated.

Meningococcal disease: A rare, serious illness caused by a bacteria (*Neisseria meningitidis*). It can cause meningitis.

Meningococcemia: A bloodstream infection caused by *N. meningitidis*.

Meningoencephalitis: A neurological condition resembling meningitis, which is the inflammation of the meninges, and encephalitis, which is the inflammation of the brain tissue.

Messenger RNA (mRNA) vaccines: A type of vaccine that uses a copy of a molecule called mRNA to produce an immune response. The vaccine delivers molecules of antigen-encoding mRNA into immune cells, which use the designed mRNA as a blueprint to build foreign proteins that a pathogen would usually produce.

Metabolic diseases: Any diseases or disorders that disrupt normal metabolism, the process of converting food to energy on a cellular level.

Microflora: A community of bacteria that exist on or inside the body and possess a unique ecological relationship with the host.

Microglia: The brain's resident immune cells constantly patrol the cerebral microenvironment to respond to pathogens and damage.

Micronutrients: A chemical element or substance required in trace amounts for living organisms' average growth and development.

Mitochondrial disease: A group of disorders that affect the mitochondria, which are tiny compartments in almost every body cell. The mitochondria's primary function is to produce energy.

Monkeypox: An infectious disease caused by the monkeypox virus. It can cause a painful rash, enlarged lymph nodes, and fever. Most people fully recover, but some get very sick.

Monoclonal antibodies: Synthetic proteins that act like human antibodies in the immune system.

Monocytes: A large, circulating white blood cell formed in the bone marrow and the spleen that ingests large foreign particles and cell debris.

Monomer: A small molecule that reacts with a similar molecule to form a larger molecule.

Mosquito-borne parasites: Diseases that are spread to people by mosquitoes include Zika virus, West Nile virus, Chikungunya virus, dengue, and malaria.

Mottling: Blotchy, red-purplish marbling of the skin. Mottling most frequently occurs on the feet and then travels up the legs. Mottling of skin before death is typical and usually occurs during the final week of life, although in some cases, it can occur earlier.

Mucin: Any of a group of mucoproteins found in human secretions and tissues (as in saliva, the lining of the stomach, and the skin).

Mucosa-associated lymphoid tissue: Initiates immune responses to specific antigens encountered on mucosal surfaces. Mucosa-associated lymphoid tissue inductive sites are secondary immune tissues where antigen sampling occurs and immune responses are initiated.

Multiple sclerosis: A chronic, typically progressive disease involving damage to the sheaths of brain and spinal cord neurons.

Multiple vaccines: Several possible meanings. A single dose of vaccine may present multiple antigens for a single disease (e.g., polio or pneumococcal vaccines) or multiple antigens for various illnesses, such as the MMR vaccine.

Mumps: A contagious disease caused by a virus that spreads from person to person. Typical symptoms of mumps include swollen salivary glands and a fever.

Mycoplasmas: Any group of tiny typically parasitic bacteria that lack cell walls and sometimes cause diseases.

Mycoses: A disease caused by infection with a fungus, such as ringworm or thrush.

Myeloid cell: A myeloid cell is a type of blood cell that originates in the bone marrow.

Myelopoiesis: Production of bone marrow or bone marrow cells.

Myoglobinuria: The presence of an excess amount of myoglobin in the urine. It is mainly caused by muscle breakdown, releasing a high amount of myoglobin in the blood. Myoglobinuria can lead to acute kidney injury.

Nasotracheal intubation: Passing an endotracheal tube through the naris, into the nasopharynx, and the trachea, most commonly after induction of general anesthesia in the operating room.

National Childhood Vaccine Injury Act: Provides compensation to people found to be injured by certain vaccines.

Necroptosis: An alternative mode of regulated cell death mimicking features of apoptosis and necrosis.

Neisseria meningitidis: A diplococcal, gram-negative, and human commensal bacterium of the upper respiratory tract. The pathogen can invade the mucosa and access the bloodstream, resulting in meningitis, severe sepsis, or localized infections in joints and heart.

Neoplasia: The uncontrolled, abnormal growth of cells or tissues in the body and the abnormal growth itself.

Neutralization: The ability of antibodies to block the site(s) of bacteria or viruses they use to enter their target cell.

Neutrophils: A type of white blood cell that acts as the immune system's first line of defense.

Nucleotides: Organic molecules comprise a nitrogenous base, a pentose sugar, polymers, and a phosphate. They serve as monomeric units of the nucleic acids: DNA and RNA.

Oophoritis: An inflammation of the ovaries.

Opportunistic infections: Infections that occur more frequently and are more severe in people with weakened immune systems, including people with human immunodeficiency virus.

Opsonins: Freely circulating serum molecules that are produced to attach to the surface of microbes, rendering them more attractive to phagocytes.

Optical coherence tomography: A noninvasive imaging test that uses light waves to take cross-section photographs of the retina.

Oral tolerance: An active process of local and systemic immune unresponsiveness to orally ingested antigens, including food.

Oral vaccines: Vaccines that are administered into the mouth.

Orchitis: The inflammation of the testicle unilaterally or bilaterally, usually caused by viruses and bacteria.

***Orthopoxvirus*:** A genus of large, brick-shaped, double-stranded DNA viruses. Smallpox is the most severe disease associated with a high mortality rate.

Ovalbumin: An essential reference protein for vaccination experiments; the protein is a significant constituent of chicken egg whites.

Palatine tonsils: Commonly referred to as tonsils, these are bundles of lymphatic tissue located in the lateral oropharynx.

Parakeratosis: Incomplete maturation of epidermal keratinocytes, resulting in abnormal retention of nuclei in the stratum corneum. It occurs in many diseases of the skin, particularly psoriasis.

Paralysis: A loss of motor function in one or more muscles. It can also be accompanied by sensory loss in the affected area if there is sensory damage.

Parotitis: An inflammation of one or both parotid glands, the major salivary glands on either side of the face, in humans.

Passive human immunization: The short-term immunity that results from introducing antibodies from another person.

Passive humoral immunity: The transfer of active humoral immunity through ready-made antibodies from one individual to another.

Pathogenesis: A disease describes the mechanisms by which it develops, progresses, and either persists or is resolved.

Perforin: A glycoprotein responsible for pore formation in cell membranes of target cells.

Peripheral immune tolerance: A noninvasive imaging method that uses reflected light to create pictures of the back of the eye.

Pertussis: Also known as whooping cough, this is a highly contagious respiratory infection caused by *Bordetella pertussis*.

Petechiae: A small red or purple spot caused by bleeding into the skin.

Peyer patches: Clusters of subepithelial lymphoid follicles found in the intestine.

Phagocytosis: Process by which specific living cells called phagocytes ingest or engulf other cells or particles.

Phagolysosome: A digestive vesicle formed within a cell by fusing a phagosome containing ingested material and a lysosome containing hydrolytic enzymes.

Phagosome: A vesicle formed around a particle engulfed by a phagocyte via phagocytosis.

Placebo: Any treatment with no active properties, such as a sugar pill.

Plasma cells: Differentiated B-lymphocyte white blood cells capable of secreting antibodies.

Plasma membrane: A microscopic membrane of lipids and proteins that forms the external boundary of the cytoplasm of a cell and regulates the passage of molecules in and out of the cytoplasm.

Plasmid: A small, circular DNA molecule found in bacteria and some other microscopic organisms.

Platelets: Also called thrombocytes, these are tiny components of the blood that help clotting.

Pneumococcal disease: Any infection caused by bacteria called *Streptococcus pneumoniae* or pneumococcus. Pneumococcal infections can range from ear and sinus infections to pneumonia and bloodstream infections. There are vaccines to help prevent pneumococcal disease.

Pneumocystis pneumonia: A severe infection caused by the fungus *Pneumocystis jirovecii*.

Poliomyelitis: A highly infectious viral disease that primarily affects children under 5 years of age. The virus is transmitted by person-to-person spread, mainly through the fecal-oral route.

Polyneuropathy: The simultaneous malfunction of many peripheral nerves throughout the body.

Polyurethane condom: A type of external condom made from plastic. The FDA approves polyurethane condoms to prevent pregnancy and sexually transmitted infections.

Postexposure prophylaxis: A dose of human rabies immune globulin and rabies vaccine is given on the day of the rabies exposure, and then a dose of vaccine is given again on days 3, 7, and 14.

Postherpetic neuralgia: A painful condition affecting the nerves and skin. It is a complica tion of shingles.

Potency: An expression of the activity of a drug in terms of the concentration or amount of the drug required to produce a defined effect, whereas clinical efficacy judges the drug's therapeutic effectiveness in humans.

Preexposure prophylaxis: Vaccine doses before coming into contact with the rabies virus. This can help protect a person against unrecognized rabies exposures or when rabies postexposure prophylaxis may be delayed.

Precipitation: The qualitative and quantitative detection of antigens and antibodies.

Probiotics: Live microorganisms intended to have health benefits when consumed or applied to the body.

Prodrome: A premonitory symptom of disease.

Prokaryotes: Organisms whose cells lack a nucleus and other organelles.

Prostaglandins: A potent, hormone-like lipid derived from fatty acids that acts as a local messenger to regulate inflammation, blood flow, muscle contraction, and labor.

Protamine sulfate: A medication used to reverse and neutralize the anticoagulant effects of heparin.

Protein-based vaccines: Using peptides or proteins as antigens to induce an immune response.

Psoriasis: A skin disease that causes a rash with itchy, scaly patches, most commonly on the knees, elbows, trunk, and scalp. Due to systemic inflammation and an immune-mediated disease.

Pulmonary edema: Excessive liquid accumulation in the lungs' tissue and air spaces (usually alveoli).

Pustules: Small, inflamed, pus-filled, blister-like lesions on the skin surface.

Pyrogens: Substances, typically produced by a bacterium, that cause fever when released into the blood.

Pyroptosis: A form of programmed cell death that occurs in immune cells in response to inflammation caused by microbial infections.

Quadrivalent vaccines: These vaccines are designed to protect against four different flu viruses, including two influenza A viruses and two influenza B viruses.

Rabies: A fatal but preventable viral disease. It can spread to people and pets if they are bitten or scratched by a rabid animal.

Reactogenicity: The physical manifestation of the inflammatory response to vaccination can include injection site pain, redness, swelling, or induration at the injection site and systemic symptoms such as fever, myalgia, or headache.

Recombinant vaccines: A vaccine produced through recombinant DNA technology. This involves inserting the DNA encoding an antigen (such as a bacterial surface protein) that stimulates an immune response into bacterial or mammalian cells, expressing the antigen in these cells, and then purifying it from them.

Regulatory T cells: A specialized subpopulation of T cells that suppress the immune response, thereby maintaining homeostasis and self-tolerance.

Reticular cells: A type of fibroblast that synthesizes collagen and uses it to produce reticular fibers.

Reticuloendothelial system: Consists of cells descending from the monocytes, which can perform phagocytosis of foreign materials and particles. Ninety percent of the reticuloendothelial system is located in the liver.

Reverse transcriptase: Also known as RNA-dependent DNA polymerase, this is a DNA polymerase enzyme that transcribes single-stranded RNA into DNA.

Reye syndrome: A rare but severe condition that causes swelling in the liver and brain. It can occur at any age but usually affects children and teenagers after a viral infection, most commonly the flu or chickenpox.

Rheumatoid arthritis: A chronic autoimmune disease that primarily affects joints. Rheumatoid arthritis occurs when the immune system attacks its tissues, which helps protect the body from infection and illness.

Rhinorrhea: An excessive mucous secretion from the nose.

Ribosomal DNA: Codes for the rRNAs used in the production of ribosomes, the sites of cellular protein synthesis.

Ribosomes: Minute particles consisting of RNA and associated proteins that function to synthesize proteins.

Rickettsia typhi: A gram-negative, aerobic, rod-shaped bacterium. It belongs to the family of Rickettsiaceae.

Rickettsialpox: A mite-borne disease that belongs to the spotted fever group of rickettsioses.

Ringworm: A common skin infection caused by a fungus that can cause a circular rash that is usually red and itchy.

Risus sardonicus: A highly characteristic, abnormal, sustained spasm of the facial muscles that appear to produce grinning. It may be caused by tetanus, strychnine poisoning, or Wilson disease and has been reported after judicial hanging.

Rocky Mountain spotted fever: A severe illness from a tick bite. It is caused by the bacterium *Rickettsia rickettsii.*

Rotavirus infection: A virus that causes symptoms of severe diarrhea, vomiting, fever, and dehydration.

Rubella: An illness caused by the virus RuV. It causes a rash, low fever, and other symptoms. It's highly contagious person-to-person. It is commonly called German measles or 3-day measles.

Salivary glands: The glands that make saliva, which aids digestion, keeps the mouth moist, and supports healthy teeth. The three pairs of major salivary glands under and behind the jaw are parotid, sublingual, and submandibular.

***Salmonella enterica* serovar Typhi:** A gram-negative bacterium that is responsible for typhoid fever. The symptoms may last for months without antibiotic treatment, and the fatality rate can be as high as 20%.

Scarlet fever: A bacterial illness that mainly affects children and causes a distinctive pink to red rash; *Streptococcus pyogenes* cause it.

Sebaceous glands: A bacterial illness that mainly affects children. It causes a distinctive pink-red rash. It is usually associated with *S. pyogenes* pharyngitis in school-age and adolescent children.

Sebum: An oily substance that protects the skin from drying out.

Selenoproteins: A protein containing selenoprotein amino acid residue.

Self-tolerance: The immune system's ability to recognize what is "self" and not react against or attack it.

Senescence-associated secretory phenotype: A crucial driver of chronic inflammation and aging phenotypes.

Senescence: The condition or process of deterioration with age.

Sepsis: A severe condition that happens when the body's immune system has an extreme response to an infection.

Septicemia: A severe bloodstream infection. It occurs when a bacterial infection enters the bloodstream from elsewhere in the body.

Serum hepatitis: Formerly known as serum hepatitis. It is an infection of the liver caused by a bloodborne virus.

Severe combined immunodeficiency: A serious primary immunodeficiency disease with a combined absence of T-lymphocyte and B-lymphocyte function.

Shingles: An acute, painful inflammation of the nerve ganglia, with a skin eruption often forming a girdle around the middle of the body. The same virus causes it as chickenpox.

Sickle cell disease: A genetic disorder caused by a mutation in the beta-globin gene that leads to a faulty hemoglobin protein called hemoglobin S. Hemoglobin S changes flexible red blood cells into rigid sickle-shaped cells. These sickle cells can block blood flow and result in pain and organ damage.

Side effects: Unwanted, undesirable effects possibly related to a drug. Side effects can vary from minor problems such as a runny nose to life-threatening events such as a heart attack or liver damage.

Smallpox: A highly contagious and often deadly disease caused by the variola virus, marked by high fever and a distinctive blistering rash.

Sporotrichosis: An infection caused by a fungus called *Sporothrix*. People get sporotrichosis by contacting the fungal spores in the environment.

Stem cells: The body's raw materials—cells from which all other cells with specialized functions are generated.

Sternum bone: A partially T-shaped vertical bone that centrally forms the anterior portion of the chest wall.

Subcutaneous injection: The injection is in the fatty tissue, just under the skin. A subcutaneous injection is the best way to give oneself certain medicines, including insulin, blood thinners, and fertility drugs.

Subunit vaccines: A vaccine that contains purified parts of the pathogen that are antigenic or necessary to elicit a protective immune response.

Surveillance systems: The ongoing and systematic collection, analysis, and interpretation of health data in describing and monitoring a health event.

Surveillance: The systematic collection, analysis, and dissemination of health data for planning, implementing, and evaluating public health programs.

Swine influenza: A respiratory disease of pigs caused by type A influenza viruses that regularly cause influenza outbreaks in pigs. There are sporadic reports of human infections with swine influenza viruses, mainly in people who had direct contact with infected pigs.

Symbiotic: Any close and long-term biological interaction between two biological organisms of different species,

T-cell transfer therapy: A type of immunotherapy that makes the immune cells better able to attack cancer.

Taxonomy: A science that deals with naming, describing, and classification of all living organisms, including plants.

Tetanus neonatorum: An illness occurring in a newborn with the average ability to suck and cry in the first 2 days of life but who loses this ability between days 3 and 28 and becomes rigid and has spasms.

Tetanus toxoid: A vaccine used in the management and treatment of tetanus. It is in the vaccine class of medications.

Tetanus: An infection caused by a bacterium called *Clostridium tetani*. Produces a toxin that causes painful muscle contractions.

Thrombocytopenia syndrome: This occurs when the vaccine produces antibodies that activate platelets, resulting in low platelets and blood clots (thrombosis).

Thrombocytopenia: A condition that occurs when the platelet count in the blood is too low.

Thrush: A fungal (yeast) infection that can grow in the mouth, throat, and other body parts.

Thymus: The organ primarily responsible for the production and maturation of immune cells.

Toll-like receptors: The essential mediators of inflammatory pathways in the gut that play a significant role in mediating the immune responses towards a wide variety of pathogen-derived ligands and link adaptive immunity with innate immunity.

Toxoid vaccines: The vaccines that use a toxin made by a pathogen that causes a disease, they create immunity to the parts of the pathogen that cause disease instead of the pathogen itself, and the immune response is targeted to the toxin.

Tracheostomy: A surgically created hole in the trachea that provides an alternative airway for breathing.

Transcytosis: A type of transcellular transport in which various macromolecules are transported across the interior of a cell.

Treatment vaccines: A type of cancer treatment called immunotherapy. They work to boost the body's immune system to fight cancer.

Triage: The prioritization of injured or sick individuals based on their need for emergency treatment.

Trismus: The restriction of the range of motion of the jaw. Initially described in the setting of tetanus, it currently refers to restricted mouth opening due to any etiology.

Trivalent vaccines: Protect against three different influenza viruses. They include components from one influenza A(H1N1) virus, one influenza A(H3N2) virus, and one influenza B/Victoria lineage virus.

Tubal tonsils: The four main tonsil groups forming the Waldeyer tonsillar ring; they are located beneath the mucosa of the eustachian tube.

Tumor necrosis factor: A critical cytokine that contributes to physiological and pathological processes.

Tumorigenesis: The production or formation of a tumor or tumors.

Tzanck smear: A simple and cheap test that relies on viewing and interpreting single cells. It is used to diagnose the pemphigus group of autoimmune bullous diseases and mucocutaneous herpesvirus infections.

Umbilical hernia: An abnormal bulge that can be seen or felt at the umbilicus.

Vaccine Safety Datalink: Technology that uses electronic health data from participating sites to monitor and assess the safety of vaccines.

Valley fever: A fungal infection caused by *Coccidioides* organisms. It can cause signs and symptoms such as a fever, cough, and tiredness.

Variable region: The primary role of the antibody variable region is to bind to the target antigen.

Varicella: A highly contagious disease caused by the varicella-zoster virus. It can cause an itchy, blister-like rash (chickenpox).

Variolation: An outdated medical technique used to protect people from smallpox.

Vastus lateralis muscle: A muscle located on the lateral, or outside, part of your thigh.

Vesicle: Small blisters, most often on the skin, can also crop up on the mucous membranes, such as the buccal mucosa.

Viral vector vaccines: Those that use a harmless virus to bring instructions for making antigens from a disease-causing virus into cells, triggering protective immunity.

Viral vector: Tools commonly used by molecular biologists to deliver genetic material into cells.

Viremia: The presence of viruses in the blood.

Virulent: An ability of an organism to infect the host and cause a disease. Virulence factors are the molecules that assist the bacterium in colonizing the host at the cellular level.

Waterhouse-Friderichsen syndrome: A group of symptoms caused by the adrenal glands failing to function normally. This occurs as a result of bleeding into the glands. Meningococcemia is a life-threatening infection that occurs when *N. meningitidis* invades the bloodstream.

West Nile virus infection: A mosquito-borne zoonosis. The virus is transmitted among birds via the bite of infected mosquitoes; incidentally, humans and other mammals may become infected.

Wilson disease: A rare autosomal recessive disorder caused by abnormal copper accumulation in the body, particularly involving the brain, liver, and cornea.

Yeasts: Eukaryotic, single-celled microorganisms classified as members of the fungus kingdom.

Yellow fever: A severe disease caused by the yellow fever virus. Most people infected with this virus do not get sick or have only mild symptoms.

Index

Note: Page numbers followed by "*f*" indicate figures, "*t*" indicate tables, and "*b*" indicate boxes.

D

E

I

N

O

P

W

Y

Z